Synaptic Plasticity: Dynamics, Development and Disease

Synaptic Plasticity: Dynamics, Development and Disease

Edited by Miles Smith

STATES
ACADEMIC PRESS
www.statesacademicpress.com

States Academic Press,
109 South 5th Street,
Brooklyn, NY 11249, USA

Visit us on the World Wide Web at:
www.statesacademicpress.com

ISBN: 978-1-63989-505-2

Cataloging-in-Publication Data

Synaptic plasticity : dynamics, development and disease / edited by Miles Smith.
p. cm.
Includes bibliographical references and index.
ISBN 978-1-63989-505-2
1. Neuroplasticity. 2. Developmental neurobiology. 3. Neurons--Growth. I. Smith, Miles.
QP363.3 .S96 2022
612.82--dc23

Table of Contents

Preface

The ability of synapses to weaken or strengthen over time in response to the decrease and increase in their activity is referred to as synaptic plasticity. It is one of the significant neurochemical foundations in memory and learning because memories are suggested to be represented by interconnections of neural circuits in the brain. Plastic change is a result of the alterations in the number of neurotransmitter receptors present on a synapse. Several mechanisms take place and cooperate in order to achieve synaptic plasticity. Some of these are alteration in the quantity of neurotransmitters releasing into a synapse, and alteration in the effectiveness of cells responding to these neurotransmitters. The topics covered in this extensive book deal with the core subjects of synaptic plasticity. It brings forth some of the most innovative concepts and elucidates the unexplored aspects of synaptic plasticity. The extensive content of this book provides the readers with a thorough understanding of the subject.

The researches compiled throughout the book are authentic and of high quality, combining several disciplines and from very diverse regions from around the world. Drawing on the contributions of many researchers from diverse countries, the book's objective is to provide the readers with the latest achievements in the area of research. This book will surely be a source of knowledge to all interested and researching the field.

In the end, I would like to express my deep sense of gratitude to all the authors for meeting the set deadlines in completing and submitting their research chapters. I would also like to thank the publisher for the support offered to us throughout the course of the book. Finally, I extend my sincere thanks to my family for being a constant source of inspiration and encouragement.

Editor

Preface

1

Synaptic Plasticity by Afferent Electrical Stimulation

Stefan Golaszewski

Abstract

The effect of afferent electrical stimulation on synaptic plasticity within the sensorimotor cortex will be discussed. Afferent electrical stimulation induces a down regulation of inhibitory neural circuits and plays a critical role in strengthening excitatory synapses. Synaptic modifications such as long-term potentiation (LTP) mechanisms could be a crucial mechanism underlying this stimulation-induced cortical plasticity. LTP and long-term depression (LTD) of synaptic transmission are crucial factors for activity-dependent changes in the strength of synaptic connections. Many studies demonstrated that these pathways play an important role in cortical synaptic plasticity. Repeated activation of excitatory synapses induces both short-term potentiation (STP) and LTP. Both types of synaptic potentiation affect N-methyl-D-aspartate glutamate receptors leading to the formation of new synapses or the unmasking of excitatory amino acid receptors on motor neurons. This increased excitability localized within the sensorimotor cortex may reflect an increase in neuronal activity as a result of a dynamic interaction of various synaptic and cellular mechanisms due to the local processing of afferent electrical input to the sensorimotor cortex. The chapter reviews also the large number of studies using fMRI and TMS to examine the effects of afferent electrical input from the hand on the excitability of human sensorimotor cortex.

Keywords: neuromodulation, afferent electrical stimulation, long-term potentiation (LTP), sensorimotor cortex, stroke rehabilitation

1. Introduction

In the development of neurobiology, it was generally thought that synapses simply transfer information between one neuron and another neuron or between one neuron and a muscle cell. Further, it was thought that established connections during development are relatively fixed in their strength. However, up to now, the current opinion in neurobiology is that most synapses are highly plastic and are able to change their strength depending on their own activity or through synaptic input from another pathway. It is generally accepted that synaptic plasticity is the basic mechanism for learning and memory and reorganization in brain damage.

Synaptic plasticity can be divided into an intrinsic and extrinsic synaptic plasticity. Intrinsic synaptic plasticity refers to changes in the strength of a synapse by its own activity. Extrinsic synaptic plasticity is a change in the strength of a synapse by synaptic input through another pathway. For this change in the strength of a synapse through input from another pathway, there is a widely accepted model in neurobiology called long-term potentiation (LTP) that links synaptic plasticity with memory and long-term depression (LTD). The chapter will discuss the effect of afferent electrical (AE) stimulation on synaptic transmission and synaptic plasticity in general and especially within the sensorimotor cortex with a special protocol using whole-hand afferent electrical stimulation with a wire glove. Results from AE stimulation provide evidence for the induction of synaptic plasticity within the sensorimotor cortex leading to a reduced short interval intracortical inhibition (SICI) and an increased intracortical facilitation (ICF) and consequently to an increased motor cortex excitability, as verified with functional magnetic resonance imaging (fMRI) and transcranial magnetic stimulation (TMS) techniques.

AE stimulation has been proven to induce changes in synaptic transmission and synaptic plasticity within the sensorimotor cortex [1]. An increased blood oxygen level dependent (BOLD) response after 30 min of AE stimulation within the sensorimotor cortex has been shown by fMRI [2]. 30 min of AE stimulation is able to modulate the corticospinal excitability as well as the activity of intracortical inhibitory and excitatory circuits that can be detected by TMS [3]. These conditioning effects could be measured up to 2 h post stimulation [2]. This exploration has strengthened the understanding that electrical peripheral nerve stimulation is a powerful tool to induce sustained excitability increases as well as rapidly evolving neuroplastic changes of the human sensorimotor cortex. Up to now, the optimal set of parameters for afferent electrical stimulation for the modulation of the corticomotor output is not exactly known [4]. Stimulation intensity appeared to have the strongest relationship to motor cortical excitability, whereas frequency has been shown to modulate motor-evoked potential (MEP) amplitudes [5]. Furthermore, different levels of afferent electrical stimulation were investigated—sham, sub-threshold (below the threshold for sensory perception)/50 Hz, sensory (above the threshold for sensory perception)/2 and 50 Hz, and motor level/2 Hz.

2. Synaptic plasticity by afferent electrical stimulation in BOLD imaging

2.1. Neurophysiology of afferent electrical stimulation

Afferent electrical stimulation generates synchronous tonic input to the brain due to depolarization of a large diameter group, Ia and Ib afferents, and to a lesser extent group II afferents of the hand, as it is the case in functional and neuromuscular electrical stimulation [6–10]. The electrical input is transmitted to the spinal cord posterior column nuclei, the ventral postero-lateral nucleus of the thalamus, and to the Brodmann areas 3a, 2, and 4 of the brain cortex [11–14]. The hand is a rich source of proprioceptive input to the brain via the afferents because the hand's intrinsic muscles have high-density muscle spindles [15, 16], a large number of joint receptors, as well as Golgi tendon organs [17, 18] with a portion of the tendons within the hand but belonging to the forearm muscles [10]. In addition, there are definite experimental findings that confirm that proprioceptive and exteroceptive somatosensory afferents of groups Ia (primary large muscle afferents), Ib (afferents from Golgi organs), and group II (slow and rapidly adapting skin afferents, secondary thin muscle afferents) have short latency projections to the contralateral sensorimotor cortex, particularly BA 3a, 1, 2, and 4 [14, 19, 20]. For the afferent route to the primary motor cortex M1, a projection from BA 3a is discussed [21]. By applying afferent electrical stimulation there will be afferents involved that "sense the body's own movement" [22]. In several positron emission tomography (PET) and fMRI studies, it was confirmed that vibration to the hand palm of healthy adult humans activates the contralateral primary sensorimotor (SM1), the supplementary motor area (SMA), and the secondary somatosensory cortex S2 bilaterally [23–25].

2.2. Methodology of afferent electrical stimulation

Continuous whole-hand afferent electrical stimulation with a wire glove (WG, **Figure 1**) is a potential tool that can induce neuromodulatory effects within the sensorimotor cortex. For ipsilateral neuromodulatory effects, cortical projections of Ia, Ib, II afferents, and transcallosal projections from the contralateral brain cortex are supposed [26, 27].

The wire glove is connected to a two-channel transcutaneous electrical nerve stimulation (TENS) stimulator. The WG acts as the anode, and carbon film surface electrodes above the tendons of the forearm flexors and extensors just proximal to the wrist act as cathodes (**Figure 1**). Before fitting the hand to the WG, conductive jelly should be applied over the whole hand. A train of 50-Hz stimuli with a pulse width of 300 μs is used for stimulation (**Figure 2**).

Depending on the skin resistance, the amplitude for the threshold of sensation lies between 2.0 and 4.0 mA and the level for supra-threshold stimulation is set to 120% of the threshold of sensation level. For sham, the stimulator is set to 0 mA, and healthy volunteers are told to be stimulated below the level of sensation. AE stimulation is applied for 30 min to the relaxed right or left hand [3]. Pulse width is set to 300 μs (**Figure 2**).

The level for sub-threshold stimulation is set to 80% of the threshold of sensation level. At the sensory level, (120% of the threshold of sensation level) electromyography (EMG) did not show any muscle contractions. For somatosensory AE stimulation, the frequency is set at 50 Hz and for motor AE stimulation at 2 Hz. The current stimulus amplitude for 50 Hz ranges from 2.0 to about 5.0 mA. For the motor level, the intensity is increased from the sensory threshold level until slight motor contractions of all small hand muscles are visible. The current stimulus amplitude for the motor level is about 10.0 mA. The sham stimulation is carried out identically, but the stimulation amplitude is set to 0 mA. Subjects are not informed about the stimulation level and are instructed to distract attention from the stimulation.

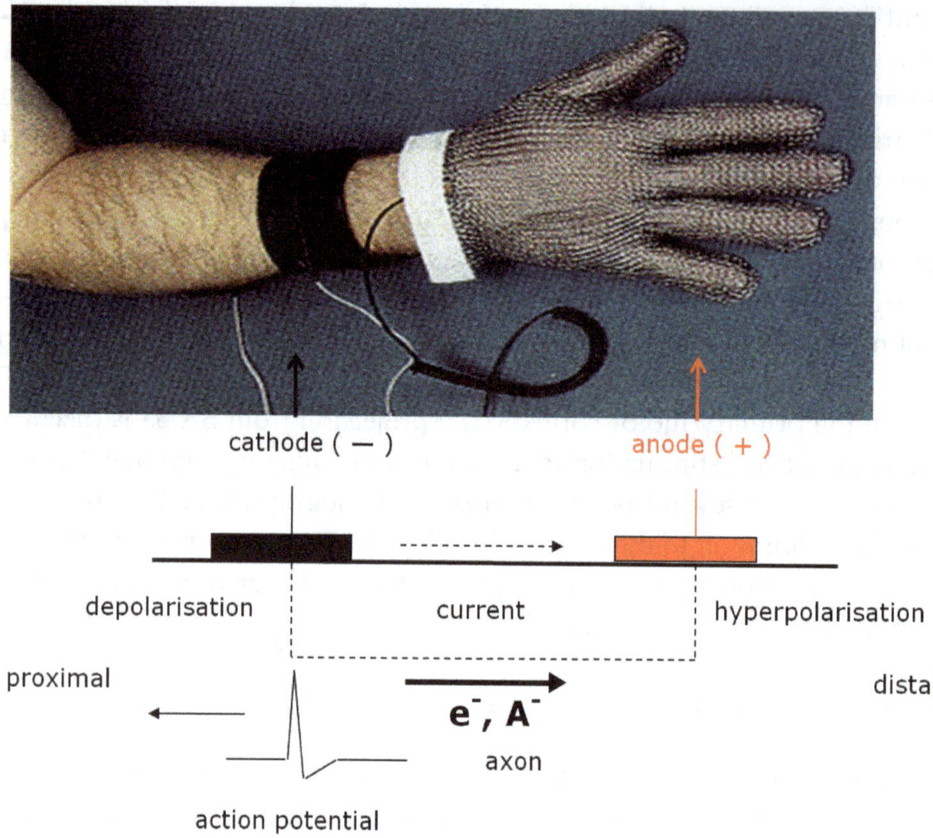

Figure 1. Wire glove: a two-channel stimulator delivers a train of 50-Hz stimuli (pulse width 300 ms) with the amplitude for somatosensory and motor stimulation, ranging from 2.0 to 10.0 MA. The wire glove acts as a common anode. The cathodes are placed over the tendons of the forearm flexors and extensors. Beneath the electrodes over the forearm flexors and extensors, the action potentials for the AE stimulation are elicited.

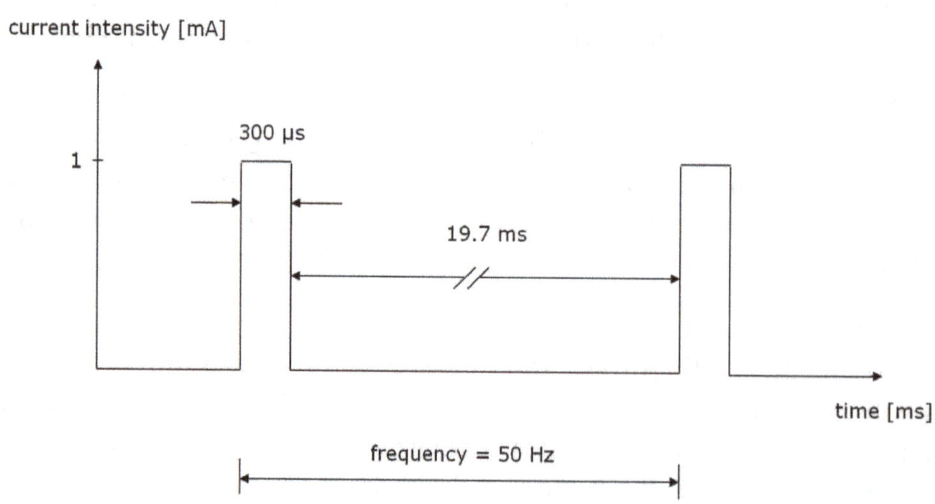

Figure 2. Current pulse: with a rectangular pulse with a width of 300 µs and a frequency of 2/50 Hz, the AE stimulation is continuous for 30 min. The current intensities range between 2 (somatosensory threshold) and 10 mA (motor threshold).

2.3. BOLD modulation by afferent electrical stimulation

Neuromodulatory effects of afferent electrical stimulation are already proven by fMRI [2, 28] applying self-paced simple finger movements. During finger-to-thumb-tapping with a frequency of about 2 Hz in fMRI movement-related BOLD responses of several brain areas are well known in the contra and ipsilateral hemisphere within the pre- and postcentral gyrus, the medial and superior frontal gyrus, and on both cerebellar hemispheres with a dominance ipsilaterally to the active left hand (**Figure 3**).

Neuronal activation within these areas is expected and has been reported by other investigators who studied the activity of human cortical motor areas during self-paced finger movements [29–31]. In a classical pre-/post-study design, a baseline finger-to-thumb tapping paradigm is run in fMRI (**Figure 4**).

Post 30 min of whole-hand afferent electrical stimulation of the tapping hand, the finger-to-thumb tapping paradigm in fMRI shows an increase of brain activation measured by the corresponding BOLD response on both hemispheres within the pre- and post-central as well as the medial frontal gyrus (**Figure 5**).

The left SMA shows augmented brain activation as well. The finding that an increase of movement-related responses is absent when the sham paradigm is applied further confirms the validity of these results. Obviously, afferent electrical stimulation can change motor cortex representation bilaterally within the primary and secondary sensorimotor cortex and consequently has the potential to induce neuroplasticity in neurorehabilitation. The detected increased BOLD responses reflect an increased neuronal activity due to augmented afferent proprioceptive and exteroceptive inputs to the sensorimotor cortex [32]. Logothetis could demonstrate a strong correlation between spatially localized BOLD response and local field potentials. AE stimulation of group Ia and Ib afferents and their

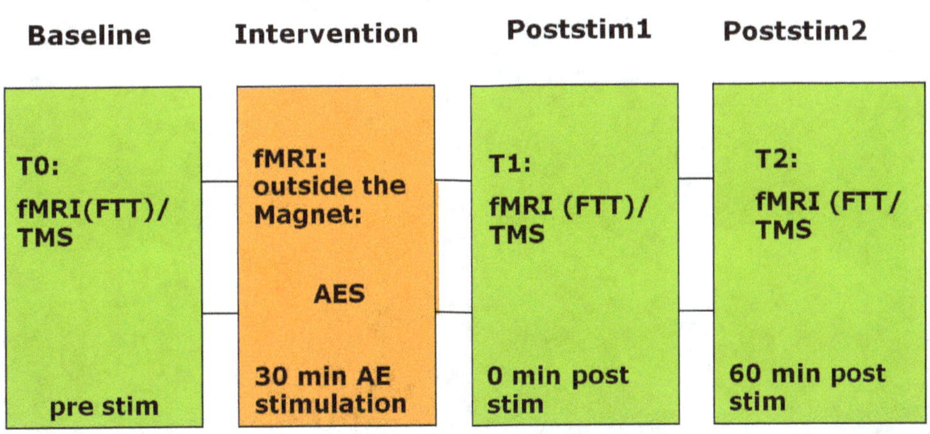

Figure 3. Classical pre-/post-design for studying synaptic plasticity: at T0 baseline measurement (finger-to-thumb tapping in fMRI, TMS) prior to 30-min AE stimulation, at T1 first measurement (fMRI/TMS) post stimulation (post stimulation 1) and at T2 60-min post-AE stimulation second measurement (fMRI/TMS) post stimulation (post stimulation 2).

direct transcallosal projections induce augmented local field potentials (LFP) for at least several minutes within the sensorimotor cortex that was already proven in somatosensory-evoked potential studies [13]. Augmented LFPs change intramotorcortical excitability with a larger recruitment by a motor task. AE stimulation addresses especially group Ia and Ib and to a lesser extent group II afferents and thus should augment sensorimotor LFPs. AE stimulation in stroke patients after a daily stimulation training program over several weeks improved motor performance [33–35], obviously by an increased motoneuron recruitment due to augmented motorcortical excitability leading to synaptic plasticity with intracortical facilitation and unmasking of preexisting silent synapses [36–41]. Horizontal connections transversing the superficial layers of the sensorimotor cortex are capable of both increases and decreases in strength and synaptic efficacy [42, 43]. A persistent high-frequency input enhances the motoneuron recruitment with probably a synaptic modification through long-term potentiation (LTP). Post-tetanic potentiation is unlikely because the neuromodulation lasts at least 2 h (**Figure 6**).

However, in the literature, there is evidence for a cortical origin of the modulation of cortical motoneuron excitability by afferent electrical input [1, 26, 44]. The multimodal integration cortex in the superior (SPL) and inferior (IPL) parietal lobule receives sensory information of

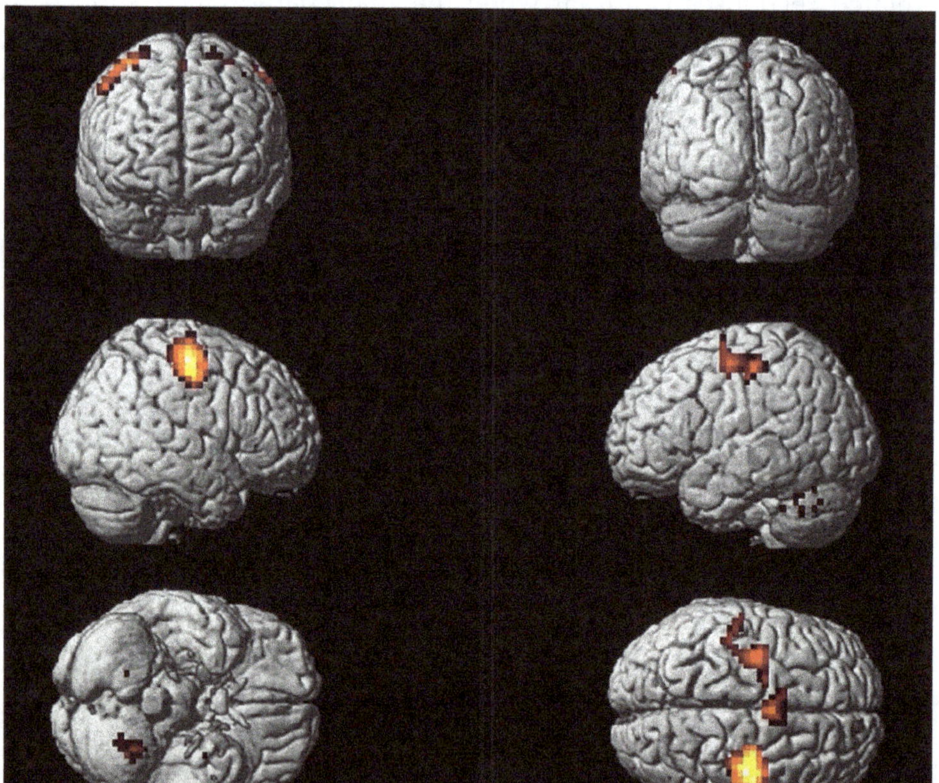

Figure 4. BOLD response during the test motor task (TMT): contra and ipsilaterally within the SM1, premotor area (PM), and SMA as well as in both cerebellar hemispheres with a dominance of the left hemisphere ipsilaterally to the stimulated hand.

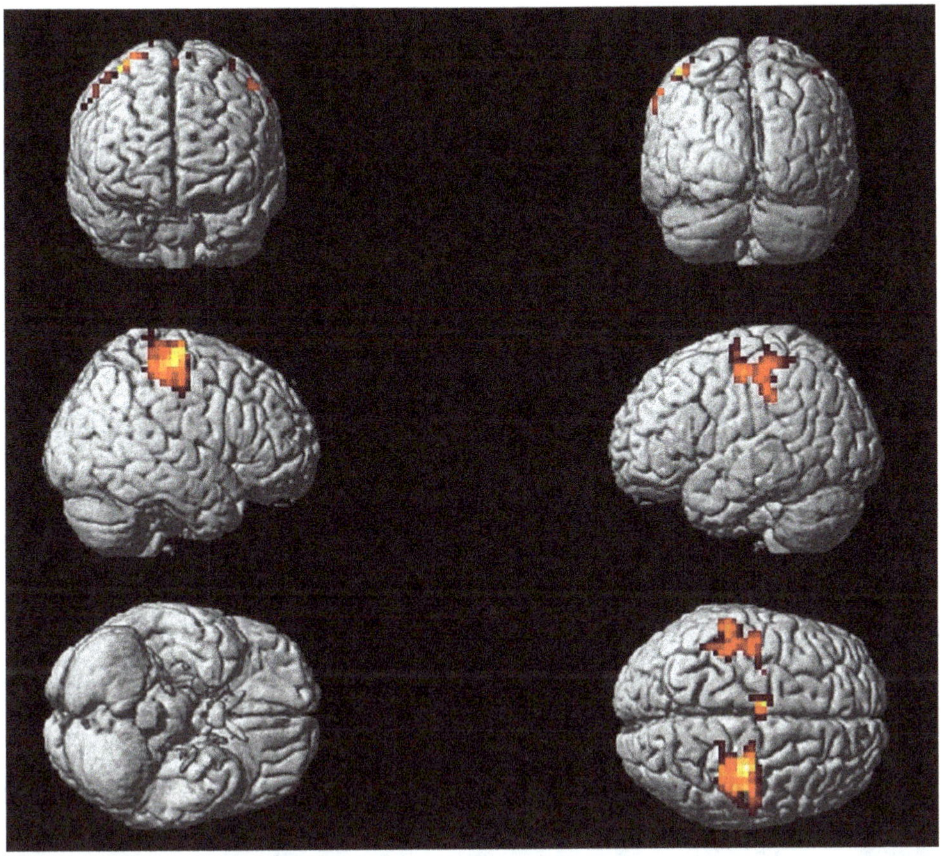

Figure 5. Between-condition analysis in fMRI: conditioned motor task at T1 (CMT1)—test motor task at T0 shows an increase of BOLD response during CMT1 of the contralateral hemisphere within SM1, PM, and IPL and of the ipsilateral hemisphere within SM1, PM, IPL, SMA, and cingulate gyrus (GC).

different modalities and transforms it into information for proper action. In IPL, proprioceptive, exterozeptive, premotor, and visual information converges during grasping with the hand. IPL is involved in sensorimotor transformations to convert retinal signals of target locations into a pattern of peripheral motor output to muscles to move the hand to the target [45, 46]. The information for these target movements will be processed primarily by the group Ia and Ib afferents, which are especially addressed by the afferent electrical stimulation. Thus, the IPL activity in the conditioned motor task immediately after the AE stimulation (CMT1) indicates direct input bilaterally to IPL that is very important for the neurorehabilitation for visually guided movements and the eye-hand coordination (**Figure 3**). Increased IPL activity after daily AE stimulation for 3 months in stroke patients concurs also with an improvement of neglect [33, 34]. Increased proprioceptive and exteroceptive input to the brain has also the potential of lowering muscle tone, which is in agreement with described beneficial effects of AE stimulation on spasticity [33, 34, 45, 46].

The increased BOLD responses were supposed to be due to a precapillary vascular response or to reduced sensorimotor network thresholds. Wu et al. [47] demonstrated in 2005 that median nerve stimulation elicited an enduring increase in task-related perfusion and BOLD responses in the cortical thumb representation in the absence of changes in baseline blood

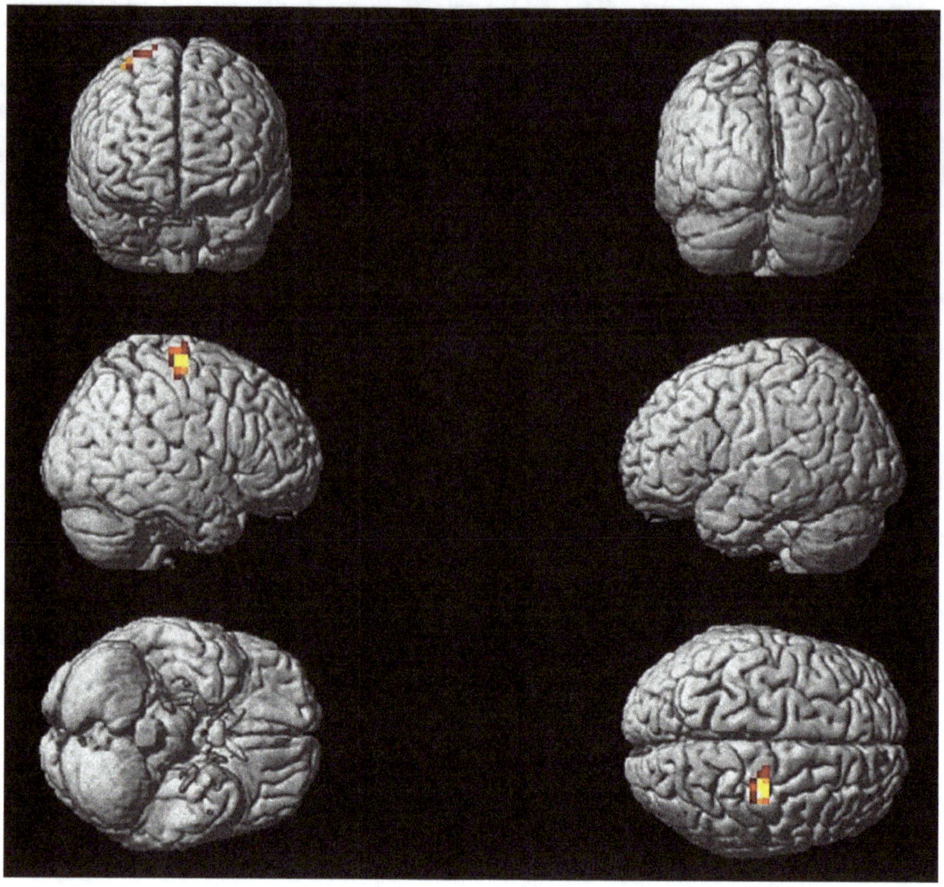

Figure 6. Between-condition analysis in fMRI: conditioned motor task at T2 (CMT2)—test motor task at T0 shows still an increase of BOLD response 2 h post stimulation with brain activation declining nearly to TMT level.

flow. Consecutively, the increased BOLD response was associated with increased cortical excitability but was still unclear.

3. Synaptic plasticity by afferent electrical stimulation in TMS

3.1. Background

With transcranial magnetic stimulation (TMS, excitatory and inhibitory circuits of the human motor cortex can be studied. Many studies have used TMS to investigate the effect of AE stimulation of the hand on motor cortex excitability with the paired-pulse technique, demonstrating a reduction of SICI [48, 49]. By a preceding electrical stimulus to a mixed or cutaneous nerve Motor Evoked Potentials (MEPs) are affected and show a smaller amplitude [48, 50–52]. AE stimulation of the hand showed conflicting results with no effect on MEP amplitudes, MEP amplitude facilitation, MEP amplitude inhibition, or both [12, 53–61], depending on the parameters used [62–65] on disparate effects of stimuli on different motoneuron pools, on different experimental settings (e.g., single pulses versus stimulus trains, various stimulus intensities, relaxed versus contracted target muscles), and on different stimulation and recording sites. Low-amplitude vibration of a muscle increased MEP amplitudes and decreased the effectiveness of SICI [66, 67].

BOLD signal intensity changes prior to and after constraint-induced movement therapy (CIMT) within the sensory and motor cortex proved a close correlation with SICI and ICF in paired-pulse TMS [68]. With TMS effects of AE stimulation on the motor system, its duration can be investigated very easily, yielding to information about the excitability of the motor cortex, and they help to clarify the physiological basis of variations in BOLD responses by AE stimulation. In case of a specific vascular response of the precapillary microvasculature independent from neuronal effects, TMS parameters should not change after afferent electrical stimulation.

3.2. TMS methodology

Again, a classical pre-/post-design is implemented (**Figure 4**) with a baseline TMS assessment (T0), AE stimulation for 30 min, a further TMS assessment (T1), a resting period for 1 h, and a third TMS assessment (T2). The experimental setup includes four different AE stimulation levels in randomized order: (1) sham, (2) sub-threshold with 50 Hz (sub-threshold/50 Hz), (3) sensory with 50 Hz (sensory/50 Hz), and (4) AE stimulation at motor level with 2 Hz (motor/2 Hz). At motor level, 2 Hz is chosen to avoid painful tetanic muscle contraction. Between sessions, there is at least an interim time of 5 days. Paired-pulse TMS is performed using a bi-stimulation module. A figure-of-eight coil with external loop diameter of 90 mm is applied for motor responses in the right first dorsal interosseus (FDI) muscle at the lowest motor threshold (MT, **Figure 7**).

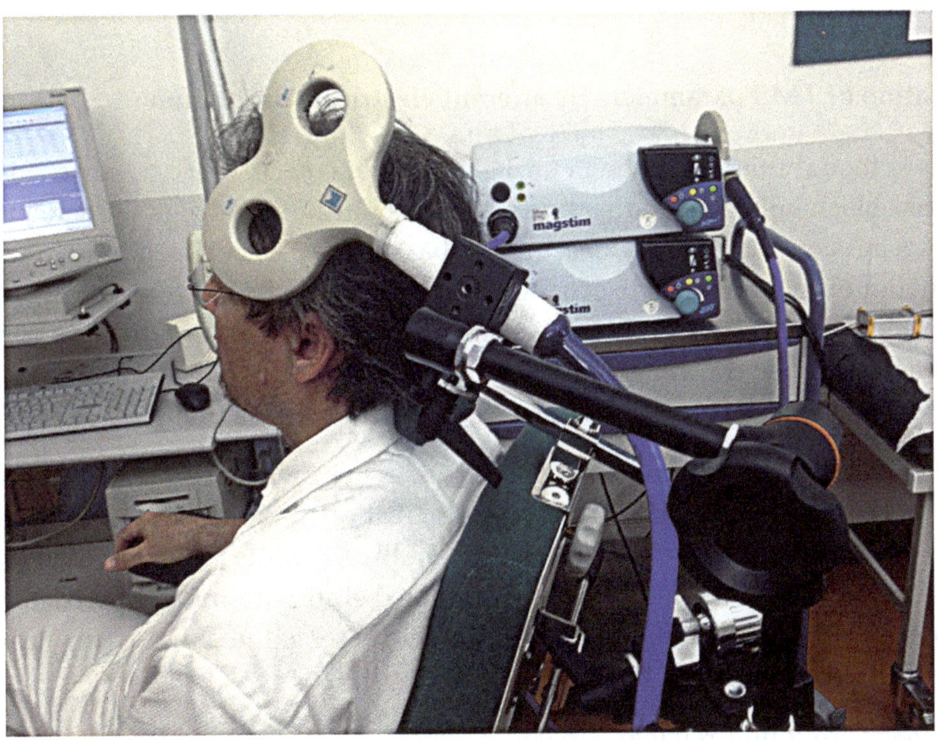

Figure 7. TMS experimental setup: a figure-of-eight coil (external loop diameter of 90 mm) is held over the left motor cortex at the optimum scalp position to elicit motor responses in the right FDI muscle at the lowest MT. The intersection of the coil is placed tangentially to the scalp with the handle pointing backward and laterally at a 45° angle away from the midline to induce postero-anterior current flow. Surface muscle responses are obtained via two 9-mm diameter of Ag-AgCl electrodes with the active electrode applied over the motor point of the muscle and the reference on the metacarpophalangeal joint of the index finger. Muscle responses are amplified and filtered (bandwidth 8–2000 Hz).

The coil is held tangentially to the scalp with a 45° angle away from the midline for postero-anterior current flow. Muscle responses are recorded with 9-mm diameter of Ag-AgCl electrodes over the belly of the first dorsal interosseus (FDI) and the metacarpophalangeal joint of the index finger and are amplified and filtered (bandwidth 8–2000 Hz). The minimum stimulus intensity that produces an MEP at rest of 50 μV in three out of five trials defines the resting motor threshold (RMT). Then MEP recruitment curve (RC) with TMS intensities of 90, 100, 110, 120, 130, 140, 150, and 160 of the MT is measured. RC is recorded in T0, T1 and T2 measurements. For each stimulator, output intensity of five pulses is delivered with randomized stimulus intensity. The first MEP for each trial is discarded because of startle and reflex responses. Short interval cortical inhibition (SICI) is performed according to the technique of paired magnetic stimulation [69]. The conditioning and the test stimuli are set at 80 and 120% of MT, respectively. Inhibitory interstimulus intervals (ISIs) of 3 ms and facilitatory ISIs with 13 ms are applied. Conditioned and unconditioned trials are randomized. If MT after T0 for the paired-pulse measurement is changed, the stimulus intensity is adjusted to the corresponding MT in T1 and T2. The actual amplitudes after correction relate to those before AE stimulation. Usually paired-pulse TMS studies are carried out in 20–30 subjects with half of the subjects assigned to the verum and half to the control group. The verum group undergoes afferent electrical stimulation and the control group undergoes sham stimulation. Subjects are seated in a comfortable reclining chair during TMS measurements, afferent electrical stimulation, and at rest. Both hands are placed relaxed on soft supports beside the body [3].

3.3. Modulation of TMS parameters by afferent electrical stimulation

MT in TMS is thought to reflect the neuronal membrane excitability because it is increased by drugs that block voltage-gated sodium channels but not by drugs influencing neuronal synaptic transmission [70–72]. MT measured at baseline varies between 37 and 45% of maximum stimulator output among subjects. As shown in **Figure 8**, AE stimulation of 30 min has a significant decreasing effect on MT. This effect is obviously related to the strong effect of AE stimulation since the control group does not show any differences in MT. Post-hoc comparisons shows reliable MT decreases immediately after and 1 h after AE stimulation [3, 73].

Compared to MT, the MEP recruitment curve assesses neurons that are intrinsically less excitable or spatially further away from the center of activation by TMS. Increasing the TMS intensities from 90, 100, 110, 120, 130, 140, 150 to 160% of the MT determined for each subject MEP recruitment curves that show an increasing left-sided shift with increasing current intensity after the 30-min period of AE stimulation. **Figure 9** presents the effect of AE stimulation on MEP recruitment curves measured at T0 and T1.

No other effects are found reliable. However, whereas the control group shows any effects on amplitudes after time and no interaction effects of "stimulus intensity" and "time", the group with verum AE stimulation shows the important reliable main effect of "time" with increased amplitudes after AE stimulation. The interaction effect does not reach significance. In both post-stimulation conditions (T1 and T2), the recruitment curve is increased compared to T0. Post-hoc comparisons at each intensity level reveal that at lower and mid-range intensities, MEP increases are significant both in T1 and T2 compared to T0. At higher stimulus

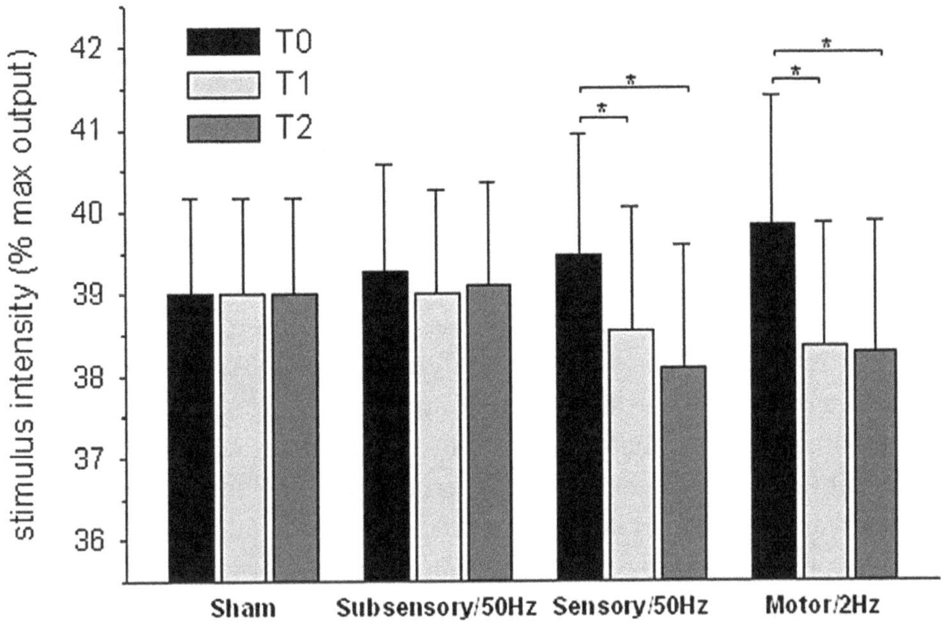

Figure 8. Resting motor threshold expressed as percentage of maximum stimulator output for the FDI muscle before (T0), immediately after (T1), and 1 h after (T2) afferent electrical stimulation with sub-sensory, sensory/50 Hz, and motor level electrical stimulation intensity as well as sham stimulation. Values plotted as mean (S.E.M). * indicates significant difference ($p < 0.05$) from T0. For sham stimulation there is no change of the resting motor threshold at T1 and T2 compared to the baseline measurement.

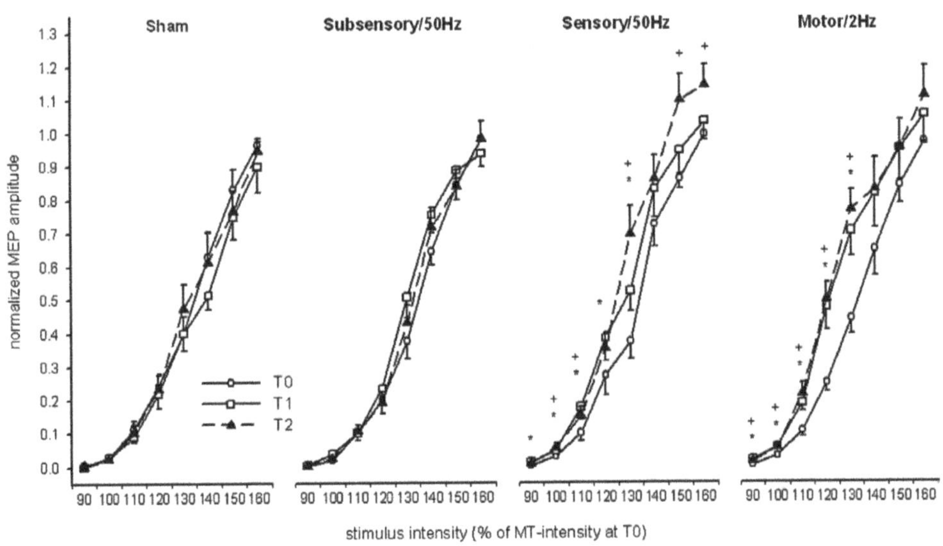

Figure 9. MEP recruitment curves before (T0), after (T1), and 1 h after (T2) AE stimulation at sub-sensory, sensory/50 Hz, motor level, and sham stimulation. MEPs are normalized to the mean MEPmax at T0. Mean (S.E.M.) of the normalized MEP amplitude is plotted for each stimulus intensity. * indicates significant difference ($p < 0.05$) between T1/T0 and (+) significant difference ($p < 0.05$) between T2/T0. A left-sided shift can be seen with increasing current intensities.

intensities (140–160% of MTT0 intensity), the tendency is partly kept although not reaching significance level (**Figure 9**). Additionally, post-hoc group comparisons of each intensity level are conducted and show reliable differences between AE and sham at T1 and T2. A two-factorial ANOVA with factors "group" and "stimulus intensity" is applied that does not reveal any difference in groups at T0.

Since paired-pulse TMS gives access to the motor cortex independently of spinal or peripheral mechanisms, it allows the evaluation of the intracortical circuits [3, 73]. There is good evidence that the interaction between a sub-threshold conditioning stimulus and a supra-threshold test stimulus at short interstimulus intervals (1–5 ms) relies on activation of c-aminobutyric acid (GABA)—in particular GABAA—circuits in the motor cortex. **Figure 10** shows the effect of AE stimulation on SICI and ICF.

Here, apart from the inherent effect of "interstimulus interval (ISI)", the three-factorial ANOVA reveals also a main effect of "time" and an interaction effect between "time" and "group". No other effects are found reliable. Follow-up ANOVAs for each group separately confirmed the effect of "ISI" for controls and AE stimulation group, respectively, but found a reliable effect of "time" only for the group who received verum AE stimulation. Other effects are not found reliable. Generally, in the verum group, the MEP inhibition at 3 ms is reduced and the facilitation at 13 ms is increased compared to T0 at T1 and T2. These changes do not reach significance for T1 but do so for T2 as post-hoc comparisons reveal. The circuit underlying intracortical facilitation is less well understood and is thought to be mediated by glutamate. Moreover, the downregulation of inhibitory neural circuits seems to play also a critical role in strengthening excitatory synapses. Current data suggest that afferent electrical stimulation also has a direct effect on the excitability of the intracortical circuits responsible for SICI and ICF at a cortical level. Conversely, no changes in spinal motor excitability (amplitude and persistence of F waves) are currently observed.

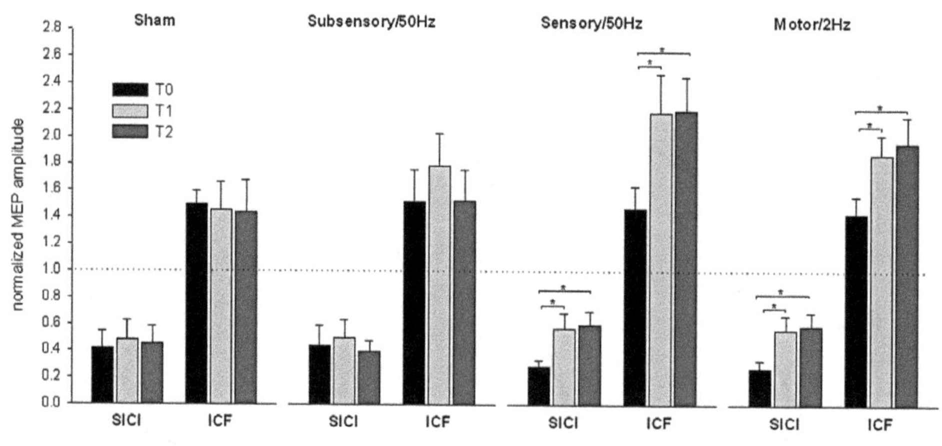

Figure 10. Paired-pulse TMS stimulation: before (T0), after (T1), and 1 h after (T2) AE stimulation at sensory/2 Hz level. The values for intracortical inhibition and ICF are normalized to their corresponding values in single-pulse stimulation for each condition and are then plotted as the mean (S.E.M). * indicates significant difference ($p < 0.05$) from T0. At T1 and T2, a decrease of SICI can be seen; ICF is significantly increased at T2.

4. Discussion

From these pre-/post-AE stimulation studies, we learn that changes in motor cortex excitability outlast AE stimulation up to 2 h and intracortical excitability is significantly enhanced 1 h after AE stimulation and not significantly increased immediately after the AE stimulation. Up to now, this late excitability enhancement remains unclear. Maybe an intracortical synaptic reorganization LTP is the underlying mechanism for the delayed facilitation. The stimulation-induced cortical plasticity may be due to synaptic modification such as LTP. LTP, as well as LTD of synaptic transmission, had been suggested to be responsible for activity-dependent changes in the strength of synaptic connections and efficiency of synaptic signal transduction since its discovery in the early 1970s of the last century [74]. But the outcome of synaptic modifications on behavioral changes induced by stimuli that drive LTP- or LTD-like processes is not well known today, especially not in patients with brain lesions. STP and LTP are induced by repeated activation of excitatory synapses with N-methyl-D-aspartate glutamate receptors leading to the formation of new synapses or the unmasking of other excitatory amino acid receptors on motor neurons [75]. Also, remote modulation of motor cortex excitability may be involved including additional cortical and subcortical structures connected with the primary motor cortex. The increased excitability may reflect an increased neuronal activity due to dynamic interaction between various synaptic and cellular mechanisms that locally process the augmented afferent proprioceptive and exteroceptive input to the sensorimotor cortex [26]. The strongest neuromodulatory changes could be achieved with stimulation of the highest intensity (motor level). Defining proper stimulation parameters, in particular with regard to stimulation intensities and frequencies, will provide an important basis for further therapeutic applications of afferent electrical stimulation in neurorehabilitation, especially in stroke patients or patients after traumatic brain injury.

In conclusion, the increased cortical excitability leads to an extension of neuronal activity. The time course of neurophysiological effects, as measured by TMS, and also seen in fMRI BOLD responses, suggests a prolonged clinical efficacy of AE stimulation. Further studies should focus on the issue whether more specialized stimulation protocols in particular with regard to stimulation intensities and frequencies can prolong the modulatory effects on the sensorimotor cortex through plastic changes in synaptic efficacy and thus can sub-serve a long-term rehabilitation process of impaired motor functions of the hand after brain lesions [76]. This finding of increased motor cortical excitability after afferent electrical stimulation can help develop new rehabilitation strategies in combination with physical and occupational therapy.

Author details

Stefan Golaszewski

Address all correspondence to: S.Golaszewski@salk.at

Department of Neurology and Neuroscience Institute, Paracelsus Medical University, Salzburg, Austria

References

[1] Kaelin-Lang A, Luft AR, Sawaki L, Burstein AH, Sohn YH, Cohen LG. Modulation of human corticomotor excitability by somatosensory input. The Journal of Physiology. 2002;**540**:623–633

[2] Golaszewski SM, Siedentopf CM, Koppelstaetter F, et al. Modulatory effects on human sensorimotor cortex by whole-hand afferent electrical stimulation. Neurology. 2004;**62**:2262–2269

[3] Golaszewski SM, Bergmann J, Christova M, et al. Increased motor cortical excitability after whole-hand electrical stimulation: A TMS study. Clinical Neurophysiology: Official Journal of the International Federation of Clinical Neurophysiology. 2010;**121**:248–254

[4] Chipchase LS, Schabrun SM, Hodges PW. Peripheral electrical stimulation to induce cortical plasticity: A systematic review of stimulus parameters. Clinical Neurophysiology: Official Journal of the International Federation of Clinical Neurophysiology. 2011;**122**:456–463

[5] Christova M, Rafolt D, Golaszewski S, Gallasch E. Outlasting corticomotor excitability changes induced by 25 Hz whole-hand mechanical stimulation. European Journal of Applied Physiology. 2011;**111**:3051–3059

[6] Dimitrijevic MM, Stokic DS, Wawro AW, Wun CC. Modification of motor control of wrist extension by mesh-glove electrical afferent stimulation in stroke patients. Archives of Physical Medicine and Rehabilitation. 1996;**77**:252–258

[7] Levin MF, Hui-Chan CW. Relief of hemiparetic spasticity by TENS is associated with improvement in reflex and voluntary motor functions. Electroencephalography and Clinical Neurophysiology. 1992;**85**:131–142

[8] Kraft GH, Fitts SS, Hammond MC. Techniques to improve function of the arm and hand in chronic hemiplegia. Archives of Physical Medicine and Rehabilitation. 1992;**73**:220–227

[9] Goldman H. Improvement of double simultaneous stimulation perception in hemiplegic patients. Archives of Physical Medicine and Rehabilitation. 1966;**47**:681–687

[10] Burne JA, Lippold OC. Reflex inhibition following electrical stimulation over muscle tendons in man. Brain. 1996;**119**(Pt 4):1107–1114

[11] Bodegard A, Geyer S, Herath P, Grefkes C, Zilles K, Roland PE. Somatosensory areas engaged during discrimination of steady pressure, spring strength, and kinesthesia. Human Brain Mapping. 2003;**20**:103–115

[12] Mariorenzi R, Zarola F, Caramia MD, Paradiso C, Rossini PM. Non-invasive evaluation of central motor tract excitability changes following peripheral nerve stimulation in healthy humans. Electroencephalography and Clinical Neurophysiology. 1991;**81**:90–101

[13] Wiesendanger M, Miles TS. Ascending pathway of low-threshold muscle afferents to the cerebral cortex and its possible role in motor control. Physiological Reviews. 1982;**62**:1234–1270

[14] Phillips CG, Powell TP, Wiesendanger M. Projection from low-threshold muscle afferents of hand and forearm to area 3a of baboon's cortex. The Journal of Physiology. 1971;**217**:419–446

[15] Prochazka A. Proprioceptive feedback and movement regulation. In: Handbook of Physiology. New York: American Physiological Society; 1996 pp. 89–127

[16] Rothwell J. Control of Human Voluntary Movement. 2nd ed. London: Chapman & Hall; 1994

[17] Jami L. Golgi tendon organs in mammalian skeletal muscle: Functional properties and central actions. Physiological Reviews. 1992;**72**:623–666

[18] Lafleur J, Zytnicki D, Horcholle-Bossavit G, Jami L. Depolarization of Ib afferent axons in the cat spinal cord during homonymous muscle contraction. The Journal of Physiology. 1992;**445**:345–354

[19] McCloskey DI. Kinesthetic sensibility. Physiological Reviews. 1978;**58**:763–820

[20] McIntyre AK, Proske U, Rawson JA. Cortical projection of afferent information from tendon organs in the cat. The Journal of Physiology. 1984;**354**:395–406

[21] Porter R, Lemon R. Corticospinal Function and Voluntary Movement. Oxford: Clarendon Press; 1993

[22] Gandevia SC. Kinesthesia: Roles for afferent signals and motor commands. In: Handbook of Physiology. New York: American Physiological Society; 1996. pp. 128–172

[23] Francis ST, Kelly EF, Bowtell R, Dunseath WJ, Folger SE, McGlone F. fMRI of the responses to vibratory stimulation of digit tips. Neuroimage. 2000;**11**:188–202

[24] Golaszewski SM, Siedentopf CM, Baldauf E, et al. Functional magnetic resonance imaging of the human sensorimotor cortex using a novel vibrotactile stimulator. Neuroimage. 2002;**17**:421–430

[25] Seitz RJ, Roland PE. Vibratory stimulation increases and decreases the regional cerebral blood flow and oxidative metabolism: A positron emission tomography (PET) study. Acta Neurologica Scandinavica. 1992;**86**:60–67

[26] Butefisch CM, Netz J, Wessling M, Seitz RJ, Homberg V. Remote changes in cortical excitability after stroke. Brain. 2003;**126**:470–481

[27] Liepert J, Storch P, Fritsch A, Weiller C. Motor cortex disinhibition in acute stroke. Clinical Neurophysiology: Official Journal of the International Federation of Clinical Neurophysiology. 2000;**111**:671–676

[28] Golaszewski S, Kremser C, Wagner M, Felber S, Aichner F, Dimitrijevic MM. Functional magnetic resonance imaging of the human motor cortex before and after whole-hand afferent electrical stimulation. Scandinavian Journal of Rehabilitation Medicine. 1999;**31**:165–173

[29] Larsson J, Gulyas B, Roland PE. Cortical representation of self-paced finger movement. Neuroreport. 1996;**7**:463–468

[30] Sanes JN, Donoghue JP, Thangaraj V, Edelman RR, Warach S. Shared neural substrates controlling hand movements in human motor cortex. Science. 1995;**268**:1775–1777

[31] Seitz RJ, Roland E, Bohm C, Greitz T, Stone-Elander S. Motor learning in man: A positron emission tomographic study. Neuroreport. 1990;**1**:57–60

[32] Logothetis NK, Pauls J, Augath M, Trinath T, Oeltermann A. Neurophysiological investigation of the basis of the fMRI signal. Nature. 2001;**412**:150–157

[33] Dimitrijevic MM. Mesh-glove. 1. A method for whole-hand electrical stimulation in upper motor neuron dysfunction. Scandinavian Journal of Rehabilitation Medicine. 1994;**26**:183–186

[34] Dimitrijevic MM, Soroker N. Mesh-glove. 2. Modulation of residual upper limb motor control after stroke with whole-hand electric stimulation. Scandinavian Journal of Rehabilitation Medicine. 1994;**26**:187–190

[35] Peurala SH, Pitkanen K, Sivenius J, Tarkka IM. Cutaneous electrical stimulation may enhance sensorimotor recovery in chronic stroke. Clinical Rehabilitation. 2002;**16**:709–716

[36] Aimonetti JM, Nielsen JB. Changes in intracortical excitability induced by stimulation of wrist afferents in man. The Journal of Physiology. 2001;**534**:891–902

[37] Donoghue JP. Plasticity of adult sensorimotor representations. Current Opinion in Neurobiology. 1995;**5**:749–754

[38] Hallett M. Motor cortex plasticity. Electroencephalography and Clinical Neurophysiology Supplement. 1999;**50**:85–91

[39] Jacobs KM, Donoghue JP. Reshaping the cortical motor map by unmasking latent intracortical connections. Science. 1991;**251**:944–947

[40] Pascual-Leone A, Torres F. Plasticity of the sensorimotor cortex representation of the reading finger in Braille readers. Brain. 1993;**116**(Pt 1):39–52

[41] Grafman J, Litvan I. Evidence for 4 forms of neuroplasticity. In: Grafman J, Christen Y, editors. Neural Plasticity: Building a Bridge from the Laboratory to the Clinic. Berlin: Springer-Verlag; 1999 pp. 131–139

[42] Hess G, Donoghue JP. Long-term potentiation of horizontal connections provides a mechanism to reorganize cortical motor maps. Journal of Neurophysiology. 1994;**71**:2543–2547

[43] Hirsch JA, Gilbert CD. Long-term changes in synaptic strength along specific intrinsic pathways in the cat visual cortex. The Journal of Physiology. 1993;**461**:247–262

[44] Ridding MC, Brouwer B, Nordstrom MA. Reduced interhemispheric inhibition in musicians. Experimental Brain Research. 2000;**133**:249–253

[45] Rizzolatti G, Fogassi L, Gallese V. Parietal cortex: From sight to action. Current Opinion in Neurobiology. 1997;**7**:562–567

[46] Sakata H, Taira M, Kusunoki M, Murata A, Tanaka Y. The TINS Lecture. The parietal association cortex in depth perception and visual control of hand action. Trends in Neuroscience. 1997;**20**:350–357

[47] Wu CW, van Gelderen P, Hanakawa T, Yaseen Z, Cohen LG. Enduring representational plasticity after somatosensory stimulation. Neuroimage. 2005;**27**:872–884

[48] Ridding MC, Rothwell JC. Afferent input and cortical organisation: A study with magnetic stimulation. Experimental Brain Research. 1999;**126**:536–544

[49] Sailer A, Molnar GF, Cunic DI, Chen R. Effects of peripheral sensory input on cortical inhibition in humans. The Journal of Physiology. 2002;**544**:617–629

[50] Deuschl G, Michels R, Berardelli A, Schenck E, Inghilleri M, Lucking CH. Effects of electric and magnetic transcranial stimulation on long latency reflexes. Experimental Brain Research. 1991;**83**:403–410

[51] Rossini PM, Tecchio F, Sabato A, Finazzi-Agro A, Pasqualetti P, Rossi S. The role of cutaneous inputs during magnetic transcranial stimulation. Muscle & Nerve. 1996;**19**:1302–1309

[52] Tokimura H, Di Lazzaro V, Tokimura Y, et al. Short latency inhibition of human hand motor cortex by somatosensory input from the hand. The Journal of Physiology. 2000;**523**(Pt 2):503–513

[53] Troni W, Cantello R, De Mattei M, Bergamini L. Muscle responses elicited by cortical stimulation in the human hand: Differential conditioning by activation of the proprioceptive and exteroceptive fibers of the median nerve. In: Rossini PM, Marsden CD, editors. Non-invasive Stimulation of the Brain and Spinal Cord: Fundamentals and Clinical Application. New York: Alan R. Liss; 1988

[54] Delwaide PJ, Olivier E. Conditioning transcranial cortical stimulation (TCCS) by exteroceptive stimulation in Parkinsonian patients. Advances in Neurology. 1990;**53**:175–181

[55] Uncini A, Kujirai T, Gluck B, Pullman S. Silent period induced by cutaneous stimulation. Electroencephalography and Clinical Neurophysiology. 1991;**81**:344–352

[56] Komori T, Watson BV, Brown WF. Influence of peripheral afferents on cortical and spinal motoneuron excitability. Muscle & Nerve. 1992;**15**:48–51

[57] Ohki Y, Suzuki T, Ugawa Y, Uesaka Y, Sakai K, Kanazawa I. Excitation of the motor cortex associated with the E2 phase of cutaneous reflexes in man. Brain Research. 1994;**633**:343–347

[58] Clouston PD, Kiers L, Menkes D, Sander H, Chiappa K, Cros D. Modulation of motor activity by cutaneous input: Inhibition of the magnetic motor evoked potential by digital electrical stimulation. Electroencephalography and Clinical Neurophysiology. 1995;**97**:114–125

[59] Inghilleri M, Berardelli A, Cruccu G, Manfredi M, Priori A, Rothwell JC. Inhibition of hand muscle motoneurones by peripheral nerve stimulation in the relaxed human

subject. Antidromic versus orthodromic input. Electroencephalography and Clinical Neurophysiology. 1995;**97**:63–68

[60] Kaneko K, Kawai S, Taguchi T, Fuchigami Y, Yonemura H, Fujimoto H. Cortical motor neuron excitability during cutaneous silent period. Electroencephalography and Clinical Neurophysiology. 1998;**109**:364–368

[61] Manconi FM, Syed NA, Floeter MK. Mechanisms underlying spinal motor neuron excitability during the cutaneous silent period in humans. Muscle & Nerve. 1998;**21**:1256–1264

[62] Palmer E, Ashby P. The transcortical nature of the late reflex responses in human small hand muscle to digital nerve stimulation. Experimental Brain Research. 1992;**91**:320–326

[63] Maertens de Noordhout A, Rothwell JC, Day BL, et al. Effect of digital nerve stimuli on responses to electrical or magnetic stimulation of the human brain. The Journal of Physiology. 1992;**447**:535–548

[64] Manganotti P, Zanette G, Bonato C, Tinazzi M, Polo A, Fiaschi A. Crossed and direct effects of digital nerves stimulation on motor evoked potential: A study with magnetic brain stimulation. Electroencephalography and Clinical Neurophysiology. 1997;**105**:280–289

[65] Kofler M, Glocker FX, Leis AA, et al. Modulation of upper extremity motoneurone excitability following noxious finger tip stimulation in man: A study with transcranial magnetic stimulation. Neuroscience Letters. 1998;**246**:97–100

[66] Rosenkranz K, Pesenti A, Paulus W, Tergau F. Focal reduction of intracortical inhibition in the motor cortex by selective proprioceptive stimulation. Experimental Brain Research. 2003;**149**:9–16

[67] Rosenkranz K, Rothwell JC. Differential effect of muscle vibration on intracortical inhibitory circuits in humans. The Journal of Physiology. 2003;**551**:649–660

[68] Hamzei F, Liepert J, Dettmers C, Weiller C, Rijntjes M. Two different reorganization patterns after rehabilitative therapy: An exploratory study with fMRI and TMS. NeuroImage. 2006;**31**:710–720

[69] Kujirai T, Caramia MD, Rothwell JC, et al. Corticocortical inhibition in human motor cortex. The Journal of Physiology. 1993;**471**:501–519

[70] Ziemann U, Lonnecker S, Steinhoff BJ, Paulus W. Effects of antiepileptic drugs on motor cortex excitability in humans: A transcranial magnetic stimulation study. Annals of Neurology. 1996;**40**:367–378

[71] Ziemann U, Lonnecker S, Steinhoff BJ, Paulus W. The effect of lorazepam on the motor cortical excitability in man. Experimental Brain Research. 1996;**109**:127–135

[72] Ziemann U, Rothwell JC, Ridding MC. Interaction between intracortical inhibition and facilitation in human motor cortex. The Journal of Physiology. 1996;**496**(Pt 3):873–881

[73] Golaszewski SM, Bergmann J, Christova M, et al. Modulation of motor cortex excitability by different levels of whole-hand afferent electrical stimulation. Clinical Neurophysiology: Official Journal of the International Federation of Clinical Neurophysiology. 2012;**123**:193–199

[74] Keller A, Pavlides C, Asanuma H. Long-term potentiation in the cat somatosensory cortex. Neuroreport. 1990;**1**:49–52

[75] Ghirardi M, Montarolo PG, Kandel ER. A novel intermediate stage in the transition between short- and long-term facilitation in the sensory to motor neuron synapse of aplysia. Neuron. 1995;**14**:413–420

[76] Weiller C, Chollet F, Friston KJ, Wise RJ, Frackowiak RS. Functional reorganization of the brain in recovery from striatocapsular infarction in man. Annals of Neurology. 1992;**31**:463–472

2

GABAergic Synapse Dysfunction and Repair in Temporal Lobe Epilepsy

Meghan A. Van Zandt and Janice R. Naegele

Abstract

Severe medial temporal lobe epilepsy (mTLE) is often associated with pharmacoresistant seizures, impaired memory and mood disorders. In the hippocampus, GABAergic inhibitory interneuron dysfunction and other neural circuit abnormalities contribute to hyperexcitability, but the mechanisms are still not well understood. Experimental approaches aimed at correcting deficits in hippocampal circuits in mTLE include attempts to replace GABAergic interneurons through neural stem cell transplantation. Evidence from studies in rodent mTLE models indicates that transplanted GABAergic progenitor cells integrate into the hippocampus, form inhibitory synapses, reduce seizures and improve cognitive deficits. Here, we review current work in this field and describe potential molecular mechanisms underlying successful transplantation.

Keywords: GABA, temporal lobe, epilepsy, hippocampus, GABAergic, interneurons, neuroligin, neurexin, seizures, inhibition, gephyrin, collybistin, cognition, spatial memory, behaviour, transplantation, therapy, stem cells

1. Introduction

Epilepsy is a brain disorder characterized by a predisposition to generate epileptic seizures that may have subsequent neurological, cognitive, psychological and social effects. Many patients with severe medial temporal lobe epilepsy (mTLE) experience intractable seizures and degenerative changes in the temporal lobes of the brain, particularly the hippocampus [1]. Pharmacological treatments for these patients may become ineffective [2–5], and chronic severe pharmacoresistant seizures in mTLE patients can lead to memory impairments, anxiety and depression. While removing epileptogenic foci provides better seizure control in these patients, surgery may not be feasible if the seizures are generated bilaterally or at multiple foci. Moreover, one of the challenges of treating mTLE is that seizures trigger neuroplastic changes in the adult hippocampus, including axonal sprouting, rewiring and abnormal migration and growth of new dentate granule cells (GCs). Which of these changes are necessary and sufficient for generating recurrent seizures that can be corrected through cell-replacement therapies is not well known.

A major focus of current research is developing rigorous protocols for deriving human neural stem cells from pluripotent stem cells (PSCs) and directing their differentiation into the specific types of neurons, including subtypes of GABAergic interneurons. Additional studies are focusing on the circuit-level and molecular mechanisms that regulate incorporation of transplanted mouse or human GABAergic interneuron progenitors into host brains. Studies of the functional impact of transplanting GABAergic interneurons into the brain and spinal cord in models of different neurological disorders are still in their infancy [6], and relatively little is known about mechanisms guiding the survival, differentiation and synaptic integration of transplanted GABAergic interneurons in the adult brain. This review focuses on current work in this field of regenerative medicine and new directions for regenerating neural circuits.

2. Pathology of medial temporal lobe epilepsy

Dentate gyrus (DG) reorganization has been extensively studied in rodent models of mTLE, particularly the chemoconvulsant models that employ kainic acid or pilocarpine injections to induce status epilepticus (SE). Prominent features of DG reorganization are the loss of glutamatergic mossy cells and subsets of GABAergic interneurons. Depletion of these neuronal populations results in loss of feed-forward inhibition of DG GCs [7–11]. Some of the principal cells of CA1 and CA3, as well as adult-generated GCs of the DG born around the time of SE, sprout excitatory axon collaterals, increasing recurrent excitatory drive between neighbouring neurons [12, 13]. Many somatostatin (SOM) -expressing GABAergic interneurons degenerate in the DG and CA1 of the hippocampus in mTLE, and some residual GABAergic interneurons form compensatory synaptic connections [10, 14–18]. Axonal sprouting by surviving hippocampal GABAergic interneurons increases the number of inhibitory synaptic puncta above control values in chronically epileptic rodents, although this response is insufficient to counter the development of spontaneous recurrent seizures typical of mTLE [15, 19]. Together, these studies suggest that replacing hippocampal GABAergic interneurons in pharmacoresistant mTLE may be a promising strategy for suppressing seizures (**Figure 1**).

GCs are a type of excitatory glutamatergic neuron in the granule cell layer (GCL) of the DG of the hippocampus, and studies suggest that they are relatively more resistant to seizure-induced injury than many other cell types in the hippocampus [32]. They form axons called the mossy fibres that project to CA3 pyramidal neurons and other cell types [1, 33–35]. GCs are generated throughout life [28, 36–41]. In rodent models of mTLE and human patients, many GCs, born around the time of SE, develop altered morphology, excitability and connectivity. These adult-generated GCs form recurrent axon collaterals in the inner molecular layer, a form of neuroplasticity termed mossy fibre sprouting (MFS) [26]. Overgrowth of mossy

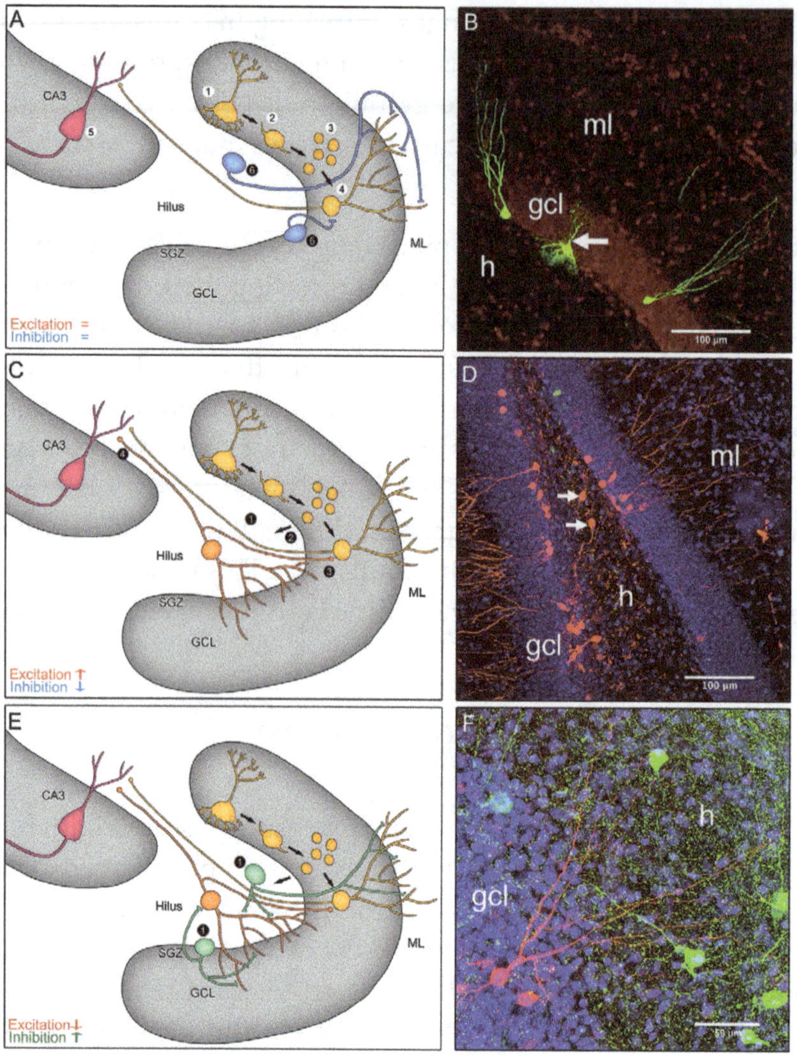

Figure 1. Studies of GABAergic interneuron transplantation are investigating whether it is feasible to replace populations of endogenous interneurons damaged by temporal lobe epilepsy. **(A)** In the non-epileptic mouse dentate gyrus (DG), self-renewing, quiescent Type 1 progenitor cells in the subgranular zone (SGZ) extend radial glial processes through the granule cell layer (GCL) (1). They divide asymmetrically to produce Type 2 progenitors (2) which further divide to generate pools of migratory Type 3 neuroblasts (3). As these neuroblasts mature, they differentiate into GCs, migrate into the GCL, extend their dendrites towards the molecular layer (ML)(4) and project axons to hilar interneurons and mossy cells and CA3 pyramidal cells (5). Inhibitory GABAergic interneurons (6) synapse with GCs and provide inhibition. GCs are shown in yellow, inhibitory interneurons in light blue and pyramidal cells in magenta. **(B)** High-resolution confocal image of retrovirally labelled GCs (green) and neuronal nuclei (NeuN, red) in the naïve mouse hippocampus. White arrow indicates a normal Type 1 progenitor cell in the SGZ. **(C)** In mTLE, some of the hilar GABAergic interneurons die, resulting in an overall loss of inhibition to GCs (1). Additionally, some adult-generated GCs undergo abnormal migration into the hilus, becoming ectopic. They typically form abnormal dendrites and sprout recurrent axonal collaterals, forming excitatory feedback projections onto other GCs (3) as well as abnormal excitatory projections to the CA3 pyramidal cells (4) [20–30]. GCs are shown in yellow; an abnormal, ectopic GC in orange; and pyramidal cells in magenta. **(D)** High-resolution confocal image of retrovirally labelled GCs (red) in the hippocampus of a mouse with mTLE. Nuclei are marked using a Nissl stain (blue). White arrows show ectopic GCs born after induction of epilepsy located in abnormal locations in the hilus. **(E)** Studies employing transplantation of GABAergic progenitors into either the normal or epileptic hippocampus show that they migrate away from the site of injection and form dense axonal arbors throughout the hilus, GCL and molecular layer. These interneurons appear to form functional synapses with hyperexcitable GCs, including those with aberrant morphologies (1), increasing synaptic inhibition in the epileptic circuit. GCs are shown in yellow; abnormal, ectopic GC in orange; transplanted GABAergic inhibitory interneurons in green; and pyramidal cells in magenta [31]. **(F)** High-resolution confocal image of a retrovirally labelled GC (red) receiving dense synaptic contacts from transplanted MGE-derived GABAergic progenitors (green). Nuclei are labelled using Nissl staining (blue) [31].

fibre recurrent collaterals onto GCs and pyramidal cells contributes to a hyperexcitable dentate environment [27, 29, 42–44].

As demonstrated by computer simulations, a few hubs of highly interconnected GCs are sufficient to create a hyperexcitable network [30, 45]. Additional epilepsy-induced neuroplastic changes to the DG include GC dispersion, formation of GC basal dendrites and ectopic migration of GCs into the hilus of the DG [23–25, 46–50]. Many adult-generated GCs born in epileptic rodents also have reduced dendritic spines and hypertrophic cell bodies [20, 21, 44, 51]. These cells often have higher baseline firing rates than normally positioned GCs in epileptic animals and non-epileptic controls and more depolarized resting membrane potentials, predisposing them to hyperexcitability [22]. Although increasing adult neurogenesis is not sufficient to cause seizures, it contributes to hyperexcitability [52, 53].

3. Cognitive changes in medial temporal lobe epilepsy

Severe mTLE is linked to a number of comorbidities including cognitive deficits, heightened anxiety, increased aggression and depression [54, 55]. Rodents with mTLE show decreased social recognition, greater preference for closed arms in the elevated zero or plus maze test for anxiety and longer periods of immobility in the forced swim test for depression [56]. Additionally, a number of studies demonstrated severe learning deficits in the Morris water maze test of spatial memory [57, 58] and other spatial memory tasks [59]. Human mTLE patients exposed to virtual environments that test spatial memory also showed memory deficits [60, 61].

Changes in the properties of hippocampal and entorhinal cortex circuits may be responsible for cognitive changes in mTLE, but the nature of these changes is not well understood. Both human and rodent spatial memory formation and recall are dependent on place cells in the hippocampus and grid cells in the entorhinal cortex. These important cells exhibit distinct, spatially specific firing patterns, forming a topographical memory map of an area as an individual moves through space [62–65]. Hippocampal inhibitory interneurons, similar to place cells, show distinct, spatially specific discharges, implicating a role in the formation and fine tuning of spatial memories [66, 67]. Studies suggest that impairments in receptive field properties of the grid and place cells may occur in mTLE [68–71].

The regulation by inhibitory interneurons of various brain rhythms may also become altered, as rodents with mTLE show distinctly lower frequency and power of theta rhythms correlated with poor performance in spatial memory tasks [72–74]. Although the exact alterations occurring in the grid-place cell network are not yet clear, it is evident that the hyperexcitable firing of GCs and the overall disinhibition of the network by loss of inhibitory interneurons severely disrupts spatial memory formation [72, 75–79]. The disinhibition of the hippocampal networks following epileptogenesis and the subsequent development of spatial memory deficits suggest that the loss of inhibitory interneurons may disrupt place fields, providing a further rationale for cell-based therapies aimed at GABAergic interneuron transplantation.

4. Seizure suppression following transplantation of medial ganglionic eminence-derived neural progenitors

Initial studies established proof of concept for cell-based therapies for treating epilepsy by demonstrating that transplants of non-neural cells engineered to release GABA non-synaptically could increase seizure thresholds [80]. Increasingly, studies have aimed to identify the functional classes of interneurons that can migrate, integrate and suppress seizures in different models of epilepsy in rodents. The large variety of functional classes of cortical inhibitory interneurons and their sites of origin in the ventricular zones of the embryonic forebrain have been extensively studied. During development, forebrain GABAergic interneurons are born in the embryonic ventricular regions called the ganglionic eminences, including the medial, lateral and caudal ganglionic eminences (MGE, LGE, CGE). These transient proliferative zones lining the forebrain lateral ventricles generate different types of GABAergic interneuron progenitors, which then migrate to their final destinations in the forebrain, including the cerebral cortex, hippocampus and striatum [81–83]. Forebrain GABAergic progenitors expressing SOM or parvalbumin (PV) emerge from the MGE in early embryonic life and migrate tangentially into the cerebral cortex and hippocampus [84].

In naïve rodents and different epilepsy models, transplanted GABAergic interneuron progenitors from the embryonic MGE have been found to be highly migratory, a prerequisite for transplantation therapies aimed at repairing large brain areas. MGE-derived GABAergic progenitors transplanted into postnatal 3–4-day old mouse cerebral cortex differentiated into inhibitory interneurons expressing markers of mature GABAergic phenotypes, including PV, SOM, calretinin (CR) and neuropeptide Y (NPY), and displayed mature firing properties characteristic of inhibitory interneurons [85]. MGE-derived PV-positive interneurons transplanted into naïve postnatal 1–2-day old pups integrated into the endogenous circuitry and, upon maturation, displayed firing properties similar to endogenous PV-expressing interneurons and formed functional synapses onto pyramidal neurons [86]. In a mouse model of mTLE generated through neurotoxin-induced ablation of GABAergic interneurons, MGE transplantation significantly increased inhibitory postsynaptic currents (IPSCs) in CA1 pyramidal cells and reduced seizure frequency and severity [87]. These grafts contained high percentages of GABAergic interneurons that co-expressed PV, NPY or CR. Transplanting MGE cells into an epilepsy model caused by mutations of the Kv1.1 potassium channel also increased IPSCs in nearby endogenous pyramidal cells [88]. Additionally, MGE cell transplants into a cyclin D2 knockout model of hippocampal disinhibition restored lost inhibitory input and normalized hyperactivity and fear conditioning [89].

The efficacy of MGE cell transplantation for controlling seizures has also been studied in chemoconvulsant models of mTLE, including the kainic acid and pilocarpine (PILO) models. In an early ground-breaking study in the rat kainic acid model, Shetty and colleagues transplanted neurospheres derived from embryonic day-14 rat MGE progenitors and found that they reduced seizure duration, total time spent in seizures and seizure severity; however, these grafts failed to improve spatial memory deficits [90]. It is important to note that the degree of cognitive impairment may differ between kainic acid or pilocarpine models, different species and even different strains of mice [91, 92].

The mouse PILO model shows a pattern of loss of hippocampal interneurons that is similar to human mTLE, making this model highly appropriate for preclinical studies investigating GABAergic interneuron transplantation [93]. Work from our laboratory showed that MGE cells transplanted into the hilus of the DG led to significant reductions in seizure frequency, duration and severity in the mouse PILO model [31]. The transplanted neurons matured into GABAergic interneurons that expressed CB, SOM or PV and formed dense networks of inhibitory synapses onto dentate GCs. Optogenetic experiments in hippocampal slices from these mice showed that light-induced depolarization of MGE transplants expressing channelrhodopsin (ChR2) triggered strong postsynaptic inhibitory currents in GCs, indicating that the transplanted neurons had integrated synaptically. These findings suggest that seizure suppression can be achieved with focal transplants into the DG. In this study, which employed continuous video-EEG recording for periods of up to 3 months, some of the mice show a reoccurrence of seizures several months after transplantation, suggesting that achieving enduring seizure suppression may require more widespread dispersion of the transplanted interneurons throughout different subfields of the hippocampus. Determining the optimal sites and cell types for permanent seizure suppression will be important for moving into clinical applications.

5. Transplantation therapy using human embryonic stem cell-derived progenitors

For treating patients with severe mTLE, sources of human interneurons are required. Previous work showed that differentiating human embryonic stem cells (hESCs) into GABAergic inhibitory interneuron progenitors can be achieved using specific combinations of signalling molecules and growth factors [94–100]. Carpentino et al. (2008) found that maturation of transplanted mouse or hESCs is highly dependent on the environment into which the cells are transplanted. For instance, in the mouse systemic kainic acid model, it was shown that ESC-derived neural progenitors transplanted in the CA3 area tended to migrate into the DG and differentiate into GCs, whereas those implanted into the fimbria tended to mature into astrocytes [101]. Lee et al. also transplanted undifferentiated hESCs into the CA3 region of the hippocampus in epileptic rats. Some of these differentiated into GABAergic interneurons (~21% of engrafted cells) and at 8 weeks post transplantation displayed immature morphology. Even with low numbers of GABAergic neurons, the animals with transplants showed reduced seizure frequency and seizure duration for 2–3 months. EEG recordings in these animals were limited to 60 hours per week, with a 2-week recording period, during daylight hours only. Additionally, when tested 3 months after transplantation, improvements in Morris water maze performance were not found [102]. More recent studies have focused on purified, fate-determined populations of hESCs for transplantation. Treating hESCs with the signalling molecule sonic hedgehog (SHH) or a sonic hedgehog agonist (SAG), in combination with modulating the WNT and FGF signalling pathways, can be used in vitro to induce ventral forebrain neural fates and MGE-like cell types [97–100, 103–106]. Ventralized hESC-derived progenitors have identities similar to that of mouse MGE-derived GABAergic interneuron progenitors, potentially allowing the large-scale *in vitro* production of human cells for therapies to treat clinical disorders [94]. However, undifferentiated hESCs can cause teratomas, making it important to develop protocols for eliminating them prior to transplantation [107].

Evidence that fate-directed human GABAergic interneuron progenitors integrate into the epileptic circuitry of the hippocampus following transplantation into the hilus has emerged in several recent studies. To reduce immune rejection of cell grafts, human and mouse ESC transplantation studies generally use immunodeficient host animals. The nonobese diabetic (NOD)-severe combined immunodeficiency (SCID) mice are an immunodeficient mouse strain lacking mature T and B cells and with reduced natural killer (NK) cell activity. Another mouse strain, the Nod-scid-gamma (NSG) triple mutant, has a mutation at the interleukin-2 receptor (IL-2R) γ-chain locus. This strain shows the highest impairment in T-cell, B-cell and NK-cell development, resulting in low graft rejection [108]. Both strains have been used to study differentiation of ESC-derived GABAergic interneurons [109].

In a recent study in which hESC-derived progenitors were differentiated in vitro into MGE-like progenitors and transplanted into NSG mice, the transplanted cells differentiated into GABAergic neurons expressing SOM, PV, CB, CR or NPY after approximately 4 months. Additionally, optogenetic stimulation of the transplanted cells produced action potentials and resulted in IPSCs in endogenous hippocampal neurons, suggesting successful synaptic integration into the existing circuitry of the hippocampus. Video-EEG monitoring of these animals 3 months post-transplant showed reduced numbers of seizures in engrafted animals [110]. However, the EEG monitoring was only for short durations of 5–10 days, which is likely too brief a period to reliably evaluate seizures in rodent chemoconvulsant models, due to the clustered and periodic nature of the spontaneous recurrent seizures.

6. Ameliorating cognitive and behavioural abnormalities in epilepsy by transplantation of GABAergic interneurons

Inconsistent results regarding spatial memory improvement have been reported following GABAergic interneuron transplantation. In the Morris water maze test of spatial memory, C57BL/6 mice with PILO induced mTLE and received mouse MGE cell transplants showed significantly reduced escape latencies in training, significantly more platform crossings in the probe trial; improved path efficiency; and a greater amount of time spent in the target quadrant than epileptic controls [111]. In another study, rats with mTLE that MGE-derived stem cell grafts showed no improvements in the Morris water maze task 8 weeks post-engraftment relative to non-engrafted mTLE controls [90]. However, transplantation took place approximately 3 months following induction of epilepsy, a longer time interval than other studies. The lack of cognitive improvement at this later transplantation time point suggests a potentially limited time window in which transplanted GABAergic interneurons must integrate to confer cognitive improvements. In a third study in NSG mice with mTLE, engrafted hESC-derived GABAergic interneuron progenitors appeared to improve performance in the Y-maze test of spatial memory and memory in the novel recognition test [110].

Behavioural tests also suggested that mTLE mice receiving interneuron grafts were less hyperactive and aggressive, compared to mTLE controls with only intrahippocampal injections of media. In the handling test of aggression, in which mice are scored for aggressive reactions to a series of increasingly uncomfortable stimuli, TLE mice with hESC or foetal mouse MGE interneuron transplants scored significantly lower in aggression ratings than controls [109, 110]. These transplants also reduced hyperactive behaviour [110]. Taken together, these results suggest that both rodent and human GABAergic interneuron transplants may ameliorate some of the psychological comorbidities in rodents with mTLE. While the Morris water maze is currently one of the standard tests in the industry for spatial memory, rodents with mTLE often exhibit a phenomenon known as thigmotaxis, in which animals will locomote or swim adjacent to the walls of an apparatus or make repeated circles [91, 112]. In such animals, it is uncertain whether the data reflect poor spatial memory or an anxiety phenotype. Therefore, alternative spatial memory tests should be used to gain a more complete understanding of how GABAergic interneuron transplantation affects cognition. An alternative test of hippocampal-dependent spatial memory is a modification of the novel object recognition test in which animals must learn to recognize that a previously familiar object has changed location. This test, called novel object location task, takes advantage of the rodent preference for novelty and desire to explore changes in its environment [113, 114]. Another test of spatial memory is the Barnes maze, consisting of an elevated platform with closed holes around the circumference. One hole is available for escape into a dark box. Remaining on the platform is unpleasant to the rodent, due to bright lights, fans and/or loud ambient noise, encouraging a swift escape to the box. As this test measures a very natural desire to escape an unpleasant environment, it is considered an effective test of normal rodent behaviour and spatial memory [115]. The Barnes maze also has no walls, eliminating thigmotaxis, although care must be taken to prevent animals from falling from the raised platform. Additional tests of spatial memory include the Y-maze, T-maze and the radial arm maze, all of which measure the ability of a rodent to remember previously travelled areas [116–121]. This extensive array of spatial memory tests can provide a more complete picture of the behavioural improvements following GABAergic interneuron transplantation in rodents with mTLE.

Currently, most testing of aggression has been done using the handling test, which, while effective, is an unnatural stimulus to the rodent [110, 111]. In addition to the handling test, the resident-intruder test can be used to analyse the response of a rodent to more natural stimuli. Male rodents are territorial, and the resident-intruder test measures the aggressive reactions to a male rival within their space. Although care must be taken to avoid injury to animals, this test measures an innate animal response and can be an effective measure of aggression in mTLE animals with transplants [122].

Although heightened anxiety is a common and well-characterized comorbidity in rodent mTLE models and human patients, surprisingly little work has been done to examine the effects of GABAergic transplants on correcting anxiety phenotypes. As rodents with mTLE have a tendency to exhibit thigmotaxis, which skews results in tests such as the open field test or the Morris water maze [91, 112], paradigms such as the elevated plus maze, elevated zero maze or the light-dark box can be used to provide more accurate measures of anxiety in rodents with mTLE [123–128].

7. GABAergic synapse formation and stability: potential mechanisms of transplanted cell integration

Relatively few studies have examined the molecular mechanisms responsible for guiding synaptic integration of transplanted cells into mature neural circuits. Previous findings suggest that cell-cell interactions mediate the formation and stabilization of both excitatory and inhibitory synapses [129–131]. The synaptic scaffolding complex between GABAergic interneurons and their postsynaptic targets in the developing brain may also guide recruitment and stabilization of the new synaptic connections formed by transplanted interneurons (**Figure 2**).

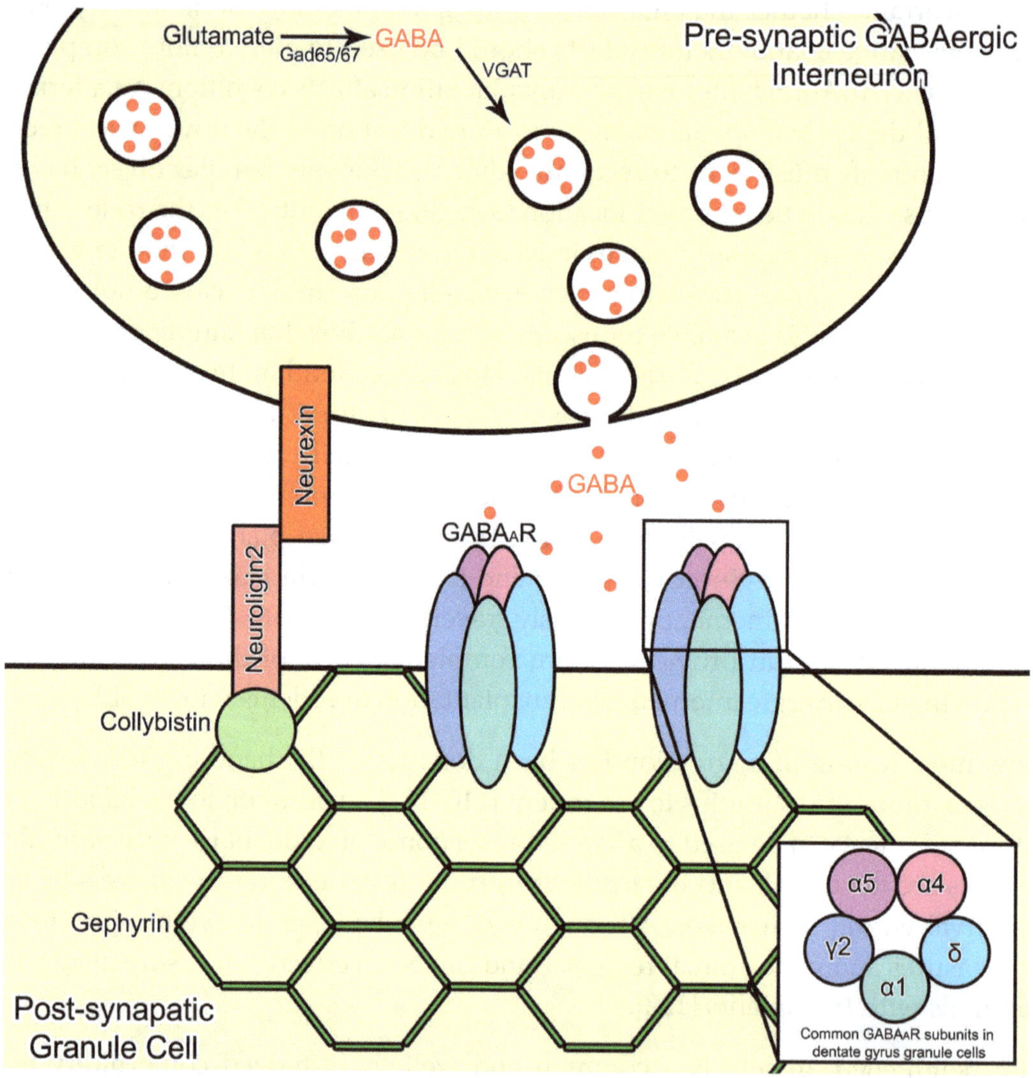

Figure 2. Interactions between cell surface molecules that are binding partners provide a potential mechanism for forming or stabilizing new synapses between transplanted GABAergic interneurons and endogenous neurons in the hippocampus. GABAergic synapse formation is coordinated by multiple molecules in the pre- and postsynaptic sites. Binding between presynaptic neurexin molecules and postsynaptic neuroligin2 (NLGN2) molecules may be important for initial formation or maintenance of GABAergic synapses. NLGN2 is associated with a postsynaptic complex containing collybistin, gephyrin and $GABA_A$Rs, which are necessary in the formation of functional inhibitory circuitry. Collybistin, gephyrin, NLGN2 or $GABA_A$R subunit γ2 deficiency results in impaired inhibitory synapses [132–141].

The synaptic scaffolding protein gephyrin is a tubulin-binding protein that forms a latticework structure of hexagonal trimers that regulate $GABA_A$ receptor clustering at synaptic sites [142, 143]. Gephyrin stabilizes inhibitory synapses and is required for proper function. Genetic reduction of the $\gamma 2$ subunit of $GABA_A$ receptors, a primary binding partner of gephyrin in GABAergic synapses, also severely reduces gephyrin and $GABA_A$ receptor clustering required for functional inhibitory synapses [132]. Repression of gephyrin expression causes a similar loss of clustering, revealing an interdependent relationship between the two synaptic binding partners necessary for proper inhibitory synapse formation and function [132, 144, 145]. Increases in endogenous gephyrin in response to compensatory surviving interneuron sprouting may also make the epileptic hippocampus a more receptive environment for new inhibitory synapses to form [146]. Gephyrin is significantly decreased in the first few weeks post-SE followed by a significant increase back towards normal levels at around 1 month post-SE [147]. Following transplantation, a majority of engrafted GABAergic interneuron synaptic boutons were associated with postsynaptic gephyrin clusters, indicating that this vital synaptic scaffolding component may be recruited to sites of new GABAergic synapse formation in the adult hippocampus [31].

Collybistin, another GABAergic synaptic scaffolding component, binds to both gephyrin and Neuroligin 2 (NLGN2) and may facilitate gephyrin-mediated clustering of $GABA_A$ receptors. Collybistin is a GDP/GTP-exchange factor that interacts directly with gephyrin in the inhibitory synaptic scaffold [131, 133, 148–150]. Collybistin-deficient mice display reduced clustering of gephyrin and $GABA_A$ receptors, reduced synaptic inhibition and altered synaptic plasticity [131, 141].

NLGN2 is part of a family of cell adhesion molecules implicated in synapse formation and stability. NLGN2 localizes only to GABAergic inhibitory synapses, where it is associated with neurexin, its presynaptic binding partner [151–153]. NLGN2 is part of the molecular scaffolding complex that includes collybistin and gephyrin [133]. NLGN2-deficient mice show decreased inhibitory function, as well as a variety of cognitive and behavioural comorbidities, such as increased anxiety, aggression and disruptions in spatial memory formation, similar to those seen in mTLE and other neurological disorders [129, 136, 137, 154–157]. Various studies have shown that binding between NLGN2 and neurexin induces inhibitory synapse formation [130, 158] and stabilization [135, 159], even in non-neuronal cell types [160].

$GABA_A$ receptor subunit composition may also play a role in the integration and stabilizing influence of transplanted inhibitory interneurons. Composition of $GABA_A$ subunits is impacted by the pathological changes induced in mTLE [161–163]. DG GCs, which are significant propagators of hyperexcitability in mTLE, are particularly enriched in the δ subunit of $GABA_A$ receptors in the normal brain; these receptors have a very high affinity for GABA and are strongly involved in tonic inhibition [164–166] at extrasynaptic sites [167]. In general, hippocampal neurons express multiple subunits, including abundant α, β, δ and γ subunits, with δ primarily restricted to GCs of the DG, with additional expression of other subunits in the CA1 and CA3 areas [168]. As such, it is apparent that $GABA_A$ receptors in the hippocampus are composed of a diverse pool of subunits that regulate inhibitory input. In mTLE, the composition of $GABA_A$ subunits becomes altered. Similar to the upregulation of gephyrin during the chronic phase of mTLE in response to compensatory interneuron sprouting, the $\gamma 2$ and α subunits also show increased expression in the hippocampus. Conversely, expression of the δ subunit decreases days after the initial epileptic event and remains depressed into the chronic stages of mTLE [169]. It is not known whether synapses formed by surviving inhibitory interneurons are capable of recruiting the necessary subunit composition for proper inhibition, considering the overall depletion of δ subunits compared to $\gamma 2$ and α. Moreover, whether transplanted, healthy GABAergic inhibitory interneurons can recruit all of the normal subunits to inhibitory synapses is not known. Further investigation of subunit composition within the epileptic hippocampus post transplantation will be necessary to investigate whether transplantation normalizes $GABA_A$ receptor composition.

8. Conclusion

While safe and effective stem cell therapies for treating neurological disorders, including severe mTLE, may be years away from the clinic, recent work has increased scientific understanding of how to derive specific types of human neurons for transplantation and how to evaluate functional changes that result. Because human neuron maturation takes many months or years, transplantation studies in rodents are limited in the kinds of information they can provide about the potential therapeutic effects of these cells in clinical populations. Recent studies have utilized a wide range of experimental tools, including electrophysiology, immunohistochemistry, optogenetics, chemogenetics and behavioural assays to assess learning, memory, anxiety, social behaviour and depression. These approaches are aiding studies to evaluate synaptic integration and functionality of human neural stem cell transplants for treating epilepsy.

Acknowledgements

We would like to thank Nicholas Woods, Bryan Luikart and Elizabeth Paquette for their assistance with retroviral labelling of GCs and confocal images. Work in our lab was supported by NINDS grant R15NS072879-01A1, Connecticut Stem Cell Established Investigator Grant and a Challenge Award from Citizens United for Research in Epilepsy (J.R.N.).

Author details

Meghan A. Van Zandt and Janice R. Naegele*

*Address all correspondence to: jnaegele@wesleyan.edu

Wesleyan University, Middletown, CT, USA

References

[1] Dulla, C.G., Coulter, D.A., and Ziburkus, J., *From molecular circuit dysfunction to disease case studies in epilepsy, traumatic brain injury, and Alzheimer's disease*. The Neuroscientist, 2016. **22**(3): pp. 295–312.

[2] Orozco-Suárez, S., Escalante-Santiago, D., Feria-Romero, I., Ureña-Guerrero, M.E., Rocha, L., Alonso-Vanegas, M.A., Villeda-Hernandez, J., Velasco, A., *Abnormalities of GABA System and Human Pharmacoresistant Epilepsy*, in *Pharmacoresistance in Epilepsy: From Genes and Molecules to Promising Therapies*, L. Rocha and E.A. Cavalheiro, Editors. 2013, Springer New York: New York, NY. pp. 127–147.

[3] Rubio-Donnadieu, F., *Pharmacoresistance and Epilepsy*, in *Pharmacoresistance in Epilepsy: From Genes and Molecules to Promising Therapies*, L. Rocha and E.A. Cavalheiro, Editors. 2013, Springer New York: New York, NY. pp. 1–9.

[4] van Vliet, E. A., Aronica, E., Gorter, J., *Role of blood–brain barrier in temporal lobe epilepsy and pharmacoresistance*. Neuroscience, 2014. 277: pp. 455–473.

[5] Alexopoulos, A.V., *Pharmacoresistant epilepsy: definition and explanation*. Epileptology, 2013. **1**(1): pp. 38–42.

[6] Tyson, J.A. and Anderson, S.A., *GABAergic interneuron transplants to study development and treat disease*. Trends in Neurosciences, 2014. **37**(3): pp. 169–177.

[7] de Lanerolle, N.C., Kim, J., Robbins, R., Spencer, D., *Hippocampal interneuron loss and plasticity in human temporal lobe epilepsy*. Brain Research, 1989. **495**(2): pp. 387–395.

[8] Tóth, K., Erőss, L., Vajda, J., Halász, P., Freund, T.F., Maglóczky, Z., *Loss and reorganization of calretinin-containing interneurons in the epileptic human hippocampus*. Brain: A Journal of Neurology, 2010. **133**(9): pp. 2763–2777.

[9] Swartz, B.E., Houser, C.R., Tomiyasu, U., Walsh, G.O., DeSalles, A., Rich, J.R., Delgado-Escueta, A., *Hippocampal cell loss in posttraumatic human epilepsy*. Epilepsia, 2006. **47**(8): pp. 1373–1382.

[10] Houser, C.R. and Esclapez, M., *Vulnerability and plasticity of the GABA system in the pilocarpine model of spontaneous recurrent seizures*. Epilepsy Research, 1996. **26**(1): pp. 207–218.

[11] Jiao, Y. and Nadler, V.J., *Stereological analysis of GluR2-immunoreactive hilar neurons in the pilocarpine model of temporal lobe epilepsy: correlation of cell loss with mossy fiber sprouting*. Experimental Neurology, 2007. **205**(2): pp. 569–582.

[12] El-Hassar, L., Esclapez, M., and Bernard, C., *Hyperexcitability of the CA1 hippocampal region during epileptogenesis*. Epilepsia, 2007. **48**(s5): pp. 131–139.

[13] Esclapez, M., Hirsch, J.C., Ben-Ari, Y., Bernard, C., *Newly formed excitatory pathways provide a substrate for hyperexcitability in experimental temporal lobe epilepsy*. Journal of Comparative Neurology, 1999. **408**(4): pp. 449–460.

[14] Maglóczky, Z., *Sprouting in human temporal lobe epilepsy: excitatory pathways and axons of interneurons*. Epilepsy Research, 2010. **89**(1): pp. 52–59.

[15] Thind, K.K., Yamawaki, R., Phanwar, I., Zhang, G., Wen, X., Buckmaster, P.S., *Initial loss but later excess of GABAergic synapses with dentate granule cells in a rat model of temporal lobe epilepsy*. Journal of Comparative Neurology, 2010. **518**(5): pp. 647–667.

[16] Peng, Z., Zhang, N., Wei, W., Huang, C., *A reorganized GABAergic circuit in a model of epilepsy: evidence from optogenetic labeling and stimulation of somatostatin interneurons*. The Journal of Neuroscience, 2013. **33**(36): pp. 14392–14405.

[17] Hofmann, G., Balgooyen, L., Mattis, J., Deisseroth, K., Buckmaster, P.S., *Hilar somatostatin interneuron loss reduces dentate gyrus inhibition in a mouse model of temporal lobe epilepsy*. Epilepsia, 2016. **57**(6): pp. 977–983.

[18] Zhang, W., Yamawaki, R., Wen, X., Uhl, J., Diaz, J., Prince, D.A., Buckmaster, P.S., *Surviving hilar somatostatin interneurons enlarge, sprout axons, and form new synapses with granule cells in a mouse model of temporal lobe epilepsy*. The Journal of Neuroscience, 2009. **29**(45): p. 14247–14256.

[19] Davenport, C.J., Brown, J.W., Babb, T.L., *Sprouting of GABAergic and mossy fiber axons in dentate gyrus following intrahippocampal kainate in the rat*. Experimental Neurology, 1990. **109**(2): pp. 180–190.

[20] Koyama, R., Tao, K., Sasaki, T., Ichikawa, J., Miyamoto, D., Muramatsu, R., Matsuki, N., Ikegaya, Y., *GABAergic excitation after febrile seizures induces ectopic granule cells and adult epilepsy*. Nature Medicine, 2012. **18**(8): pp. 1271–1278.

[21] Pierce, J.P., McCloskey D.P., and Scharfman H.E., *Morphometry of hilar ectopic granule cells in the rat*. The Journal of Comparative Neurology, 2011. **519**(6): pp. 1196–1218.

[22] Althaus, A.L., Sagher, O., Parent, J.M., Murphy, G.G., *Intrinsic neurophysiological properties of hilar ectopic and normotopic dentate granule cells in human temporal lobe epilepsy and a rat model*. Journal of Neurophysiology, 2015. **113**(4): pp. 1184–1194.

[23] Cameron, M.C., Zhan R.Z., and Nadler V.J., *Morphologic integration of hilar ectopic granule cells into dentate gyrus circuitry in the pilocarpine model of temporal lobe epilepsy*. The Journal of Comparative Neurology, 2011. **519**(11): pp. 2175–2192.

[24] Scharfman, H.E. and Pierce J.P., *New insights into the role of hilar ectopic granule cells in the dentate gyrus based on quantitative anatomic analysis and three-dimensional reconstruction*. Epilepsia, 2012. **53**(s1): pp. 109–115.

[25] Shapiro, L.A. and Ribak, C.E., *Integration of newly born dentate granule cells into adult brains: hypotheses based on normal and epileptic rodents*. Brain Research Reviews, 2005. **48**(1): pp. 43–56.

[26] Buckmaster, P.S., Zhang, G., and Yamawaki, R., *Axon sprouting in a model of temporal lobe epilepsy creates a predominantly excitatory feedback circuit*. The Journal of Neuroscience: The Official Journal of the Society for Neuroscience, 2002. **22**(15): pp. 6650–6658.

[27] Danzer, S.C., He, X., Loepke, A.W., McNamara, J.O., *Structural plasticity of dentate granule cell mossy fibers during the development of limbic epilepsy*. Hippocampus, 2010. **20**(1): pp. 113–124.

[28] Ide, Y., Fujiyama, F., Okamoto-Furuta, K., Tamamaki, N., Kaneko, T., Hisatsune, T., *Rapid integration of young newborn dentate gyrus granule cells in the adult hippocampal circuitry*. European Journal of Neuroscience, 2008. **28**(12): pp. 2381–2392.

[29] Tauck, D.L. and Nadler, J.V., *Evidence of functional mossy fiber sprouting in hippocampal formation of kainic acid-treated rats*. The Journal of Neuroscience, 1985. **5**(4): pp. 1016–1022.

[30] Zhang, W., Huguenard, J.R., and Buckmaster, P.S., *Increased excitatory synaptic input to granule cells from hilar and CA3 regions in a rat model of temporal lobe epilepsy*. The Journal of Neuroscience, 2012. **32**(4): pp. 1183–1196.

[31] Henderson, K.W., Gupta, J., Tagliatela, S., Litvina, E., Zheng, X., Van Zandt, M.A., Woods, N., Grund, E., Lin, D., Royston, S., Yanagawa, Y., Aaron, G.B., Naegele, J.R., *Long-term seizure suppression and optogenetic analyses of synaptic connectivity in epileptic mice with hippocampal grafts of GABAergic interneurons*. The Journal of Neuroscience: The Official Journal of the Society for Neuroscience, 2014. **34**(40): pp. 13492–13504.

[32] Meldrum, B., *Protection Against Ischemic Brain Damage by Excitatory Amino Acid Antagonists.* , in *Neurochemical Correlates of Cerebral Ischemia*, N.G. Bazan, P. Braquet, and M.D. Ginsberg, Editors. 1992, Springer US: Boston, MA. p. 245-263.

[33] Amaral, D.G. and Witter, M.P., *The three-dimensional organization of the hippocampal formation: A review of anatomical data*. Neuroscience, 1989. **31**(3): pp. 571–591.

[34] Witter, M.P. and Amaral, D.G., *Entorhinal cortex of the monkey: V. Projections to the dentate gyrus, hippocampus, and subicular complex*. Journal of Comparative Neurology, 1991. **307**(3): pp. 437–459.

[35] Witter, M.P. and D.G. Amaral, *CHAPTER 21 - Hippocampal Formation A2 - Paxinos, George, in The Rat Nervous System (THIRD EDITION)*. 2004, Academic Press: Burlington. pp. 635–704.

[36] Ambrogini, P., Cuppini, R., Lattanzi, D., Ciuffoli, S., Frontini, A., Fanelli, M., *Synaptogenesis in adult-generated hippocampal granule cells is affected by behavioral experiences*. Hippocampus, 2010. **20**(7): pp. 799–810.

[37] Kirschen, G.W., A. Di Antonio, and S. Ge., *Chapter 2 - Physiology and Plasticity A2 - Canales, Juan J, in Adult Neurogenesis in the Hippocampus*. 2016, Academic Press: San Diego. pp. 19–40.

[38] van Praag, H., Schinder, A.F., Christie, B.R., Toni, N., Palmer, T.D., Gage, F.H., *Functional neurogenesis in the adult hippocampus*. Nature, 2002. **415**(6875): pp. 1030–1034.

[39] Drew, L.J., Fusi, S., and Hen, R., *Adult neurogenesis in the mammalian hippocampus: why the dentate gyrus*? Learning & Memory, 2013. **20**(12): pp. 710–729.

[40] Gross, C.G., *Neurogenesis in the adult brain: death of a dogma*. Nature Reviews Neuroscience, 2000. **1**(1): pp. 67–73.

[41] Ma, D.K., Marchetto, M.C., Guo, J.U., Ming, G., Gage, F.H., Song, H., *Epigenetic choreographers of neurogenesis in the adult mammalian brain*. Nature Neuroscience, 2010. **13**(11): pp. 1338–1344.

[42] Buckmaster, P.S. and Lew, F.H., *Rapamycin suppresses mossy fiber sprouting but not seizure frequency in a mouse model of temporal lobe epilepsy*. The Journal of Neuroscience: The Official Journal of the Society for Neuroscience, 2011. **31**(6): pp. 2337–2347.

[43] Lew, F.H. and Buckmaster, P.S., *Is there a critical period for mossy fiber sprouting in a mouse model of temporal lobe epilepsy*? Epilepsia, 2011. **52**(12): pp. 2326–2332.

[44] Murphy, B.L., Pun, R., Yin, H., Faulkner, C., *Heterogeneous integration of adult-generated granule cells into the epileptic brain*. The Journal of Neuroscience, 2011. **31**(1): pp. 105–117.

[45] Case, M.J. and Soltesz, I., *Computer Modeling of Epilepsy*, in *Jasper's Basic Mechanisms of the Epilepsies [Internet]*, Noebels J.L., et al., Editors. 2012, National Center for Biotechnology Information (US): Bethesda, MD.

[46] Hester, M.S. and Danzer, S.C., *Accumulation of abnormal adult-generated hippocampal granule cells predicts seizure frequency and severity*. The Journal of Neuroscience: The Official Journal of the Society for Neuroscience, 2013. **33**(21): pp. 8926–8936.

[47] Parent, J.M., *Adult neurogenesis in the intact and epileptic dentate gyrus*. Progress in Brain Research, 2007. **163**: pp. 529–817.

[48] Shapiro, L.A. and Ribak, C.E., *Newly born dentate granule neurons after pilocarpine-induced epilepsy have hilar basal dendrites with immature synapses*. Epilepsy Research, 2006. **69**(1): pp. 53–66.

[49] Dashtipour, K., Wong, A.M., Obenaus, A., Spigelman, I., Riback, C.E., *Temporal profile of hilar basal dendrite formation on dentate granule cells after status epilepticus*. Epilepsy Research, 2003. **54**(2–3): pp. 141–151.

[50] Spigelman, I., Yan, X.X., Obenaus, A., Lee, E.Y.S., Wasterlain, C.G., Ribak, C.E., *Dentate granule cells form novel basal dendrites in a rat model of temporal lobe epilepsy*. Neuroscience, 1998. **86**(1): pp. 109–120.

[51] Singh, S.P., LaSarge, C.L., An, A., McAuliffe, J.J., Danzer, S.C., *Clonal analysis of newborn hippocampal dentate granule cell proliferation and development in temporal lobe epilepsy*. eNeuro, 2015. **2**(6): pp. 1–13.

[52] Botterill, J.J., Brymer, K.J., Caruncho, H.J., Kalynchuk, L.E., *Aberrant hippocampal neurogenesis after limbic kindling: relationship to BDNF and hippocampal-dependent memory*. Epilepsy & Behavior: E&B, 2015. **47**: pp. 83–92.

[53] Korn, M.J., Mandle, Q.J., and Parent, J.M., *Conditional disabled-1 deletion in mice alters hippocampal neurogenesis and reduces seizure threshold*. Frontiers in Neuroscience, 2016. **10**(63): pp. 1–12.

[54] Boulogne, S., Catenoix, H., Ryvlin, P, Rheims, S., *Long-lasting seizure-related anxiety in patients with temporal lobe epilepsy and comorbid psychiatric disorders*. Epileptic Disorders: International Epilepsy Journal with Videotape, 2015. **17**(3): pp. 340–344.

[55] Rocha, L., Alonso-Vanegas, M., Martínez-Juárez, I.E., Orozco-Suárez, S., Escalante-Santiago, D., Feria-Romero, I.A., Zavala-Tecuapetla, C., Cisneros, J.M.M., Buentello-García, R.M., Cienfuegos, J., *GABAergic alterations in neocortex of patients with pharmacoresistant temporal lobe epilepsy can explain the comorbidity of anxiety and depression: the potential impact of clinical factors*. Frontiers in Cellular Neuroscience, 2014. **8**: pp. 442.

[56] Lopes, M.W., Lopes, S., Santos, D., Costa, A., Gonçalves, F., de Mello, N., Prediger, R., Farina, M., Walz, R., Leal, R., *Time course evaluation of behavioral impairments in the pilocarpine model of epilepsy*. Epilepsy & Behavior: E&B, 2016. **55**: pp. 92–100.

[57] Liu, Z., Gatt, A., Werner, S.J., Mikati, M.A., Holmes, G.L., *Long-term behavioral deficits following pilocarpine seizures in immature rats*. Epilepsy Research, 1994. **19**(3): pp. 191–204.

[58] Titiz, A.S., Mahoney, J.M., Testorf, M.E., Holmes, G.L., Scott, R.C., *Cognitive impairment in temporal lobe epilepsy: role of online and offline processing of single cell information*. Hippocampus, 2014. **24**(9): pp. 1129–1145.

[59] Lin, H., Holmes, G.L., Kubie, J.L., Muller, R.U., *Recurrent seizures induce a reversible impairment in a spatial hidden goal task*. Hippocampus, 2009. **19**(9): pp. 817–827.

[60] Weniger, G., Ruhleder, M., Lange, C., Irle, E., *Impaired egocentric memory and reduced somatosensory cortex size in temporal lobe epilepsy with hippocampal sclerosis*. Behavioural Brain Research, 2012. **227**(1): pp. 116–124.

[61] Astur, R.S., Taylor, L.B., Mamelak, A.N., Philpott, L., Sutherland, R.J., *Humans with hippocampus damage display severe spatial memory impairments in a virtual Morris water task*. Behavioural Brain Research, 2002. **132**(1): pp. 77–84.

[62] Ekstrom, A.D., Kahana, M.J., Caplan, J.B., Fields, T.A., Isham, E.A., Nnewman, E.L., Fried, I., *Cellular networks underlying human spatial navigation*. Nature, 2003. **425**(6954): pp. 184–188.

[63] O'Keefe, J. and Dostrovsky, J., *The hippocampus as a spatial map. Preliminary evidence from unit activity in the freely-moving rat*. Brain Research, 1971. **34**(1): pp. 171–175.

[64] Zhang, S., Ye, J., Couey, J.J., Witter, M., Moser, E.I., Moser, M., *Functional connectivity of the entorhinal-hippocampal space circuit*. Philosophical Transactions of the Royal Society of London. Series B, Biological Sciences, 2014. **369**(1635): pp. 20120516.

[65] Hafting, T., Fyhn, M., Molden, S., Moser, M., Moser, E.I., *Microstructure of a spatial map in the entorhinal cortex*. Nature, 2005. **436**(7052): pp. 801–806.

[66] Wilent, W.B. and Nitz, D.A., *Discrete place fields of hippocampal formation interneurons*. Journal of Neurophysiology, 2007. **97**(6): pp. 4152–4161.

[67] Ego-Stengel, V. and Wilson, M.A., *Spatial selectivity and theta phase precession in CA1 interneurons*. Hippocampus, 2007. **17**(2): pp. 161–174.

[68] Rosas, K., Parrón, I., Serrano, P., Cimadevilla, J.M.M., *Spatial recognition memory in a virtual reality task is altered in refractory temporal lobe epilepsy*. Epilepsy & Behavior, 2013. **28**(2): pp. 227–231.

[69] Amlerova, J., Laczo, J, Vlcek, K, Javurkova, A., Andel, R., Marusic, P., *Risk factors for spatial memory impairment in patients with temporal lobe epilepsy*. Epilepsy & Behavior, 2013. **26**(1): pp. 57–60.

[70] Cánovas, R., León, I., Serrano, P., Roldán, M.D., Cimadevilla, J.M.M., *Spatial navigation impairment in patients with refractory temporal lobe epilepsy: evidence from a new virtual reality-based task*. Epilepsy & Behavior, 2011. **22**(2): pp. 364–369.

[71] Bohbot, V.D., Kalina, M., Stepankova, K., Spackova, N., Petrides, M., Nadel, L., *Spatial memory deficits in patients with lesions to the right hippocampus and to the right parahippocampal cortex*. Neuropsychologia, 1998. **36**(11): pp. 1217–1238.

[72] Chauvière, L., Rafrafi, N., Thinus-Blanc, C, Bartolomei, F, Esclapez, M., Bernard, C., *Early deficits in spatial memory and theta rhythm in experimental temporal lobe epilepsy*. The Journal of Neuroscience, 2009. **29**(17): pp. 5402–5410.

[73] Inostroza, M., Brotons-Mas, J.R., Laurent, F., Cid, E., de la Prida, L., *Specific impairment of "what-where-when" episodic-like memory in experimental models of temporal lobe epilepsy*. The Journal of Neuroscience, 2013. **33**(45): pp. 17749–17762.

[74] Richard, G.R., Titiz, A., Tyler, A., Holmes, G.L., Scott, R.C., Lenck-Santini, P., *Speed modulation of hippocampal theta frequency correlates with spatial memory performance*. Hippocampus, 2013. **23**(12): pp. 1269–1279.

[75] Sloviter, R.S., Bumanglag, A.V., Schwarcz, R., Frotscher, M., *Abnormal dentate gyrus network circuitry in temporal lobe epilepsy*. Epilepsia, 2010. **51**(s5): pp. 41–41.

[76] Müller, C.J., Gröticke, I., Bankstahl, M., Löscher, W., *Behavioral and cognitive alterations, spontaneous seizures, and neuropathology developing after a pilocarpine-induced status epilepticus in C57BL/6 mice*. Experimental Neurology, 2009. **219**(1): pp. 284–297.

[77] Orbán-Kis, K., Mihály, I., Lukács, I., Kiss, R., Izsák, J., Száva, I., Metz, J., Szilágyi, T., *Spatial memory deficits in juvenile rats with pilocarpine induced temporal lobe epilepsy*. Acta Medica Marisiensis, 2014. **60**(5): pp. 191–195.

[78] Pearson, J.N., Schulz, K.M., and Patel, M., *Specific alterations in the performance of learning and memory tasks in models of chemoconvulsant-induced status epilepticus*. Epilepsy Research, 2014. **108**(6): pp. 1032–1040.

[79] Gröticke, I., Hoffmann, K., and Löscher, W., *Behavioral alterations in a mouse model of temporal lobe epilepsy induced by intrahippocampal injection of kainate*. Experimental Neurology, 2008. **213**(1): pp. 71–83.

[80] Gernert, M., Thompson, K.W., Löscher, W., Tobin, A.J., *Genetically engineered GABA-producing cells demonstrate anticonvulsant effects and long-term transgene expression when transplanted into the central piriform cortex of rats*. Experimental Neurology, 2002. **176**(1): pp. 183–192.

[81] Xu, Q., Cobos, I., Cruz, E., Rubenstein, J.L., Anderson, S.A., *Origins of cortical interneuron subtypes*. The Journal of Neuroscience, 2004. **24**(11): pp. 2612–2622.

[82] Wichterle, H., Turnbull, D.H., Nery, S., Fishell, G., Alvarez-Buylla, A. , *In utero fate mapping reveals distinct migratory pathways and fates of neurons born in the mammalian basal forebrain*. Development, 2001 **128**: pp. 3759–3771.

[83] Anderson, S.A., Marin, O., Horn, C., Jennings, K., Rubenstein, J.L.R., *Distinct cortical migrations from the medial and lateral ganglionic eminences*. Development, 2001 **128**: pp. 353–363.

[84] Wichterle, H., Garcia-Verdugo, J., Herrera, D.G., Alvarez-Buylla, A., *Young neurons from medial ganglionic eminence disperse in adult and embryonic brain*. Nature Neuroscience, 1999. **2**(5): pp. 461–466.

[85] Alvarez-Dolado, M., Calcagnotto, M., Karkar, K.M., Southwell, D.G., Jones-Davis, D.M., Estrada, R.C., Rubenstein, J.L.R., Alvarez-Buylla, A., Baraban, S.C., *Cortical inhibition modified by embryonic neural precursors grafted into the postnatal brain*. The Journal of Neuroscience: The Official Journal of the Society for Neuroscience, 2006. **26**(28): pp. 7380–7389.

[86] Howard, M.A. and Baraban, S.C., *Synaptic integration of transplanted interneuron progenitor cells into native cortical networks*. Journal of Neurophysiology, 2016. **116**(2): pp. 472–478.

[87] Calcagnotto, M.E., Zipancic, I., Piquer-Gil, M., Mello, L.E., Álvarez-Dolado, M., *Grafting of GABAergic precursors rescues deficits in hippocampal inhibition*. Epilepsia, 2010. **51**(Suppl 3): pp. 66–70.

[88] Baraban, S.C., Southwell, D.G., Estrada, R.C., Jones, D.L., Sebe, J.Y., Alfaro-Cervello, C., García-Verdugo, J.M., Rubenstein, J.L., Alvarez-Buylla, A., *Reduction of seizures by transplantation of cortical GABAergic interneuron precursors into Kv1.1 mutant mice*. Proceedings of the National Academy of Sciences of the United States of America, 2009. **106**(36): pp. 15472–15477.

[89] Gilani, A.I., Chohan, M.O., Inan, M., Schobel, S.A., Chaudhury, N.H., Paskewitz, S., Chuhma, N., Glickstein, S., Merker, R.J., Xu, Q., Small, S.A., Anderson, S.A., Ross, M.E., Moore, H., *Interneuron precursor transplants in adult hippocampus reverse psychosis-relevant features in a mouse model of hippocampal disinhibition*. Proceedings of the National Academy of Sciences of the United States of America, 2014. **111**(20): pp. 7450–7455.

[90] Waldau, B., Hattiangady, B., Kuruba, R., Shetty, A.K., *Medial ganglionic eminence-derived neural stem cell grafts ease spontaneous seizures and restore GDNF expression in a rat model of chronic temporal lobe epilepsy*. Stem Cells (Dayton, Ohio), 2010. **28**(7): pp. 1153–1164.

[91] Inostroza, M., Cid, E., Brotons-Mas, J., Gal, B., Aivar, P., Uzcategui, Y.G., Sandi, C., de la Prida, L., *Hippocampal-dependent spatial memory in the water maze is preserved in an experimental model of temporal lobe epilepsy in rats*. PloS One, 2011. **6**(7): e22372.

[92] Mohajeri, M.H., Madani, R., Saini, K., Lipp, H.P., Nitsch, R.M., Wolfer, D.P., *The impact of genetic background on neurodegeneration and behavior in seizured mice*. Genes, Brain and Behavior, 2004 **3**(4): pp. 228–239.

[93] Kumar, S.S. and Buckmaster, P.S., *Hyperexcitability, Interneurons, and loss of GABAergic synapses in entorhinal cortex in a model of temporal lobe epilepsy*. The Journal of Neuroscience, 2006. **26**(17): pp. 4613–4623.

[94] Germain, N.D., Banda, E.C., Becker, S., Naegele, J.R., Grabel, L.B., *Derivation and isolation of NKX2.1-positive basal forebrain progenitors from human embryonic stem cells*. Stem Cells and Development, 2013. **22**(10): pp. 1477–1489.

[95] Liu, Y., Huisheng, L, Sauvey, C., Yao, L., Zarnowska, E.D., Zhang, S., *Directed differentiation of forebrain GABA interneurons from human pluripotent stem cells*. Nature Protocols, 2013. **8**(9): pp. 1670–1679.

[96] Tyson, J.A., Goldberg, E.M., Maroof, A.M., Xu, Q., Petros, T.I., Anderson, S.A., *Duration of culture and sonic hedgehog signaling differentially specify PV versus SST cortical interneuron fates from embryonic stem cells*. Development, 2015. **142**(7): pp. 1267–1278.

[97] Nicholas, C.R., Chen, J., Tang, Y., Southwell, D.G., Chalmers, N., Vogt, D., Arnold, C.M., Chen, Y.J., Stanley, E.G., Elefanty, A.G., Sasai, Y., Alvarez-Buylla, A., Rubenstein, J., Kriegstein, A.R. , *Functional maturation of hPSC-derived forebrain interneurons requires an extended timeline and mimics human neural development*. Cell Stem Cell, 2013. **12**(5): pp. 573–586.

[98] Kim, T.G., Yao, R., Monnel, T., Cho, J., Vasudevan, A., Koh, A., Peeyush, K.T., Moon, M., Datta, D., Bolshakov, V.Y., Kim, K., Chung, S., *Efficient specification of interneurons from human pluripotent stem cells by dorsoventral and rostrocaudal modulation*. Stem Cells, 2014. **32**(7): pp. 1789–1804.

[99] Maroof, A.M., Keros, S., Tyson, J.A., Ying, S., Ganat, Y.M., Merkle, F.T., Liu, B., Goulburn, A., Stanley, E.G., Elefanty, A.G., Widmer, H., Eggan, K., Goldstein, P.A., Anderson, S.A., Studer, L., *Directed differentiation and functional maturation of cortical interneurons from human embryonic stem cells*. Cell Stem Cell, 2013. **12**(5): pp. 559–572.

[100] Ahn, S., Kim, T., Kim, K., Chung, S., *Differentiation of human pluripotent stem cells into medial ganglionic eminence vs caudal ganglionic eminence cells*. Methods, 2016. **101**: pp. 103–112.

[101] Carpentino, J.E., Hartman, N.W., Grabel, L.B., Naegele, J.R., *Region-specific differentiation of embryonic stem cell-derived neural progenitor transplants into the adult mouse hippocampus following seizures*. Journal of Neuroscience Research, 2008. **86**(3): pp. 512–524.

[102] Lee, H., Yun, S., Kim, I., Lee, I., Shin, J., Park, S., Kim, W., Park, K., *Human fetal brain-derived neural stem/progenitor cells grafted into the adult epileptic brain restrain seizures in rat models of temporal lobe epilepsy*. PloS One, 2014. **9**(8): e104092.

[103] Chen, C.Y., Plocik, A., Anderson, N.C., Moakley, D., Boyi, T., Dundes, C., Lassiter, C., Graveley, B.R., Grabel, L., *Transcriptome and in vitro differentiation profile of human embryonic stem cell derived NKX2.1-positive neural progenitors*. Stem Cell Reviews and Reports, 2016. **12**(6): pp. 744–756.

[104] Goulburn, A.L., Alden, D., Davis, R.P., Micallef, S.J., Ng, E.S., Yu, Q.C., Lim, S.M., Soh, C.L., Elliott, D.A., Hatzistavrou, T., Bourke, J., Watmuff, B., Lang, R.J., Haynes, J.M., Pouton, C.W., Giudice, A., Trounson, A.O., Anderson, S.A., Stanley, E.G., Elefanty, A.G., *A targeted NKX2.1 human embryonic stem cell reporter line enables identification of human basal forebrain derivatives*. Stem Cells, 2011. **29**(3): pp. 462–473.

[105] Tyson, J.A., Goldberg, E.M., Maroof, A.M., Xu, Q., Petros, T.J., Anderson, S.A., *Duration of culture and sonic hedgehog signaling differentially specify PV versus SST cortical interneuron fates from embryonic stem cells*. Development (Cambridge, England), 2015. **142**(7): pp. 1267–1278.

[106] Petros, T.J., Maurer, C.W., and Anderson, S.A., *Enhanced derivation of mouse ESC-derived cortical interneurons by expression of Nkx2.1*. Stem Cell Research, 2013. **11**(1): pp. 647–656.

[107] Germain, N.D., Hartman, N.W., Cai, C., Becker, S., Naegele, J.R., Grabel, L.B., *Teratocarcinoma formation in embryonic stem cell-derived neural progenitor hippocampal transplants*. Cell Transplantation, 2012. **21**(8): pp. 1603.

[108] Shultz, L.D., Ishikawa, F., and Greiner, D.L., *Humanized mice in translational biomedical research*. Nature Reviews. Immunology, 2007. **7**(2): pp. 118–130.

[109] Maisano, X., Litvina, E., Tagliatela, S., Aaron, G.B., Grabel, L.B., Naegele, J.R., *Differentiation and functional incorporation of embryonic stem cell-derived GABAergic interneurons in the dentate gyrus of mice with temporal lobe epilepsy*. The Journal of Neuroscience: The Official Journal of the Society for Neuroscience, 2012. **32**(1): pp. 46–61.

[110] Cunningham, M., Cho, J., Leung, A., Savvidis, G., Ahn, S., Moon, M., Lee, P., Han, J.J., Azimi, N., Kim, K., Bolshakov, V.Y., Chung, S., *hPSC-derived maturing GABAergic interneurons ameliorate seizures and abnormal behavior in epileptic mice*. Cell Stem Cell, 2014. **15**(5): pp. 559–573.

[111] Hunt, R.F., Girskis, K.M., Rubenstein, J.L., Alvarez-Buylla, A., Baraban, S.C., *GABA progenitors grafted into the adult epileptic brain control seizures and abnormal behavior*. Nature Neuroscience, 2013. **16**(6): pp. 692–697.

[112] Faure, J.B., Akimana, G., Carneiro, J.E.M., Cosquer, B., Ferrandon, A., Geiger, K., Koning, E., Penazzi, L., Cassel, J., Nehlig, A., *A comprehensive behavioral evaluation in the lithium–pilocarpine model in rats: effects of carisbamate administration during status epilepticus*. Epilepsia, 2013. **54**(7): pp. 1203–1213.

[113] Antunes, M. and Biala, G., *The novel object recognition memory: neurobiology, test procedure, and its modifications*. Cognitive Processing, 2012. **13**(2): pp. 93–110.

[114] Ennaceur, A. and Delacour, J., *A new one-trial test for neurobiological studies of memory in rats. 1: behavioral data*. Behavioural Brain Research, 1988. **31**(1): pp. 47–59.

[115] Rosenfeld, C.S. and Ferguson, S.A., *Barnes maze testing strategies with small and large rodent models*. Journal of Visualized Experiments, 2014. **84**: e51194.

[116] Levin, E.D., *Psychopharmacological effects in the radial-arm maze*. Neuroscience & Biobehavioral Reviews, 1988. **12**(2): pp. 169–175.

[117] Hodges, H., *Maze procedures: the radial-arm and water maze compared*. Cognitive Brain Research, 1996. **3**(3–4): pp. 167–181.

[118] Levy, A., Kluge, P.B., and Elsmore, T.F., *Radial arm maze performance of mice: acquisition and atropine effects*. Behavioral and Neural Biology, 1983. **39**(2): pp. 229–240.

[119] Brown, M.F., Rish, P.A., VonCulin, J.E., Edberg, J.A., *Spatial guidance of choice behavior in the radial-arm maze*. Journal of Experimental Psychology Animal Behavior Processes, 1993. **19**(3): pp. 195–214.

[120] Deacon, R.M.J. and Rawlins, N.J.P., *T-maze alternation in the rodent*. Nature Protocols, 2006. **1**(1): pp. 7–12.

[121] Gong, D.-Y. and Choi, Y.-S., *Development of new analytical method evaluating working memory on Y maze*. Journal of Life Science, 2016. **26**(2): pp. 234–240.

[122] Koolhaas, J.M., Coppens, C.M., de Boer, S.F., Buwalda, B., Meerlo, P., Timmermans, P., *The resident-intruder paradigm: a standardized test for aggression, violence and social stress*. Journal of Visualized Experiments, 2013. **77**: e4367.

[123] Komada, M., Takao, K., and Miyakawa, T., *Elevated plus maze for mice*. Journal of Visualized Experiments, 2008. **22**: e1088.

[124] Sidor, M.M., Rilett, K., and Foster, J.A., *Validation of an automated system for measuring anxiety-related behaviours in the elevated plus maze*. Journal of Neuroscience Methods, 2010. **188**(1): pp. 7–13.

[125] Shepherd, J.K., Grewal, S.S., Fletcher, A., Bill, D.J., Dourish, C.T., *Behavioural and pharmacological characterisation of the elevated "zero-maze" as an animal model of anxiety*. Psychopharmacology, 1994. **116**(1): pp. 56–64.

[126] Kulkarni, S.K., Singh, K., and Bishnoi, M., *Elevated zero maze: a paradigm to evaluate antianxiety effects of drugs*. Methods and Findings in Experimental and Clinical Pharmacology, 2007. **29**(5): pp. 343–348.

[127] Misslin, R., Belzung, C., and Vogel, E., *Behavioural validation of a light/dark choice procedure for testing anti-anxiety agents*. Behavioural Processes, 1989. **18**(1–3): pp. 119–132.

[128] Kulesskaya, N. and Voikar, V., *Assessment of mouse anxiety-like behavior in the light–dark box and open-field arena: role of equipment and procedure*. Physiology & Behavior, 2014. **133**: pp. 30–38.

[129] Südhof, T.C., *Neuroligins and neurexins link synaptic function to cognitive disease*. Nature, 2008. **455**(7215): pp. 903–911.

[130] Craig, A.M. and Kang, Y., *Neurexin-neuroligin signaling in synapse development*. Current Opinion in Neurobiology, 2007. **17**(1): pp. 43–52.

[131] Papadopoulos, T. and Soykan, T., *The role of collybistin in gephyrin clustering at inhibitory synapses: facts and open questions*. Frontiers in Cellular Neuroscience, 2011. **5**: pp. 11.

[132] Essrich, C., Lorez, M., Benson, J.A., Fritschy, J.M., Lüscher, B., *Postsynaptic clustering of major GABAA receptor subtypes requires the gamma 2 subunit and gephyrin*. Nature Neuroscience, 1998. **1**(7): pp. 563–571.

[133] Poulopoulos, A., Aramuni, G., Meyer, G., Soykan, T., Hoon, M., Papadopoulos, T., Zhang, M., Paarmann, I., Fuchs, C., Harvey, K., Jedlicka, P., Schwarzacher, S.W., Betz,

H., Harvey, R.J., Brose, N., Zhang, W., Varoqueaux, F., *Neuroligin 2 drives postsynaptic assembly at perisomatic inhibitory synapses through gephyrin and collybistin.* Neuron, 2009. **63**(5): pp. 628–642.

[134] Jacob, T.C., Bogdanov, Y.D., Magnus, C., Saliba, R.S., Kittler, J.T., Haydon, P.G., Moss, S.J., *Gephyrin regulates the cell surface dynamics of synaptic GABAA receptors.* The Journal of Neuroscience, 2005. **25**(45): pp. 10469–10478.

[135] Varoqueaux, F., Aramuni, G., Rawson, R.L., Mohrmann, R., Missler, M., Gottmann, K., Zhang, W., Südhof, T.C., Brose, N., *Neuroligins determine synapse maturation and function.* Neuron, 2006. **51**(6): pp. 741–754.

[136] Babaev, O., Botta, P., Meyer, E., Müller, C., Ehrenreich, H., Brose, N., Lüthi, A., Krueger-Burg, D., *Neuroligin 2 deletion alters inhibitory synapse function and anxiety-associated neuronal activation in the amygdala.* Neuropharmacology, 2016. **100**: pp. 56–65.

[137] Gibson, J.R., Huber, K.M., and Südhof, T.C., *Neuroligin-2 deletion selectively decreases inhibitory synaptic transmission originating from fast-spiking but not from somatostatin-positive interneurons.* The Journal of Neuroscience: The Official Journal of the Society for Neuroscience, 2009. **29**(44): pp. 13883–13897.

[138] Jedlicka, P., Hoon, M., Papadopoulos, T., Vlachos, A., Winkels, R., Poulopoulos, A., Betz, H., Deller, T., Brose, N., Varoqueaux, F., Schwarzacher, S.W., *Increased dentate gyrus excitability in neuroligin-2-deficient mice in vivo.* Cerebral Cortex, 2011. **21**(2): pp. 357–367.

[139] Hines, R.M., Wu, L., Hines, D.J., Steenland, H., Mansour, S., Dahlhaus, R., Singaraja, R.R., Cao, X., Sammler, E., Hormuzdi, S.G., Zhuo, M., El-Husseini, A., *Synaptic imbalance, stereotypies, and impaired social interactions in mice with altered neuroligin 2 expression.* The Journal of Neuroscience, 2008. **28**(24): pp. 6055–6067.

[140] Liang, J., Xu, W., Hsu, Y.T., Yee, A.X., Chen, L., Südhof, T.C., *Conditional neuroligin-2 knockout in adult medial prefrontal cortex links chronic changes in synaptic inhibition to cognitive impairments.* Molecular Psychiatry, 2015. **20**(7): pp. 850–859.

[141] Papadopoulos, T., Korte, M., Eulenburg, V., Kubota, H., Retiounskaia, M., Harvey, R.J., Harvey, K., O'Sullivan, G.A., Laube, B., Hülsmann, S., Geiger, J.R.R., Betz, H., *Impaired GABAergic transmission and altered hippocampal synaptic plasticity in collybistin-deficient mice.* The EMBO Journal, 2007. **26**(17): pp. 3888–3899.

[142] Prior, P., Schmitt, B., Grenningloh, G., Pribilla, I., Multhaup, G., Beyreuther, K., Maulet, Y., Werner, P., Langosch, D., Kirsch, J., Betz, H., *Primary structure and alternative splice variants of gephyrin, a putative glycine receptor-tubulin linker protein.* Neuron, 1992. **8**(6): pp. 1161–1170.

[143] Tyagarajan, S.K. and Fritschy, J.-M.M., *Gephyrin: a master regulator of neuronal function?* Nature Reviews. Neuroscience, 2014. **15**(3): pp. 141–156.

[144] Kneussel, M., Brandstätter, J.H., Laube, B., Stahl, S., Müller, U., Betz, H., *Loss of postsynaptic GABA(A) receptor clustering in gephyrin-deficient mice.* The Journal of Neuroscience: The Official Journal of the Society for Neuroscience, 1999. **19**(21): pp. 9289–9297.

[145] Lüscher, B. and Keller, C.A., *Regulation of GABAA receptor trafficking, channel activity, and functional plasticity of inhibitory synapses*. Pharmacology & Therapeutics, 2004. **102**(3): pp. 195–221.

[146] Thind, K.K., Yamawaki, R., Phanwar, I., Zhang, G., Wen, X., Buckmaster, P.S., *Initial loss but later excess of GABAergic synapses with dentate granule cells in a rat model of temporal lobe epilepsy*. Journal of Comparative Neurology, 2010. **518**(5): pp. 647–677.

[147] Fang, M., Shen, L., Yin, H., Pan, Y., Wang, L., Chen, D., Xi, Z., Xiao, Z., Wang, X., Zhou, S., *Downregulation of gephyrin in temporal lobe epilepsy neurons in humans and a rat model*. Synapse (New York, N.Y.), 2011. **65**(10): pp. 1006–1014.

[148] Kins, S., Betz, H., and Kirsch, J., *Collybistin, a newly identified brain-specific GEF, induces submembrane clustering of gephyrin*. Nature Neuroscience, 2000. **3**(1): pp. 22–29.

[149] Harvey, K., Duguid, I.C., Alldred, M.J., Beatty, S.E., Ward, H., Keep, N.H., Lingenfelter, S.E., Pearce, B.R., Lundgren, J., Owen, M.J., Smart, T.G., Lüscher, B., Rees, M.I., Harvey, R.J., *The GDP-GTP exchange factor collybistin: an essential determinant of neuronal gephyrin clustering*. The Journal of Neuroscience: The Official Journal of the Society for Neuroscience, 2004. **24**(25): pp. 5816–5826.

[150] Saiepour, L., Fuchs, C., Patrizi, A., Sassoè-Pognetto, M., Harvey, R.J., Harvey, K., *Complex role of collybistin and gephyrin in GABAA receptor clustering*. Journal of Biological Chemistry, 2010. **285**(38): pp. 29623–29631.

[151] Varoqueaux, F., Jamain, S., and Brose, N., *Neuroligin 2 is exclusively localized to inhibitory synapses*. European Journal of Cell Biology, 2004. **83**(9): pp. 449–456.

[152] Dean, C. and Dresbach, T., *Neuroligins and neurexins: linking cell adhesion, synapse formation and cognitive function*. Trends in Neurosciences, 2006. **29**(1): pp. 21–29.

[153] Siddiqui, T.J. and Craig, A.M., *Synaptic organizing complexes*. Current Opinion in Neurobiology, 2011. **21**(1): pp. 132–143.

[154] Blundell, J., Tabuchi, K., Bolliger, M.F., Blaiss, C.A., Brose, N., Liu, X., Südhof, T.C., Powell, C.M., *Increased anxiety-like behavior in mice lacking the inhibitory synapse cell adhesion molecule neuroligin 2*. Genes, Brain, and Behavior, 2009. **8**(1): pp. 114–126.

[155] Maćkowiak, M., Mordalska, P., and Wędzony, K., *Neuroligins, synapse balance and neuropsychiatric disorders*. Pharmacological Reports: PR, 2014. **66**(5): pp. 830–835.

[156] van der Kooij, M.A., Fantin, M., Kraev, I., Korshunova, I., Grosse, J., Zanoletti, O., Guirado, R., Garcia-Mompó, C., Nacher, J., Stewart, M.G., Berezin, V., Sandi, Carmen., *Impaired hippocampal neuroligin-2 function by chronic stress or synthetic peptide treatment is linked to social deficits and increased aggression*. Neuropsychopharmacology: Official Publication of the American College of Neuropsychopharmacology, 2014. **39**(5): pp. 1148–1158.

[157] Sun, C., Cheng, M., Qin, R., Liao, D., Chen, T., Koong, F., Chen, G., Chen, Chia., *Identification and functional characterization of rare mutations of the neuroligin-2 gene*

(NLGN2) associated with schizophrenia. Human Molecular Genetics, 2011. **20**(15): pp. 3042–3051.

[158] Graf, E.R., Zhang, X., Jin, S., Linhoff, M.W., Craig, A., *Neurexins induce differentiation of GABA and glutamate postsynaptic specializations via neuroligins*. Cell, 2004. **119**(7): pp. 1013–1026.

[159] Zhang, C., Atasoy, D., Araç, D., Yang, X., Fucillo, M.V., Robison, A.J., Ko, J., Brunger, A.T., Südhof, T.C., *Neurexins physically and functionally interact with GABA(A) receptors*. Neuron, 2010. **66**(3): pp. 403–416.

[160] Dong, N., Qi, J., and Chen, G., *Molecular reconstitution of functional GABAergic synapses with expression of neuroligin-2 and GABAA receptors*. Molecular and Cellular Neuroscience, 2007. **35**(1): pp. 14–23.

[161] Loup, F., Wieser, H.G., Yonekawa, Y., Aguzzi, A., Fritschy, J.M., *Selective alterations in GABAA receptor subtypes in human temporal lobe epilepsy*. The Journal of Neuroscience: The Official Journal of the Society for Neuroscience, 2000. **20**(14): pp. 5401–5419.

[162] Poulter, M.O., Brown, L.A., Tynan, S., Willick, G., William, R., McIntyre, D.C., *Differential expression of alpha1, alpha2, alpha3, and alpha5 GABAA receptor subunits in seizure-prone and seizure-resistant rat models of temporal lobe epilepsy*. The Journal of Neuroscience: The Official Journal of the Society for Neuroscience, 1999. **19**(11): pp. 4654–4661.

[163] Rice, A., Rafiq, A., Shapiro, S.M., Jakoi, E.R., Coulter, D.A., DeLorenzo, R.J., *Long-lasting reduction of inhibitory function and gamma-aminobutyric acid type A receptor subunit mRNA expression in a model of temporal lobe epilepsy*. Proceedings of the National Academy of Sciences of the United States of America, 1996. **93**(18): pp. 9665–9669.

[164] Brown, N., Kerby, J., Bonnert, T.P., Whiting, P.J., Wafford, K.A., *Pharmacological characterization of a novel cell line expressing human alpha(4)beta(3)delta GABA(A) receptors*. British Journal of Pharmacology, 2002. **136**(7): pp. 965–974.

[165] Saxena, N.C. and Macdonald, R.L., *Assembly of $GABA_A$ receptor subunits: role of the delta subunit*. The Official Journal of the Society for Neuroscience, 1994. **14**(11): pp. 7077–7086.

[166] Stell, B.M., Brickley, S.G., and Tang, C.Y., *Neuroactive steroids reduce neuronal excitability by selectively enhancing tonic inhibition mediated by δ subunit-containing $GABA_A$ receptors*. Proceedings of the National Academy of Sciences United States of America, 2003. **100**(24): pp. 14439–14444.

[167] Wu, X., Wu, Z., Ning, G., Guo, Y., Ali, Rashid., Macdonald, R.L., Blas, A.L., Luscher, B., Chen, G., *γ-aminobutyric acid type A (GABAA) receptor α subunits play a direct role in synaptic versus extrasynaptic targeting*. Journal of Biological Chemistry, 2012. **287**(33): pp. 27417–27430.

[168] Wisden, W., Laurie, D.J., Monyer, H., Seeburg, P.H., *The distribution of 13 GABAA receptor subunit mRNAs in the rat brain. I. Telencephalon, diencephalon, mesencephalon*. The

Journal of Neuroscience: The Official Journal of the Society for Neuroscience, 1992. **12**(3): pp. 1040–1062.

[169] Peng, Z., Huang, C.S., Stell, B.M., Mody, I., Houser, C.R., *Altered expression of the delta subunit of the GABAA receptor in a mouse model of temporal lobe epilepsy*. The Journal of Neuroscience: The Official Journal of the Society for Neuroscience, 2004. **24**(39): pp. 8629–8639.

3

Molecular Mechanisms of Drug-Induced Plasticity

Robert J Oliver and Nora I Perrone-Bizzozero

Abstract

Substance-use disorders (SUDs) are a significant societal burden. Like many other conditions, SUDs are characterized by chronic relapse after periods without symptoms. Alterations in synaptic plasticity have been documented after acute and addiction-related behavioral exposures to drugs of abuse. These synaptic alterations are persistent and similar to the chronic relapse state of patients with SUDs, suggesting that reversing these synaptic alterations may prevent relapse. Additionally, many of these synaptic features of addiction mirror those found in other forms of learning and memory. These features suggest that the etiology of this disorder stems from persistent modifications in corticolimbic synaptic plasticity mediated by drug-induced alterations in addiction-related gene (ARG) expression. Understanding the regulation of addiction-related genes and their impact on synaptic plasticity and behavior may inform new pharmacological treatments that reverse these aberrant drug-evoked forms of plasticity in favor of remission.

Keywords: addiction, substance-use disorders, Fos, CREB, ADAR, BDNF, Mef2, miR-212, miR-9, FMRP, HuD, ELAVL

1. Introduction

Substance-use disorders (SUDs), or more colloquially known as drug addiction, are a significant societal burden both financially, incurring an estimated $193 billion in costs (www.justice.gov/ndic, 2011), and emotionally devastating to patients and their families. In opposition to more controlled, casual drug use, SUDs are characterized by uncontrollable bouts of drug consumption in spite of negative life consequences. Patients with this disorder appear to lose interest in normal prosocial activities, instead directing their energy toward the pursuit of these substances. Since addiction is a chronic, relapsing condition, this disorder has been notoriously difficult to manage. A complete review of pharmacological mechanisms of drugs of abuse understanding of the molecular, physiological, and behavioral mechanisms involved in the disorder is necessary for the discovery and implementation of more effective treatments.

The mesolimbic dopamine system is the most well-studied and implicated circuit associated with the disorder. Naturally, this neurocircuit may have evolved as an information-processing center to direct behavior toward environmentally important stimuli predicting the presence of vital resources, for example, food and water. Synaptic plasticity within these regions is implicated in associative learning of these stimuli to guide behavior necessary to receive these rewarding resources. Depending on the frequency and accuracy that a particular stimulus may predict a natural reward, goal-directed behavior toward this stimulus with the intention of obtaining the reward may become habitual. Thus, if an exogenous substance were to recruit this same neurocircuitry, this may elicit similar goal-directed behavior toward obtaining these compounds.

Structurally, drugs of abuse are highly varied and have many specific protein targets within the body (for a review of pharmacological mechanisms of drugs of abuse, see [1]). However, all pharmacological mechanisms of drugs of abuse cause excessive dopamine release originating from the ventral tegmental area within the nucleus accumbens (VTA, NAc; [2, 3]). Not only are these regions involved in this disorder, they also appear to be crucial mediators of appropriate goal-directed behavior toward natural rewards. Dopaminergic projections from VTA neurons are important in regulating motivation to perform integral, evolutionarily conserved behaviors such as feeding and reproduction [4, 5]. Drug-elicited synaptic plasticity also occurs within this region, possibly through similar mechanisms as natural rewards. Mirroring a classical symptom of addiction, the synaptic alterations induced by drugs of abuse inhibit the ability of other non-drug-related experiences to elicit synaptic plasticity [6, 7]. As such, it has been hypothesized that drugs of abuse cause a heightened form of plasticity-dependent associative memory leading to habit formation and addiction-like behaviors [8].

Although drug use is required for the development of addiction, it is most certainly not sufficient to cause this disorder. For example, around 176.6 million Americans from the age of 12 and up drink alcohol but only 17 million are classified as having an alcohol-use disorder (SAMSHA, 2013). Drugs are metabolized and eventually cleared from the body, thus, the drug's pharmacological effect is not sufficient. In addition, SUDs are classically characterized by chronic relapse after periods without symptoms [9]. This may occur many years after a patient's last reported use of a drug, suggesting that some stable functional alteration has occurred within the brain. Repeated drug exposure is required for an accumulation of molecular events that alter plasticity within specific regions affecting the functioning of the entire circuit. These synaptic alterations are persistent and similar to the chronic relapse state of patients with SUDs, suggesting that reversing these synaptic alterations may prevent relapse [9, 10]. Additionally, they appear to be protein-synthesis-dependent forms of plasticity [11–13]. Thus, the molecular mechanisms regulating gene expression ending with the translation into functional protein may play a role in the etiology of this disorder and thus may stem from persistent modifications in region-specific synaptic plasticity mediated by drug-induced alterations in addiction-related gene (ARG) expression.

Regulation of these molecules can occur at many different steps. The DNA in the genome is organized into small compact three-dimensional units assembled by histones into nucleosomes, which form the structure of chromatin. As such, basal transcription is necessarily stagnant in the absence of the regulation of gene accessibility. Modifications to the accessibility of genes, by regulation of these structures, are termed epigenetic regulation and have also been found to be an integral component in the development of addiction. Given that the epigenetic control of drug addiction has been elegantly reviewed in previous work [14–17], this chapter focuses on other aspects of gene expression control starting at the level of transcription.

2. Transcriptional regulation of addiction-related genes

Transcriptional regulation occurs through transcription factors, which are proteins that respond to intracellular changes leading to association with specific elements in target genes. Since the promoter region where the transcription factor binds to is outside of the coding region of that gene, these sequences are also termed cis-regulatory elements.

2.1. The Fos family transcription factors are differentially altered by drugs of abuse and contribute to addiction-related plasticity and behavior

Although altered transcription of various genes had been suggested by earlier work [18], it was not until the discovery that morphine caused increased striatal expression of a transcription factor, c-Fos, that it was shown that transcription factors may regulate this drug-induced gene expression [19]. Although first found to be regulated by acute morphine treatment, it was found that other drugs of abuse cause specific, dopamine-dependent, alterations in the expression of this transcription factor within addiction-related regions [20–22]. Important for the study of relapse, it was found that c-Fos was upregulated in mesolimbic structures following withdrawal, suggesting that it may play a role in the intense drug craving present in this disorder [23]. c-Fos is part of the Fos family of transcription factors, including FosB and ΔFosB, which all heterodimerize with Jun to form the AP-1 transcription factor complex [24]. This complex then associates its specific cyclic AMP response element (CRE), the AP-1 binding site, leading to increased transcription of genes downstream of these sequences.

Fos genes are considered immediate early genes (IEGs), or factors that are basally expressed at low levels but elevated rapidly by specific stimuli (first reviewed in the context of neuronal cells [25]). Since it was upregulated by other plasticity and memory-inducing events, it was hypothesized that c-Fos, and possibly other IEGs, may alter gene expression involved in memory formation [26]. As expected, the upregulation of c-Fos, FosB, ΔFosB, and Jun leads to increased AP-1-mediated transcription within addiction-related regions such as the NAc rapidly after acute drug administration [27]. Due to its regional specificity, it was hypothesized that alterations in these genes may provide a mechanism for reorganization of functional interactions between these brain regions in addiction [28]. Although c-Fos is rapidly upregulated and returns to basal levels quickly, AP-1 binding continues in the absence of elevated c-Fos mRNA or protein expression suggesting that other Fos proteins may replace c-Fos and accumulate during chronic use of drugs. This may provide a molecular trace of chronic drug use in the absence of drug itself. This tolerance to initial c-Fos upregulation appears to be drug agnostic, as acute alcohol exposure blocked the previously observed acute cocaine upregulation of c-Fos, also suggesting that this molecular trace persists for the use of all different drugs [29].

To more specifically test the role of specific transcription factors in addiction, transgenic mice with specific mutations were engineered. The first experiment to utilize this approach used a transgenic mouse with a mutant *fosB* gene that prevented the production of ΔFosB. It is important to consider that this mutant *fosB* gene was not targeted to any specific cell type or even to the brain, but throughout the body. These mutant mice showed attenuated chronic induction of AP-1-binding activity, suggesting that the previously observed AP-1 binding without c-Fos upregulation was probably due to ΔFosB [30]. Additionally, this study was the first to link transcriptional regulation with altered addiction-like behavior. These researchers used a model of drug-seeking behavior termed conditioned place preference (CPP), where animals are trained to associate one environment with an experimenter-administered drug and a separate environment with saline [31]. Over time, animals will seek out the drug-paired cues associated with the environment where they received the drug. These fosB-mutant mice showed increased CPP compared to wild-type controls, suggesting that normal ΔFosB AP-1 binding might be involved in a compensatory or adaptive response to drugs. Fos family members have also been found to be upregulated after exposure to drug-paired cues in the absence of the drug itself, suggesting that this CPP effect may be due to the interaction between drug and cues soliciting the availability of the drug, an importance facet in addiction research [32].

Although certain molecular factors may cause increased addiction-like behavior or plasticity within one set of cells, it may cause an opposite effect on these measures in another. Cellular specificity is an important point that has been discussed in neuroscience for some time. In an experiment complimentary to this performed by Schroeder and colleagues, researchers developed an inducible system to specifically overexpress ΔFosB within D1 neurons in the striatum [33]. Neurons within the striatum are primarily GABAergic medium-spiny neurons that mostly express D1 or D2 dopamine receptors. Since D1 receptors are G_s GPCRs, they activate the neuron leading to increased GABA release, while D2 receptors are G_i and are inhibited by dopamine binding. Since drugs of abuse cause hyperdopaminergic conditions within the striatum, both D1 and D2 containing neurons play important but dissociable roles in the development of addiction. Targeted ΔFosB overexpression in D1 neurons showed a similar effect on increased CPP behavior at low doses (5 and 15 mg/kg), but normal CPP behavior at higher doses (20 mg/kg). This suggests that cocaine-induced ΔFosB expression within these cells is necessary and sufficient to promote addiction-like behaviors. Furthermore, GABAergic inhibition from these cells may play a role in CPP behavior. Finally, this is physiologically relevant, as drugs of abuse and to a lesser extent natural rewards cause upregulation of ΔFosB in this specific neuronal subtype [28, 34]. In a similar experiment, nonspecific deletion of ΔFosB throughout the body caused the same behavioral alteration, increased CPP behavior to lower doses of cocaine [30]. Although this finding may seem contradictory, when taken together with previous data, this points to the existence of other regions or possibly neuronal subtypes that act in opposition to D1 neurons. Following up on this, overexpression of ΔFosB within D2 expressing neurons in the striatum produced no effects, illustrating the cellular specificity of these drug-induced alterations [35]. Thus, ΔFosB within these regions or cells may not play a role, or possibly inhibit, the plasticity required for the development of these behaviors.

Another behavioral model frequently used to study addiction is self-administration of drugs [36]. In this model, an intravenous catheter will infuse cocaine into the animal once it has completed a specific behavioral response, usually pressing an active lever in opposition to an inactive lever that produces no effect. This can be used to study motivation to consume drugs, as the requirement for lever pressing can be made harder by increasing the number of presses required to receive an infusion of drug. Animals with a similar inducible ΔFosB genotype as used by Kelz and colleagues showed increased motivation to self-administer cocaine [37]. This was also the first experiment to show that this alteration specifically affected motivation toward drugs and not naturally rewards such as a food pellet.

Transcription factors elicit changes in the expression of genes; thus this work suggests that there must be some downstream targets of Fos proteins that are mediating these effects on addiction-related behavior. Kelz and colleagues first described a downstream target that may alter plasticity involved in these behavioral alterations [33]. Striatal neurons are normally quiescent, even with dopamine input, and thus require glutamate which is an important neurotransmitter in addiction-like behaviors to alter their firing (reviewed in [38]). Kelz and colleagues found that ΔFosB overexpression caused an increase in a specific AMPAR subunit, GluR2 which could lead to altered plasticity [39]. Additionally, they could recapitulate their effects on behavior by viral-mediated overexpression of this subunit in the striatum. Overall, many ΔFosB targets are genes that appear to be previously linked to addiction-like behaviors such as CDK5 and NFkB.

2.2. CREB, a transcription factor well established in learning and memory associated plasticity, plays a role in addiction

Drugs of abuse can cause acute regulation of molecular-signaling cascades that can modify transcription factor activity. For example, many drugs of abuse can cause acute upregulation of the second messenger cAMP within many addiction-associated brain regions [40–46]. cAMP response element-binding protein (CREB) is phosphorylated in response to cAMP upregulation by a kinase sensitive to cAMP, protein kinase A (PKA; [47, 48]), calcium-calmodulin dependent kinases (CaMK) and other kinases [49]. The role of CREB in other forms of plasticity-associated memory has been well elucidated [48]. Once phosphorylated, CREB can enter the nucleus and bind to its response element, the cyclic AMP response element (CRE). CREB was first implicated in drug-induced alterations in response to acute and chronic morphine treatment within the locus coeruleus, another brain region associated with addiction [50]. Later, it was found that chronic, but not acute, morphine caused a decrease in CREB within the NAc [51]. Cocaine self-administration was found to be sensitive to PKA inhibition, an upstream regulator of CREB, by increasing lever pressing [52]. Following this experiment, it was later found that NAc overexpression of CREB caused a decrease in cocaine-CPP behavior [41]. Conversely, overexpression of a mutant CREB containing a single-point mutation, alanine for serine at residue 133, that prevents its phosphorylation and blocks its ability to regulate transcription acting as a dominant negative form of CREB, caused an increase in cocaine-CPP behavior. Further correlating the role of this transcription factor in the association of drug cues, researchers found that re-exposure to the original drug-paired environment in CPP without drug caused increased phosphorylation of CREB [53]. Highlighting the differences of behavioral tasks, it was found that NAc overexpression of CREB caused an increase in self-administration behavior [54]. This gene has also been studied in human patients. Researchers found that opioid-dependent patients were more likely to have a polymorphism in a protein that associates with CREB, CREB-binding protein, within a region associated with its activation by phosphorylation [55]. Altogether, it appears that CREB expression is involved in many aspects of addiction-related behavior.

CREB is a nuclear transcription factor that binds to CRE upstream of target genes. CREB regulation has been found to cause upregulation of ARG mRNA such as *c-fos*, *Fosb*, brain-derived neurotropic factor (*BDNF)*, and *TrkB* (e.g., in methamphetamine self-administration [56]). BDNF and its receptor TrkB have a very long history in the study of addiction-related behaviors as well as general plasticity occurring within the brain [57]. Further implicating CREB as a regulator of plasticity, it has been found to be involved in late-phase forms of long-term potentiation (LTP [58]). As mentioned before, NAc neurons are normally quiescent and require glutamate activation with or without dopamine stimulation to fire. CREB has been associated with the regulation of this feature of NAc neuronal membrane excitability [59]. It was found that increased CREB activity leads to enhanced NMDAR-mediated currents, an important receptor for causing action potentials as well as for learning and memory. This regulation increases NAc neuronal-firing probability through enhancement of the membrane excitability. This may partially explain the effect of NAc CREB on behaviors such as self-administration. Thus, CREB regulates the expression of many genes associated with plasticity and addiction-related behaviors.

CREB and ΔFosB are very well-documented addiction-related transcription factors but, undoubtedly, there are many more transcriptional factors that alter addiction-related plasticity and ultimately behavior. Myocyte-enhancing factor 2 (MEF2) was found to be involved in cocaine-induced structural plasticity [60]. Interestingly, it was necessary and sufficient to increase the number of dendritic spines. Structural plasticity or the alteration of the physical synaptic shape has been associated with electrophysiological measurements of plasticity [61–63] specifically in addiction [63]. Additionally, it was found that MEF2 regulates a wide network of plasticity-associated genes opening up further exploration into its role in addiction-related plasticity and behavior [64]. Overall, transcriptional regulation of ARG expression can lead to modifications in drug-evoked synaptic plasticity and behavior [65, 66].

3. Posttranscriptional regulation of plasticity and addiction-related transcripts can promote addiction-like behaviors

Posttranscriptional regulation occurs after transcription until the mRNA is translated into a functional protein. Posttranscriptional regulation takes many forms such as mRNA processing, splicing, editing, stability, and translation. mRNA stability and translation have been the most well-characterized posttranscriptional mechanism in plasticity, especially in addiction. Additionally, it appears that mRNA stability may be especially important in the brain, as nearly 20% of brain-expressed genes have been predicted to be controlled through this mechanism [67].

3.1. miRNAs destabilize specific mRNAs which could lead to diminished expression of genes involved in addiction

Stability can be influenced by direct binding of factors to discrete recognition sites. One group of factors involved in this type of mRNA stability are small noncoding RNAs, termed microRNAs (miRNAs). miRNAs are ~20–22 oligonucleotide molecules that are encoded within the genome and make up nearly 2–3% of transcribed genes but are not translated into protein. miRNAs target specific mRNAs through binding of complementary sequences within the miRNA, termed seed regions, to the 3′ untranslated region (UTR) of the mRNA. Association of miRNAs with the 5′UTR of mRNA has also been discovered [68] leading to different cellular effects, but most studies within the brain have focused on the 3′UTR. Accordingly, the rest of this section focuses on this mechanism.

Although the miRNA may associate directly with the mRNA target, the aftereffects of this binding are mediated through a large, supporting protein complex, the RNA-induced-silencing complex or RISC. Through associating with the RISC, an miRNA can target specific mRNAs for degradation or translational repression [69]. This complex contains a multitude of auxiliary proteins, with the most important being Argonaute (Ago; [70]). Ago is the component most directly involved in regulating the mRNA. There are many Ago isoforms, but generally they are separated into those containing nuclease "slicer" activity and those without. Thus, Ago is important for the well-characterized miRNA-induced destruction of mRNA.

Although one miRNA has one specific seed region to bind to mRNAs, mRNAs may have numerous sites complementary for multiple miRNAs. This suggests that a single miRNA targets many mRNAs, affecting a myriad of cellular processes and pathways. This is reminiscent of transcriptional regulation, as one transcription factor may regulate a specific sequence that is upstream of various types of genes. This opens the possibility for an miRNA that may regulate a network of plasticity-associated genes. For example, miR-9-3p was found to diminish *Dmd* and *Sap97* mRNA [71]. These genes are negatively associated with LTP expression, thus miRNA-induced silencing of these mRNAs would reverse this effect. A hippocampal LTP-dependent behavior, the Morris water maze, was also found to be regulated by the expression of this miRNA.

Similar to a group of plasticity- and addiction-associated transcription factors, miRNA expression patterns appear to be similar to IEGs in their temporal- and activity-dependent regulation [72–74]. As demonstrated before, many of these IEGs play integral roles in general plasticity and addiction-related plasticity. Similar to IEGs, miRNAs have been associated with neural development, synaptic plasticity, and even behavior [73–79].

The role of miRNA-induced posttranscriptional regulation in addiction was first studied in the regulation of the large-conductance-calcium-and-voltage-activated potassium channel (BK). This channel is integral to plasticity by affecting excitability, firing, and transmitter release from neurons [80]. It is also one of the many protein targets of alcohol within the brain, for the most part potentiating its conductance [81]. This channel has been well studied in its role in tolerance to alcohol in the striatum, requiring larger amounts to exert similar effects [82]. This seems to be mediated by decreased BK channel expression in the membrane. A single gene can produce multiple mRNAs with the same coding region but with different 3′UTRs through the inclusion or exclusion of different exons [83]. Research has shown that the alpha subunit of this BK channel is alternatively spliced both in the coding region and in the 3′ UTR in response to neuronal activity [82, 84]. These researchers also found that alcohol caused a decrease in one specific BK mRNA that has an miR-9-binding site in its 3′ UTR. Given that this isoform of the BK channel mRNA is the most abundant in the striatum and miR-9 expression is increased by alcohol exposure, alcohol tolerance seems to be mediated at least in part by this miRNA [82]. As mentioned before, miRNAs target many mRNAs that contain a complementary sequence in the 3′UTR. Thus, these authors also proposed that miR-9 targets many other mRNAs such as the beta subunit of the GABA receptor, GABRB2, and the D2 receptor. Overall, this suggests that alcohol-mediated upregulation of miR-9 leads to the development of an alcohol-specific regulation of mRNAs associated with plasticity and addiction.

When animals are given extended access to drugs of abuse in a self-administration model, they undergo a specific behavioral response termed escalation of drug use. Uncontrollable use of large amount of drugs is an important facet in the human condition. With this, researchers sought out an miRNA that may be increased by this behavior and found that miR-212, an activity-dependent miRNA regulated by CREB, was upregulated in the dorsal striatum of these animals after extended access [85]. One of the targets of miR-212 is Sprout-related, EVH1 domain containing 1 (SPRED1), a corepressor of serine-threonine protein kinase Raf1, which increases the activity of adenylate cyclase by promoting its phosphorylation. Thus, upregulation of miR-212 during escalated drug use diminishes SPRED1 levels, potentiating cAMP production and CREB activity leading to increased miR-212 expression. When miR-212 was overexpressed within the dorsal striatum, rats in extended access showed decreased levels of cocaine infusions. Oppositely, blocking of miR-212 by a locked nucleic acid (LNA) caused an increase in cocaine infusions. Thus, extended access to cocaine may recruit miR-212 leading to a positive feedback loop that effectively diminishes stereotypical escalation of drug intake. Overall, this suggests miR-212 acts on a pathway involving CREB to enhance its signaling, possibly in a compensatory, protective manner.

3.2. RNA-binding proteins bind to mRNAs and can bidirectionally regulate addiction-associated mRNA translation into protein

RNA-binding proteins (RBPs) are another group of regulators of mRNA stability and translation. Some RBPs recognize discrete sequences in the 3′UTR, such as the AU-rich instability conferring elements (AREs [86]). As with miRNAs, there is potential for a single RBP to affect multiple downstream processes leading to miRNAs and RBPs to be termed "master switches" of gene regulation [87, 88]. This is especially important in the brain, as around 15–20% of brain-specific transcripts contain AREs suggesting these genes are regulated by this type of posttranscriptional regulation [67]. Fragile x-mental retardation protein (FMRP) is an RBP that regulates the translation of nearly 850 brain mRNAs, many associated with synaptic function [89]. One of its regulatory targets are the group I metabotropic glutamate receptors mGluR1 and mGluR5 [90–92]. These receptors have been associated with cocaine-evoked behaviors [93, 94]. Thus, Smith and colleagues tested the role of FMRP in addiction-related behaviors [95]. They found that *Fmr1* KO mice were deficient in cocaine locomotor sensitization and conditioned place preference. The effect on conditioned place preference was reversed by genetic reduction in mGluR5, suggesting that FMRPs effect on drug-evoked behaviors was due to mGluR5 activity. Finally, they found that FMRP caused a reduction in cocaine-induced structural plasticity suggesting that these behavioral deficits may be caused by this aberrant plasticity.

Although FMRP is the only RBP specifically studied in addiction-like behaviors, many more have been associated with these behaviors [96]. One such family of RBPs is the Hu, or embryonic lethal abnormal vision-like (ELAV-L) proteins. Hu proteins are brain and neuronal specific and are homologous to the *Drosophila* protein ELAV protein [97, 98]. HuD expression and function is activity dependent, suggesting it may regulate IEGs and other activity-dependent genes associated with plasticity [99–101]. In confirmation of this idea, our laboratory has shown that HuD is critical for stabilizing U-rich containing mRNAs during neuronal development and synaptic plasticity [101]; work from our laboratory reviewed in [102, 103]. HuD is a critical regulator of multiple plasticity-associated genes, thus suggesting that it may be involved in addiction-related altered gene expression, plasticity, and ultimately behavior. Overall, post-transcriptional regulation may emerge as an important player tying drug-evoked molecular alterations with behavior.

3.3. mRNA editing can alter the sequence or expression of an addiction-related mRNA leading to alterations in addiction-related plasticity and behavior

mRNA editing is another posttranscriptional regulatory mechanism. The most common mechanism for RNA editing is through covalent modifications of a specific nucleotide, without the alteration of the original DNA-encoded gene. This would generate multiple alternative forms of a protein which may be important in different cellular contexts.

The most common mRNA modification leading to editing is the removal of an amino group and its replacement with an oxygen, termed deamination. This occurs on the N6 position of adenosine nucleotides, converting this nucleotide into an inosine. This position directly contributes to conventional Watson-Crick base pairing, thus allowing inosine to pair with cytosine similar to guanosine. Translationally, this leads to the original adenosine to be read as a guanine, effectively causing an A→G site-directed mutagenesis. This modification is catalyzed by adenosine deaminase that acts on RNA (ADAR) enzymes [104–108].

Specific mRNA editing in a neurophysiological context was first described in the GluRA2 subunit of AMPAR [109]. As mentioned before, editing of mRNA is a rapid mechanism to generate multiple alternative forms of a protein depending on environmental circumstances. These receptors are integral to excitatory synaptic signaling, especially in plasticity. Thus, AMPAR editing generates channels that are impermeable to calcium and displays faster recovery rates from desensitization. In terms of drug-induced plasticity, a recent study demonstrated that GluA2 editing by ADAR2 in the NAc of rats regulates cocaine seeking [110]. These researchers studied reinstatement, a specific stage of drug self-administration [36]. Animals first need to learn the required instrumental behavior to receive a reward in self-administration. When the animal reaches an experimenter-determined criterion, then the animal is said to have "acquired" self-administration behavior. If the animal is then presented with the same context and levers, but rewards are withdrawn, the animal will eventually override the previously learned reward-driven behavior. Eventually, the animal will no longer perform the task required for the reward, which is termed extinction. Finally, when an animal is exposed to cues associated with the reward or the reward itself, the animal will reinstate its behavior to receive the reward. Reinstatement is thought to be analogous to relapse in human-addiction patients. In this study, they found that abstinence from cocaine was associated with a decrease in NAc-edited calcium-impermeable AMPAR as well as ADAR2. Next, Schmidt and colleagues overexpressed ADAR2 within the NAc. They found that this diminished cocaine-primed reinstatement of self-administration behavior, suggesting that ADAR2 within the NAc is important for the regulation of relapse-like behavior. Overall, there are many avenues for mRNA editing in drug-induced plasticity and addiction-like behaviors [111].

Another posttranscriptional mRNA modification is the covalent modification of adenosine to N6-methyladenosine (m^6A). This modification is carried out by a methyltransferase complex, containing WTAP, METTL14, and KIAA1429. Hence, this complex is usually thought of as the "writers" of m^6A modifications. In opposition to the activity of this complex, enzymes have been discovered that promote the demethylation of mRNA, or the "erasers" of these modifications. These modifications have been studied for many years as a stable, unalterable modification. However, with the discovery of m^6A demethylases this shifted opinion to suggest that this modification is dynamic and thus could be regulated by physiological conditions (reviewed in [112]). For example, it was reported that regulation of m^6A was important to the normal functioning of the circadian rhythm in mammals [113]. Thus, m^6A is physiologically relevant in behavior.

The first m^6A demethylase to be discovered was the fat mass and obesity-associated protein (FTO). As the name suggests, it was identified as the strongest genetic variation to predispose patients to obesity [114–117]. At the opening of this chapter, evidence was presented to show that addiction-related neurocircuitry originally evolved to elicit goal-directed behavior toward food, suggesting this gene may also be involved in other forms of goal-directed behavior. The first study to link these findings was performed in alcoholic patients, finding that the genotype associated with obesity (rs9939609) was inversely correlated with general alcohol consumption, measures of alcohol dependence, as well as cigarette use [118].

Later work found that this gene is expressed in dopaminergic neurons within the midbrain and is increased by acute cocaine administration (20 mg/kg [119]). Cocaine, and to a lesser extent amphetamines, inhibits the dopamine transporter (DAT), leading to increased synaptic dopamine. This in turn leads to hyperactivation of dopamine receptors on both sides of the synapse. The presynaptic terminal contains D2 and D3 receptors, which are inhibitory GPCRs. Thus, the presynaptic dopaminergic neuron will show increased suppression of firing in response to cocaine. In the next set of experiments, these researchers found that Fto-deficient dopaminergic neurons showed diminished cocaine-induced suppression of firing rate, suggesting that signaling through D2/D3 receptors is regulated by Fto. As expected, it was found that protein expression of these downstream targets (DRD3, GIRK2, and NMDAR1) was reduced by Fto deficiency. Functionally, Fto deficiency led to a reduction in GIRK currents, possibly detailing a mechanism for the diminished cocaine-induced suppression of firing rate in dopaminergic neurons. Finally, Fto-deficient mice showed attenuated acute cocaine-induced locomotor activity, suggesting that these genetic and electrophysiological measures translate into this behavioral modification.

4. Conclusion

As shown here, there are many avenues for regulation of ARGs at the transcriptional or the posttranscriptional level. These regulatory mechanisms all have been implicated in the development of this disorder and thus may be involved in the vulnerability of some individuals to substance-use disorders. Understanding the regulation of addiction-related genes and their impact on synaptic plasticity and behavior may inform new pharmacological treatments that reverse these aberrant drug-evoked forms of plasticity in favor of remission.

Author details

Robert J Oliver and Nora I Perrone-Bizzozero*

*Address all correspondence to: nbizzozero@salud.unm.edu

Department of Neurosciences, University of New Mexico School of Medicine, Albuquerque, NM, USA

References

[1] Lüscher C, Ungless MA. The mechanistic classification of addictive drugs. PLoS Med. 2006;3:2005–10.

[2] Di Chiara G, Imperato A. Drugs abused by humans preferentially increase synaptic dopamine concentrations in the mesolimbic system of freely moving rats. Proc Natl Acad Sci U S A. 1988;85(July):5274–8.

[3] Nestler EJ. Is there a common molecular pathway for addiction? Nat Neurosci. 2005;8(11):1445–9. Available from: http://www.ncbi.nlm.nih.gov/pubmed/16251986

[4] Kelley AE, Berridge KC. The neuroscience of natural rewards: relevance to addictive drugs. J Neurosci. 2002;22(9):3306–11.

[5] Bromberg-Martin ES, Matsumoto M, Hikosaka O. Dopamine in motivational control: rewarding, aversive, and alerting. Neuron. 2010;68:815–34.

[6] Kolb B, Gorny G, Li Y, Samaha A-N, Robinson TE. Amphetamine or cocaine limits the ability of later experience to promote structural plasticity in the neocortex and nucleus accumbens. Proc Natl Acad Sci U S A. 2003;100(18):10523–8.

[7] Hamilton D a, Kolb B. Differential effects of nicotine and complex housing on subsequent experience-dependent structural plasticity in the nucleus accumbens. Behav Neurosci. 2005;119(2):355–65.

[8] Stuber GD, Klanker M, de Ridder B, Bowers MS, Joosten RN, Feenstra MG, et al. Reward-predictive cues enhance excitatory synaptic strength onto midbrain dopamine neurons. Science. 2008 (5896):1690–2. Available from: http://www.ncbi.nlm.nih.gov/entrez/query.fcgi?cmd=Retrieve&db=PubMed&dopt=Citation&list_uids=18802002

[9] McLellana T, Lewis DC, O'Brien CP, Kleber HD. Drug dependence, a chronic medical illness. JAMA J Am Med Assoc. 2000;284(13):1689.

[10] Shen H, Toda S, Moussawi K, Bouknight A, Zahm DS, Kalivas PW. Altered dendritic spine plasticity in cocaine-withdrawn rats. J Neurosci. 2009;29(9):2876–84.

[11] Montiel T, Almeida D, Arango I, Calixto E, Casasola C, Brailowsky S. Long-lasting effects of GABA infusion into the cerebral cortex of the rat. Neural Plast. 2000;7(1–2):1–8. Available from: http://www.pubmedcentral.nih.gov/articlerender.fcgi?artid=2565370&tool=pmcentrez&rendertype=abstract

[12] Hernandez PJ, Sadeghian K, Kelley AE. Early consolidation of instrumental learning requires protein synthesis in the nucleus accumbens. Nat Neurosci. 2002;5(12):1327–31.

[13] Scheyer AF, Wolf ME, Tseng KY. A protein synthesis-dependent mechanism sustains calcium-permeable AMPA receptor transmission in nucleus accumbens synapses during withdrawal from cocaine self-administration. J Neurosci. 2014;34(8):3095–100. Available from: http://www.ncbi.nlm.nih.gov/pubmed/24553949

[14] Bastle RM, Neisewander JL. Epigenetics and drug. In: Bastle RM, Neisewander JL, William Meil, editors. Recent Advances in Drug Addiction Research and Clinical Applications. InTech, Rijeka, Croatia; 2016. Available from: http://www.intechopen.com/books/recent-advances-in-drug-addiction-research-and-clinical-applications/epigenetics-and-drug-abuse

[15] Cadet JL, McCoy MT, Jayanthi S. Epigenetics and addiction. Clin Pharmacol Ther. 2016;99(5):502–11. Available from: http://dx.doi.org/10. 1002/cpt.345

[16] Tuesta LM, Zhang Y. Mechanisms of epigenetic memory and addiction. EMBO J. 2014 Apr 28;33(10):1091 LP-1103. Available from: http://emboj.embopress.org/content/33/10/1091.

[17] Robison AJ, Nestler EJ. Transcriptional and epigenetic mechanisms of addiction. Nat Rev Neurosci. 2011;12(11):623–37. Available from: http://dx.doi.org/10. 1038/nrn3111

[18] Fleming EW, Woodson ME, Tewari S. Ethanol and cycloheximide alter protein and RNA synthesis of Cox astrocytoma cells in culture. J Neurosci Res. 1981;6(4):511–24. Available from: http://dx.doi.org/10. 1002/jnr.490060408

[19] Chang SL, Squinto SP, Harlan RE. Morphine activation of c-fos expression in rat brain. Biochem Biophys Res Commun. 1988;157(2):698–704. Available from: http://www.sciencedirect.com/science/article/pii/S0006291X88803061

[20] Graybiela M, Moratalla R, Robertson HA. Amphetamine and cocaine induce drug-specific activation of the c-fos gene in striosome-matrix compartments and limbic subdivisions of the striatum. Proc Natl Acad Sci U S A. 1990;87(17):6912–6.

[21] Young ST, Porrino LJ, Iadarola MJ. Cocaine induces striatal c-fos-immunoreactive proteins via dopaminergic D1 receptors. Proc Natl Acad Sci U S A. 1991;88(4):1291–5.

[22] Persico AM, Schindler CW, O'Hara BF, Brannock MT, Uhl GR. Brain transcription factor expression: effects of acute and chronic amphetamine and injection stress. Mol Brain Res. 1993;20(1–2):91–100.

[23] Hayward MD, Duman RS, Nestler EJ. Induction of the c-fos proto-oncogene during opiate withdrawal in the locus coeruleus and other regions of rat brain. Brain Res. 1990;525(2):256–66.

[24] Milde-Langosch K. The Fos family of transcription factors and their role in tumourigenesis. Eur J Cancer. 2005;41(16):2449–61. Available from: http://www.ncbi.nlm.nih.gov/pubmed/16199154

[25] Sheng M, Greenberg ME. The regulation and function of c-fos and other immediate early genes in the nervous system. Neuron. 1990;4(4):477–85.

[26] Curran T, Morgan JI, Butler S. Memories of fos. BioEssays. 1987;7(6):255–8.

[27] Hope BT, Kosofsky B, Hyman SE, Nestler EJ. Regulation of immediate early gene expression and AP-1 binding in the rat nucleus accumbens by chronic cocaine. Proc Natl Acad Sci U S A. 1992;89(13):5764–8. Available from: http://www.ncbi.nlm.nih.gov/entrez/query.fcgi?cmd=Retrieve&db=PubMed&dopt=Citation&list_uids=1631058

[28] Moratalla R, Vallejo M, Elibol B, Graybiel AM. D1-class dopamine receptors influence cocaine-induced persistent expression of Fos-related proteins in striatum. Neuroreport. 1996;8(1):1–5. Available from: http://www.ncbi.nlm.nih.gov/entrez/query.fcgi?cmd=Retrieve&db=PubMed&dopt=Citation&list_uids=9051741

[29] Torres G. Acute administration of alcohol blocks cocaine-induced striatal c-fos immunoreactivity protein in the rat. Synapse. 1994;18(2):161–7.

[30] Hiroi N, Brown JR, Haile CN, Ye H, Greenberg ME, Nestler EJ. FosB mutant mice: loss of chronic cocaine induction of Fos-related proteins and heightened sensitivity to cocaine's psychomotor and rewarding effects. Proc Natl Acad Sci U S A. 1997;94(19):10397–402. Available from: http://www.ncbi.nlm.nih.gov/pubmed/9294222\nhttp://www.pubmedcentral.nih.gov/articlerender.fcgi?artid=PMC23374

[31] Tzschentke TM. Measuring reward with the conditioned place preference (CPP) paradigm: update of the last decade. Addict Biol. 2007;12(3–4):227–462.

[32] Schroeder BE, Holahan MR, Landry CF, Kelley AE. Morphine-associated environmental cues elicit conditioned gene expression. Synapse. 2000;37(2):146–58.

[33] Kelz MB, Chen J, Carlezon WA, Whisler K, Gilden L, Beckmann AM, et al. Expression of the transcription factor ΔFosB in the brain controls sensitivity to cocaine. Nature. 1999;401(6750):272–6. Available from: http://www.nature.com/nature/journal/v401/n6750/abs/401272a0. html\npapers3://publication/uuid/F51CD165-BEAE-4D11-BDAB-02B1F29A79C5

[34] Nye HE, Hope BT, Kelz MB, Iadarola M, Nestler EJ. Pharmacological studies of the regulation of chronic FOS-related antigen induction by cocaine in the striatum and nucleus accumbens. J Pharmacol Exp Ther. 1995;275(3):1671–80. Available from: http://www.ncbi.nlm.nih.gov/entrez/query.fcgi?cmd=Retrieve&db=PubMed&dopt=Citation&list_uids=8531143

[35] Zachariou V, Bolanos CA, Selley DE, Theobald D, Cassidy MP, Kelz MB, et al. An essential role for DeltaFosB in the nucleus accumbens in morphine action. Nat Neurosci. 2006;9(2):205–11. Available from: http://www.ncbi.nlm.nih.gov/entrez/query.fcgi?cmd=Retrieve&db=PubMed&dopt=Citation&list_uids=16415864

[36] Roberts DCS, Morgan D, Liu Y. How to make a rat addicted to cocaine. Prog Neuro-Psychopharmacol Biol Psychiatry. 2007;31(8):1614–24.

[37] Colby CR, Whisler K, Steffen C, Nestler EJ, Self DW. Striatal cell type-specific overexpression of DeltaFosB enhances incentive for cocaine. J Neurosci. 2003;23(6):2488–93. Available from: http://www.jneurosci.org/content/23/6/2488. abstract\nhttp://www.ncbi.nlm.nih.gov/pubmed/12657709

[38] van Huijstee AN, Mansvelder HD. Glutamatergic synaptic plasticity in the mesocorticolimbic system in addiction. Front Cell Neurosci. 2015;8(January):1–13. Available from: http://journal.frontiersin.org/journal/10. 3389/fncel.2014. 00466/abstract

[39] Kauer J a, Malenka RC. Synaptic plasticity and addiction. Nat Rev Neurosci. 2007;8(11):844–58.

[40] Cole RL, Konradi C, Douglass J, Hyman SE. Neuronal adaptation to amphetamine and dopamine: Molecular mechanisms of prodynorphin gene regulation in rat striatum. Neuron. 1995;14(4):813–23.

[41] Carlezon Jr. WA, Thome J, Olson VG, Lane-Ladd SB, Brodkin ES, Hiroi N, et al. Regulation of cocaine reward by CREB. Science. 1998;282(5397):2272–5. Available from: http://www.ncbi.nlm.nih.gov/entrez/query.fcgi?cmd=Retrieve&db=PubMed&dopt=Citation&list_uids=9856954

[42] Berke JD, Hyman SE. Addiction, dopamine, and the molecular mechanisms of memory. Neuron. 2000;25(3):515–32.

[43] Nestler EJ. Molecular basis of long-term plasticity underlying addiction. Nat Rev Neurosci. 2001;2(2):119–28.

[44] Shaw-Lutchman TZ, Barrot M, Wallace T, Gilden L, Zachariou V, Impey S, et al. Regional and cellular mapping of cAMP response element-mediated transcription during naltrexone-precipitated morphine withdrawal. J Neurosci. 2002;22(9):3663–72. Available from: http://www.ncbi.nlm.nih.gov/pubmed/11978842\nhttp://www.jneurosci.org/content/22/9/3663. full.pdf

[45] Shaw-Lutchman TZ, Impey S, Storm D, Nestler EJ. Regulation of CRE-mediated transcription in mouse brain by amphetamine. Synapse. 2003;48(1):10–7.

[46] Walters CL, Kuo YC, Blendy JA. Differential distribution of CREB in the mesolimbic dopamine reward pathway. J Neurochem. 2003;87(5):1237–44.

[47] Shaywitz AJ, Greenberg ME. CREB: a stimulus-induced transcription factor activated by a diverse array of extracellular signals. Annu Rev Biochem. 1999;68:821–61.

[48] Mayr B, Montminy M. Transcriptional regulation by the phosphorylation-dependent factor CREB. Nat Rev Mol Cell Biol. 2001;2(8):599–609. Available from: http://www.ncbi.nlm.nih.gov/pubmed/11483993

[49] Sheng M, Thompson MA, Greenberg ME. CREB: a Ca^{2+}-regulated transcription factor phosphorylated by calmodulin-dependent kinases. Science. 1991;252:1427–30.

[50] Guitart X, Thompson M a, Mirante CK, Greenberg ME, Nestler EJ. Regulation of cyclic AMP response element-binding protein (CREB) phosphorylation by acute and chronic morphine in the rat locus coeruleus. J Neurochem. 1992;58:1168–71.

[51] Widnell KL, Self DW, Lane SB, Russell DS, Vaidya VA, Miserendino MJ, et al. Regulation of CREB expression: in vivo evidence for a functional role in morphine action in the nucleus accumbens. J Pharmacol Exp Ther. 1996;276(1):306–15. Available from: http://www.ncbi.nlm.nih.gov/pubmed/8558448

[52] Self DW, Genova LM, Hope BT, Barnhart WJ, Spencer JJ, Nestler EJ. Involvement of cAMP-dependent protein kinase in the nucleus accumbens in cocaine self administration and relapse of cocaine-seeking behavior. J Neurosci. 1998;18:1848–59. Available from: http://www.jneurosci.org/content/18/5/1848.

[53] Tropea TF, Kosofsky BE, Rajadhyaksha AM. Enhanced CREB and DARPP-32 phosphorylation in the nucleus accumbens and CREB, ERK, and GluR1 phosphorylation in the dorsal hippocampus is associated with cocaine-conditioned place preference behavior. J Neurochem. 2008;106(4):1780–90.

[54] Larson EB, Graham DL, Arzaga RR, Buzin N, Webb J, Green T a., et al. Overexpression of CREB in the nucleus accumbens shell increases cocaine reinforcement in self-administering rats. J Neurosci. 2011;31(45):16447–57.

[55] Kumar D, Deb I, Chakraborty J, Mukhopadhyay S, Das S. A polymorphism of the CREB binding protein (CREBBP) gene is a risk factor for addiction. Brain Res. 2011;1406:59–64.

[56] Krasnova IN, Chiflikyan M, Justinova Z, McCoy MT, Ladenheim B, Jayanthi S, et al. CREB phosphorylation regulates striatal transcriptional responses in the self-administration model of methamphetamine addiction in the rat. Neurobiol Dis. 2013;58:132–43.

[57] Li X, Wolf ME. Multiple faces of BDNF in cocaine addiction. Behav Brain Res. 2015;279:240–54. Available from: http://dx.doi.org/10. 1016/j.bbr.2014. 11. 018

[58] Barco A, Alarcon JM, Kandel ER. Expression of constitutively active CREB protein facilitates the late phase of long-term potentiation by enhancing synaptic capture. Cell. 2002;108(5):689–703.

[59] Huang YH, Lin Y, Brown TE, Han MH, Saal DB, Neve RL, et al. CREB modulates the functional output of nucleus accumbens neurons: a critical role of N-methyl-D-aspartate glutamate receptor (NMDAR) receptors. J Biol Chem. 2008;283(5):2751–60.

[60] Pulipparacharuvil S, Renthal W, Hale CF, Taniguchi M, Xiao G, Kumar A, et al. Cocaine regulates MEF2 to control synaptic and behavioral plasticity. Neuron. 2008;59(4):621–33.

[61] Yagishita S, Hayashi-Takagia., Ellis-Davies GCR, Urakubo H, Ishii S, Kasai H. A critical time window for dopamine actions on the structural plasticity of dendritic spines. Science. 2014;345(6204):1616–20.

[62] Alvarez V a, Sabatini BL. Anatomical and physiological plasticity of dendritic spines. Annu Rev Neurosci. 2007;30:79–97.

[63] Russo SJ, Dietz DM, Dumitriu D, Morrison JH, Malenka RC, Nestler EJ. The addicted synapse: mechanisms of synaptic and structural plasticity in nucleus accumbens. Trends Neurosci. 2010;33(6):267–76. Available from: http://dx.doi.org/10. 1016/j.tins.2010. 02. 002

[64] Flavell SW, Kim TK, Gray JM, Harmin DA, Hemberg M, Hong EJ, et al. Genome-wide analysis of MEF2 transcriptional program reveals synaptic target genes and neuronal activity-dependent polyadenylation site selection. Neuron. 2008;60(6):1022–38.

[65] Persico AM, Uhl GR. Transcription factors: potential roles in drug-induced neuroplasticity. Rev Neurosci. 1996;7(4):233–75.

[66] Nestler EJ. Transcriptional mechanisms of drug addiction. Clin Psychopharmacol Neurosci. 2012;10(3):136–43. Available from: http://www.pubmedcentral.nih.gov/articlerender.fcgi?artid=3569166&tool=pmcentrez&rendertype=abstract

[67] Bolognani F, Contente-Cuomo T, Perrone-Bizzozero NI. Novel recognition motifs and biological functions of the RNA-binding protein HuD revealed by genome-wide identification of its targets. Nucleic Acids Res. 2009;38(1):117–30.

[68] Panda AC, Sahu I, Kulkarni SD, Martindale JL, Abdelmohsen K, Vindu A, et al. MiR-196b-mediated translation regulation of mouse insulin2 via the 5'UTR. PLoS One. 2014;9(7):1–11.

[69] Bartel DP. MicroRNAs: genomics, biogenesis, mechanism, and function. Cell. 2004;116(2):281–97.

[70] Sontheimer EJ. Assembly and function of RNA silencing complexes. Nat Rev Mol Cell Biol. 2005;6(2):127–38.

[71] Sim S-E, Lim C-S, Kim J-I, Daekwan Seo X, Chun H, Nam-Kyung Yu X, et al. Cellular/molecular the brain-enriched MicroRNA miR-9-3p regulates synaptic plasticity and memory. 2016;36(33):8641–52.

[72] Nudelman AS, Dirocco DP, Lambert TJ, Garelick MG, Le J, Nathanson NM, et al. Neuronal activity rapidly induces transcription of the CREB-regulated microRNA-132, in vivo. Hippocampus. 2010;20(4):492–8.

[73] Krol J, Busskamp V, Markiewicz I, Stadler MB, Ribi S, Richter J, et al. Characterizing light-regulated retinal microRNAs reveals rapid turnover as a common property of neuronal microRNAs. Cell. 2010;141(4):618–31.

[74] Joilin G, Guévremont D, Ryan B, Claudianos C, Cristino AS. Rapid regulation of microRNA following induction of long-term potentiation in vivo. Front Mol Neurosci. 2014;7:98.

[75] Vo N, Klein ME, Varlamova O, Keller DM, Yamamoto T, Goodman RH, et al. A cAMP-response element binding protein-induced microRNA regulates neuronal morphogenesis. Proc Natl Acad Sci U S A. 2005;102(45):16426–31.

[76] Kosik KS. The neuronal microRNA system. Nat Rev Neurosci. 2006;7(12):911–20.

[77] Schratt GM, Tuebing F, Nigh E a, Kane CG, Sabatini ME, Kiebler M, et al. A brain-specific microRNA regulates dendritic spine development. Nature. 2006;439(7074):283–9.

[78] Kim J, Inoue K, Ishii J, Vanti WB, Voronov S V, Murchison E, et al. A MicroRNA feedback circuit in midbrain dopamine neurons. Science. 2007;317(5842):1220–4. Available from: http://www.sciencemag.org/content/317/5842/1220. abstract

[79] Fiore R, Siegel G, Schratt G. MicroRNA function in neuronal development, plasticity and disease. Biochim Biophys Acta Gene Regul Mech. 2008;1779(8):471–8.

[80] Storm JF. Potassium currents in hippocampal pyramidal cells. Prog Brain Res. 1990;83:161–87.

[81] Butler A, Tsunoda S, McCobb DP, Wei A, Salkoff L. mSlo, a complex mouse gene encoding "maxi" calcium-activated potassium channels. Sci (New York, NY). 1993;261(5118):221–4. Available from: http://eutils.ncbi.nlm.nih.gov/entrez/eutils/elink.fcgi?dbfrom=pubmed&id=7687074&retmode=ref&cmd=prlinks\npapers3://publication/uuid/DAB5A528-4A25-49DE-8BE9-051FDF21F823

[82] Pietrzykowski AZ, Martin GE, Puig SI, Knott TK, Lemos JR, Treistman SN. Alcohol tolerance in large-conductance, calcium-activated potassium channels of CNS terminals is intrinsic and includes two components: decreased ethanol potentiation and decreased channel density. J Neurosci. 2004;24(38):8322–32. Available from: http://www.ncbi.nlm.nih.gov/pubmed/15385615

[83] Legendre M, Ritchie W, Lopez F, Gautheret D. Differential repression of alternative transcripts: a screen for miRNA targets. PLoS Comput Biol. 2006;2(5):333–42.

[84] Xie J, McCobb DP. Control of alternative splicing of potassium channels by stress hormones. Science. 1998;280(5362):443–6.

[85] Im H-I, Hollander J a, Bali P, Kenny PJ. MeCP2 controls BDNF expression and cocaine intake through homeostatic interactions with microRNA-212. Nat Neurosci. 2010;13(9):1120–7. Available from: http://dx.doi.org/10. 1038/nn.2615

[86] Bakheet T, Williams BRG, Khabar KSA. ARED 3. 0: the large and diverse AU-rich transcriptome. Nucleic Acids Res. 2006;34 (suppl 1):D111–4.

[87] Deschênes-Furry J, Perrone-Bizzozero N, Jasmin BJ. The RNA-binding protein HuD: a regulator of neuronal differentiation, maintenance and plasticity. BioEssays. 2006;28(8):822–33.

[88] Keene JD. RNA regulons: coordination of post-transcriptional events. Nat Rev Genet. 2007;8(7):533–43.

[89] Darnell JC, Van Driesche SJ, Zhang C, Hung KYS, Mele A, Fraser CE, et al. FMRP stalls ribosomal translocation on mRNAs linked to synaptic function and autism. Cell. 2011;146(2):247–61.

[90] Ceman S, O'Donnell WT, Reed M, Patton S, Pohl J, Warren ST. Phosphorylation influences the translation state of FMRP-associated polyribosomes. Hum Mol Genet. 2003;12(24):3295–305.

[91] Nalavadi VC, Muddashetty RS, Gross C, Bassell GJ. Dephosphorylation-induced ubiquitination and degradation of FMRP in dendrites: a role in immediate early mGluR-stimulated translation. J Neurosci. 2012;32(8):2582–7.

[92] Narayanan U, Nalavadi V, Nakamoto M, Pallas DC, Ceman S, Bassell GJ, et al. FMRP phosphorylation reveals an immediate-early signaling pathway triggered by group I mGluR and mediated by PP2A. J Neurosci. 2007;27(52):14349–57.

[93] Chiamulera C, Epping-Jordan MP, Zocchi A, Marcon C, Cottiny C, Tacconi S, et al. Reinforcing and locomotor stimulant effects of cocaine are absent in mGluR5 null mutant mice. Nat Neurosci. 2001;4(9):873–4. Available from: http://www.ncbi.nlm.nih.gov/entrez/query.fcgi?cmd=Retrieve&db=PubMed&dopt=Citation&list_uids=11528416

[94] Olsen CM, Childs DS, Stanwood GD, Winder DG. Operant sensation seeking requires metabotropic glutamate receptor 5 (mGluR5). PLoS One. 2010;5(11).

[95] Smith LN, Jedynak JP, Fontenot MR, Hale CF, Dietz KC, Taniguchi M, et al. Fragile X mental retardation protein regulates synaptic and behavioral plasticity to repeated cocaine administration. Neuron. 2014;82(3):645–58. Available from: http://linkinghub.elsevier.com/retrieve/pii/S089662731400258X

[96] Bryant CD, Yazdani N. RNA binding proteins, neural development and the addictions. Genes Brain Behav. 2015;15(1):169–86. Available from: http://www.ncbi.nlm.nih.gov/pubmed/26643147

[97] Szabo A, Dalmau J, Manley G, Rosenfeld M, Wong E, Henson J, et al. HuD, a paraneoplastic encephalomyelitis antigen, contains RNA-binding domains and is homologous to Elav and Sex-lethal. Cell. 1991;67(2):325–33.

[98] Yao KM, Samson ML, Reeves R, White K. Gene elav of Drosophila melanogaster: a prototype for neuronal-specific RNA binding protein gene family that is conserved in flies and humans. J Neurobiol. 1993;24:723–39.

[99] Bolognani F, Tanner DC, Nixon S, Okano HJ, Okano H, Perrone-Bizzozero NI. Coordinated expression of HuD and GAP-43 in hippocampal dentate granule cells during developmental and adult plasticity. Neurochem Res. 2007;32(12):2142–51.

[100] Tiruchinapalli DM, Ehlers MD, Keene JD. Activity-dependent expression of RNA binding protein HuD and its association with mRNAs in neurons. RNA Biol. 2008;5(3):157–68.

[101] Vanevski F, Xu B. HuD Interacts with Bdnf mRNA and is essential for activity-induced BDNF synthesis in dendrites. PLoS One. 2015;10(2):e0117264. Available from: http://dx.plos.org/10. 1371/journal.pone.0117264

[102] Perrone-Bizzozero N, Bolognani F. Role of HuD and other RNA-binding proteins in neural development and plasticity. J Neurosci Res. 2002;68(2):121–6.

[103] Bolognani F, Perrone-Bizzozero NI. RNA-protein interactions and control of mRNA stability in neurons. J Neurosci Res. 2008;68:481–9.

[104] Bass BL, Weintraub H. An unwinding activity that covalently modifies its double-stranded RNA substrate. Cell. 1988;55(6):1089–98.

[105] Kim U, Wang Y, Sanford T, Zeng Y, Nishikura K. Molecular cloning of cDNA for double-stranded RNA adenosine deaminase, a candidate enzyme for nuclear RNA editing. Proc Natl Acad Sci U S A. 1994;91(24):11457–61. Available from: http://www.ncbi.nlm.nih.gov/entrez/query.fcgi?cmd=Retrieve&db=PubMed&dopt=Citation&list_uids=7972084

[106] Kim U, Garner TL, Sanford T, Speicher D, Murray JM, Nishikura K. Purification and characterization of double-stranded-RNA adenosine deaminase from bovine nuclear extracts. J Biol Chem. 1994;269:13480–9.

[107] Melcher T, Maas S, Herba, Sprengel R, Seeburg PH, Higuchi M. A mammalian RNA editing enzyme. Nature. 1996;379:460–4.

[108] Wagnert RW, Smitht JE, Coopermant BS, Nishikurat K. A double-stranded RNA unwinding activity introduces structural alterations by means of adenosine to inosine conversions in mammalian cells. Proc Natl Acad Sci. 1989;86:2647–51.

[109] Lomeli H, Mosbacher J, Melcher T, Höger T, Geiger JR, Kuner T, et al. Control of kinetic properties of AMPA receptor channels by nuclear RNA editing. Science. 1994;266(5191):1709–13.

[110] Schmidt HD, McFarland KN, Darnell SB, Huizenga MN, Sangrey GR, Cha J-HJ, et al. ADAR2-dependent GluA2 editing regulates cocaine seeking. Mol Psychiatry. 2014;(February):1–7. Available from: http://www.nature.com/doifinder/10. 1038/mp.2014.134

[111] Rosenthal JJC. The emerging role of RNA editing in plasticity. J Exp Biol. 2015;218: 1812–21.

[112] Cao G, Li H-B, Yin Z, Flavell RA. Recent advances in dynamic m^6A RNA modification. Open Biol. 2016;6(4):160003. Available from: http://rsob.royalsocietypublishing.org/content/6/4/160003

[113] Fustin JM, Doi M, Yamaguchi Y, Hida H, Nishimura S, Yoshida M, et al. RNA-methylation dependent RNA processing controls the speed of the circadian clock. Cell. 2013:155(4):793–806.

[114] Frayling TM, Timpson NJ, Weedon MN, Zeggini E, Freathy RM, Lindgren CM, et al. A common variant in the FTO gene is associated with body mass index and predisposes to childhood and adult obesity. Science. 2007;316(5826):889–94. Available from: http://www.pubmedcentral.nih.gov/articlerender.fcgi?artid=2646098&tool=pmcentrez&rendertype=abstract

[115] Dina C, Meyre D, Gallina S, Durand E, Körner A, Jacobson P, et al. Variation in FTO contributes to childhood obesity and severe adult obesity. Nat Genet. 2007;39(6):724–6. Available from: http://www.nature.com/doifinder/10. 1038/ng2048

[116] Cecil JE, Tavendale R, Watt P, Hetherington MM, Palmer CNA, Ph D, et al. An obesity-associated FTO gene variant and increased energy intake in children. N Engl J Med. 2008;359(24):2558–66. Available from: http://www.ncbi.nlm.nih.gov/pubmed/19073975

[117] Wardle J, Carnell S, Haworth CMA, Farooqi IS, O'Rahilly S, Plomin R. Obesity associated genetic variation in FTO is associated with diminished satiety. J Clin Endocrinol Metab. 2008;93(9):3640–3.

[118] Sobczyk-Kopciol A, Broda G, Wojnar M, Kurjata P, Jakubczyk A, Klimkiewicz A, et al. Inverse association of the obesity predisposing FTO rs9939609 genotype with alcohol consumption and risk for alcohol dependence. Addiction. 2011;106(4):739–48. Available from: http://www.ncbi.nlm.nih.gov/pubmed/21182554

[119] Hess ME, Hess S, Meyer KD, Verhagen L a W, Koch L, Brönneke HS, et al. The fat mass and obesity associated gene (Fto) regulates activity of the dopaminergic midbrain circuitry. Nat Neurosci. 2013;16(8):1042–8. Available from: http://www.ncbi.nlm.nih.gov/pubmed/23817550

4

Post-Transcriptional Mechanisms of Neuronal Translational Control in Synaptic Plasticity

Dylan Kiltschewskij and Murray J. Cairns

Abstract

The dynamic complexity of synaptic function is matched by extensive multidimensional regulation of neuronal mRNA translation which is achieved by a number of post-transcriptional mechanisms. The first key aspect of this regulatory capacity is mRNA distal trafficking through RNA-binding proteins, which governs the transcriptomic composition of post-synaptic compartments. Small non-coding microRNA and associated machinery have the capacity to precisely coordinate neural gene networks in space and time by providing a flexible specificity dimension to translational regulation. This RNA-guided subcellular fine-tuning of protein synthesis is an exquisite mechanism used in neurons to exert control of synaptic properties. Emerging evidence also implicates brain-enriched long non-coding RNA and novel circular RNA in posttranscriptional regulation of gene expression through the modulation of both mRNA and miRNA functions, thereby exemplifying the complex nature of neuronal translation. Herein, we review current knowledge of these regulatory systems and analyse how these mechanisms of transcriptomic regulation may be linked together to achieve high-order spatiotemporal control of post-synaptic translation.

Keywords: translation, mRNA trafficking, messenger ribonucleoprotein, microRNA, P-bodies, circular RNA

1. Introduction

The early phases of long-term potentiation (LTP) and long-term depression (LTD) are characterised by post-translational modification and trafficking of AMPA glutamate receptors, modifying reactivity of the post-synaptic membrane following an appropriate inducing stimulus [1]. While this is an effective means of altering synaptic transmission in the short term, consolidation of these changes into late-phase synaptic plasticity requires a substantially deeper response, driven by novel transcription and translation of messenger RNA (mRNA) [2]. Translation is a particularly interesting aspect of this system as discrete foci of polyribosomes have been observed in dendritic spines engaging in protein synthesis, indicating a role for localised distal translation in dendritic function which has since proven critical in synaptic plasticity, and indeed, learning and memory [2–5].

Considering the importance of dendritic translation in strengthening alterations to the post-synaptic compartment, the role of mRNA in connecting neuronal transcription and distal translation is crucial and understandably subject to significant modulation. To this extent, neurons exploit a variety of post-transcriptional regulatory mechanisms to ensure an array of over 2500 unique, dendritically localised mRNAs are only translated when appropriate [5]. At present, it is clear that a variety of mRNA-binding proteins (RBPs) act to selectively distribute mRNAs to individual dendritic spines and may additionally act as enhancers or inhibitors of translation. Non-coding RNA, specifically microRNA (miRNA), provides a potent and specific dimension to translational control, which themselves may be regulated by other novel, brain-enriched, non-coding RNA.

Despite extensive investigation of neuronal mechanisms of translation control, we still lack a clear understanding of how these systems work both individually and synergistically to regulate the localisation and appropriate timing of translation. This chapter therefore explores recent advances in the field of neuronal post-transcriptional translational regulation, with particular focus on miRNA and how these small non-coding RNAs interact with a variety of intermediates to exert precise control over neuronal protein synthesis.

2. Intracellular trafficking supplies dendrites with mRNA

2.1. Cis-acting factors

Neuronal subcellular compartments such as dendritic spines rely on distal trafficking of mRNA from the soma to provide a stockpile of transcripts for protein synthesis. Considering the functional similarity and close proximity of these compartments, precise localisation of mRNA is critical for modulation of the dendritic transcriptome, which influences translation in response to stimuli such as synaptic transmission. This raises a key question; how can thousands of unique mRNAs successfully localise in functionally similar subcellular neuronal compartments?

Part of the answer lies within the mRNA itself as its 3′ UTR is encoded with *cis*-acting sequences known as localisation elements (LE), which signal the desired site of transcript localisation. LEs were initially observed in chicken embryonic myoblasts whereby isoform-specific 3′ UTR sequences were shown to direct the accumulation of α-actin and β-actin in peripheral and perinuclear regions, respectively [6]. Dendrite-specific LEs have since been identified in key mediators of synaptic plasticity, including AMPA receptors, MAP2, αCaMKII and BDNF [7–10], indicating LEs play a critical role in the post-synaptic localisation of specific mRNAs. The AMPA receptor is a particularly interesting example as "flip" and "flop" splice variants have been shown to respectively localise in dendrites and the soma [7], revealing alternative splicing may serve to edit LE expression and subcellular localisation through removal of undesirable LEs in specific transcript splice variants. Furthermore, MAP2 long and short 3′ UTR variants generated by alternative polyadenylation have been shown to, respectively, target the dendrites and soma [9], implicating polyadenylation as another possible mechanism through which LE expression may be altered.

Following the discovery of LEs, a subset of studies has focussed on identifying a mechanistic basis through which these sequences facilitate selective mRNA trafficking. Considering the role of proteins in physically transporting mRNA (covered next), a distinct possibility is "digital" LEs form secondary structures to facilitate "analogue" recognition by RNA-binding proteins (RBP) [11]. This proposed mechanism of LE function is strongly supported by the identification of 3′ UTR stem-loop LEs required for the transport of K10, ASH1 and Oskar mRNAs in non-neuronal models [12–14]. In the context of synaptic function, a 5′ UTR stem-loop motif has recently been shown to direct sensorin mRNA to the synapse in *Aplysia*, both demonstrating the role of stem-loops in moderating synaptic mRNA localisation and revealing that LEs may not be purely confined to the 3′ UTR [15].

2.2. Trans-acting factors

While encoding mRNAs with LEs constitutes an elegant mechanism by which transcripts may be directed to subcellular compartments, neurons require an efficient physical mechanism of mRNA distribution to ensure all dendrites and their spines are adequately supplied with transcripts. Such a system is provided by a specialised group of RBPs, the neuronal microtubule network and associated motor proteins, all of which act in concert to facilitate mRNA trafficking from the soma to far distal regions of the neuron.

Current evidence heavily implicates neuronal messenger ribonucleoprotein (mRNP) granules as the primary vehicles of neuronal mRNA trafficking as observed through their translocation in neurites and mRNA/protein enrichment [16, 17]. These granules are composed of aggregated mRNA-RBP complexes, which are hypothesised to form upon *cis-trans* interaction between RBPs and target mRNA LEs (**Figure 1**), conferring specificity to this system while additionally providing a means of translationally repressing mRNAs during transport [18, 19]. At present, the neuronally enriched fragile X mental retardation protein (FMRP) and Staufen family proteins are the chief candidate RBPs involved in neuronal mRNA trafficking as evidenced by their enrichment within mRNP granules while complexed with a variety of plasticity-relevant mRNAs including CaMKIIα, MAP1b, β-actin and poly(A)-binding protein (PABP) [20–25]. An important aspect of these studies is that neuronal RBPs clearly target a variety of unique mRNAs, therefore suggesting RBPs recognise a number of different LEs, or alternatively, LEs for the same subcellular compartment share similar structural properties. Regardless, the key advantage of this system is the need for relatively few unique RBPs relative to the number of mRNAs requiring transport. In contrast to this observation, zipcode-binding protein 1 (ZBP1) specifically engages in activity-dependent trafficking of β-actin mRNA to the axon and dendrites through recognition of a 54nt LE within the 3′ UTR [26, 27]. While other binding partners may exist, it is possible that ZBP1 acts as a highly specific mediator of β-actin expression due to the high demand for this protein in neuronal cytoskeletal remodelling [28].

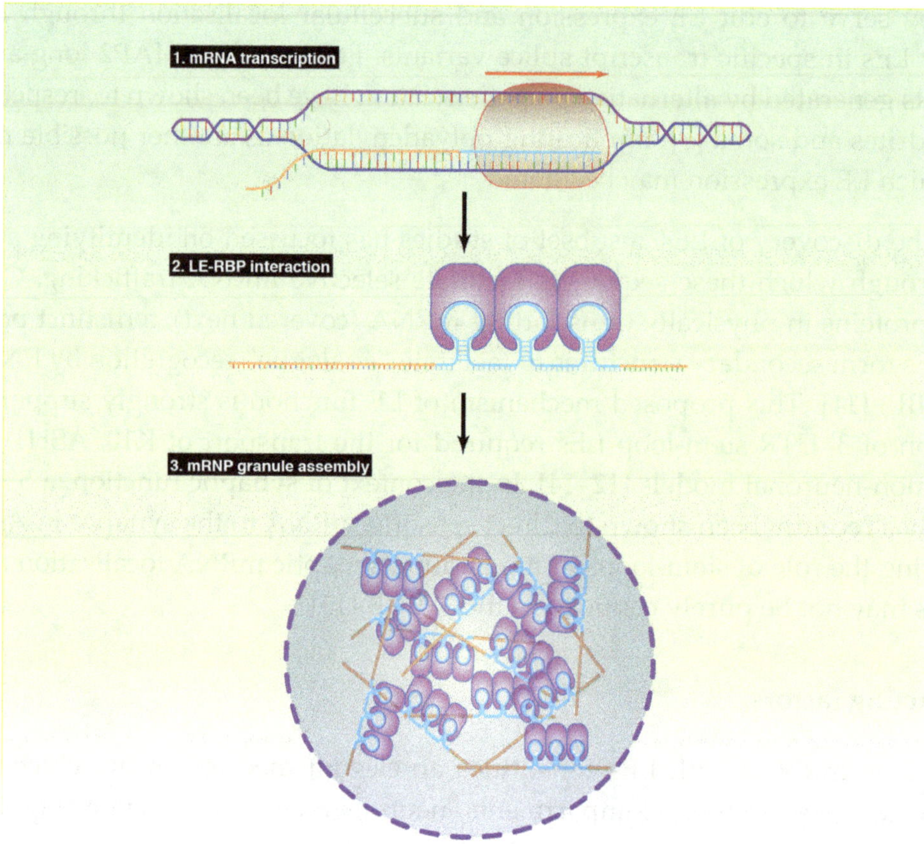

Figure 1. Assembly of neuronal messenger ribonucleoprotein granules. (1) During transcription, mRNAs are inherently encoded with cis-acting localisation elements in the 3′ UTR. (2) These sequences form secondary structures such as stem-loops, facilitating recognition by RNA-binding proteins. (3) Aggregation of multiple mRNA-RBP complexes results in the formation of neuronal mRNP granules, which transport mRNAs to distal locations in a translationally repressed state.

The overall significance of RBPs in neuronal mRNA trafficking is further exemplified by their hypothesised role as adaptors, linking transcripts to motor proteins for distal transport via microtubules. Supporting this view, mRNP granule-associated FMRP has been shown to directly interact with KIF3c and KIF5 kinesin motor protein subunits [22, 29], while similarly, ZPB1 directly binds the tail domain of KIF11 while complexed with β-actin mRNA [30]. The role of microtubules in this process has been further elucidated by the observed microtubule-dependent translocation of Staufen granules to the dendrites in response to synaptic activity as seen through GFP-fusion experiments [31]. It is interesting to note that Dynein is another candidate motor protein involved in mRNA microtubular trafficking; however, its role is currently only described in *Drosophila* embryonic extracts [32].

2.3. "Synaptic Tag and Capture" and "Sushi Belt" theories

Evidence pertaining the activity-dependent migration of neuronal mRNP granules to the dendrites implies that these granules bear functional significance in the regulation of activity-dependent translation [31, 33]. However, despite our extensive knowledge of neuronal mRNA trafficking, it is still unclear how specific neuronal mRNP granules are successfully delivered to individual dendritic spines following stimuli such as synaptic transmission. A commonly accepted model regarding this question was initially proposed in 1997 by Frey and Morris, who presented the "Synaptic Tag and Capture" theory in the context of LTP [34, 35] which has since received significant attention, and indeed, refinement [36–38]. At the core of this theory, strong synaptic stimuli capable of inducing late-phase LTP "tags" specific dendritic spines, signalling for the uptake of plasticity-related proteins and mRNAs from dendritic shafts and the soma [34]. While evidence obtained since the original proposal of this model has supported synaptic tag and capture, the identity of the tag, whether a single molecule or state of the synapse, has yet to be elucidated [38].

More recently, Doyle and Kiebler [18] have proposed an alternate "Sushi Belt" theory of dendritic mRNA trafficking with stronger emphasis on neuronal mRNP granules. This theory suggests that mRNPs constitutively circulate dendritic shafts through microtubules and motor proteins, analogous to a sushi conveyor belt. Application of a potentiating stimulus to any particular spine "tags" it, resulting in recruitment of mRNP granules to that spine through the action of dynamic microtubules when novel translation is required. Importantly, this theory accounts for both basal and activity-dependent mRNP transport in addition to anterograde and retrograde mRNP translocation, which has previously been observed [16]. Considering current knowledge of mRNA dendritic transport, however, it remains a distinct possibility that facets from both of these models may likely underlie the true mechanism behind both basal and activity-dependent neuronal mRNA trafficking.

3. microRNAs specifically and potently regulate post-synaptic translation

MicroRNAs (miRNAs) are a class of short, ~22nt non-coding RNAs that function as target-specific guides in the degradation and translational repression of mRNA. Since their initial discovery in 1993 [39, 40], the role of miRNA in providing combinatorial specificity to translational regulation has been highlighted through the discovery of more than 3700 unique miRNA participating in over 366,000 experimentally supported miRNA-target interactions [41]. Profiling studies have further identified the CNS as a source of significant miRNA enrichment whereby a subset of miRNA and associated factors regulate synaptic plasticity and are subject to activity-dependent turnover, indicating a key role in the maintenance of synaptic function [42]. Consequently, dysregulation of miRNA function is thought to contribute to the pathogenesis of complex neurological diseases, in particular, neuropsychiatric conditions characterised by impairments in learning and memory [43].

3.1. miRNA biogenesis and target interaction

miRNAs are derived from the transcription and processing of miRNA genes (**Figure 2**) located in a diverse array of genomic locations, including coding, non-coding and intergenic regions [44, 45]. Transcription of miRNA genes by RNA polymerase II yields primary miRNA (pri-miR), which house one (monocistronic) or multiple (polycistronic) miRNA species and are post-transcriptionally supplemented with 5′ methylguanosine cap and 3′ poly(A)

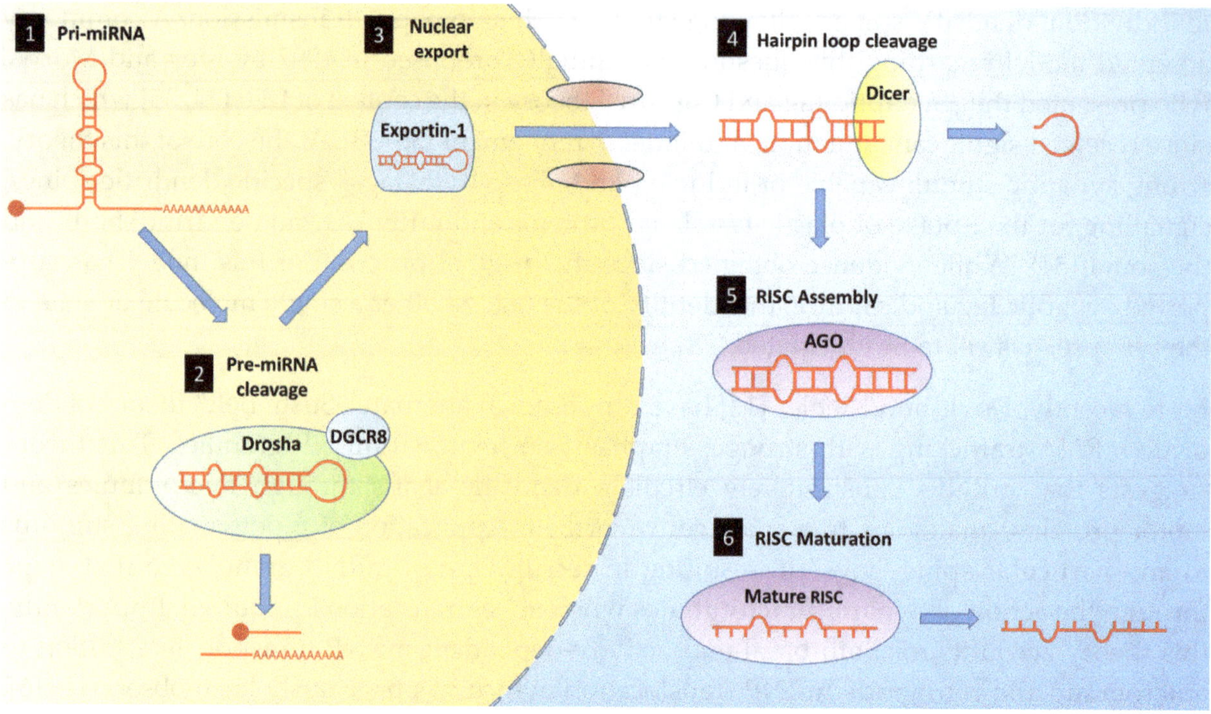

Figure 2. miRNA biogenesis. (1) Transcription of miRNA genes yields pri-miRNA, which adopt a hairpin secondary structure and contain 5′ cap and 3′ poly(A) tail similarly to mRNA. (2) These structures are cleaved from the pri-miRNA by Drosha and cofactor DGCR8, yielding a ~70nt pre-miRNA which is (3) transported to the cytosol through exportin-5. (4) Further processing by dicer cleaves the pre-miRNA hairpin loop, leaving a miRNA duplex which is (5) loaded into one of four human argonaute proteins. (6) The RISC is considered mature following selection of a guide strand and subsequent ejection of the passenger strand.

tail structures [46–48]. Complementary base pairing between the miRNA sequence and its antisense counterpart forms a secondary hairpin structure which is liberated from the primary transcript via cleavage, mediated by the nuclear microprocessor Drosha and co-factor DGCR8 [49]. The resultant ~70nt miRNA precursor (pre-miR) is exported to the cytoplasm through the action of Exportin-5 in a Ran-GTP-dependent manner [50, 51] wherein the cytoplasmic RNase III Dicer cleaves the hairpin loop structure from this pre-miR [52, 53]. This produces a ~22nt double-stranded miRNA duplex which associates with one of four orthologues of the Argonaute (AGO) protein family, thereby forming an immature RNA-induced silencing complex (RISC) [54]. Maturation of this complex is achieved through positive selection of a 5′ uridine containing "guide" [55] strand from the miRNA duplex and subsequent ejection of the antisense "passenger" strand from the RISC [56–58]. Incomplete Watson-Crick base complementarity between the miRNA seed region (nucleotides 2–8) and miRNA recognition elements encoded in the mRNA 3′ UTR (and occasionally, 5′ UTR and CDS) subsequently acts as a targeting mechanism for the RISC, facilitating translational repression and degradation of specific mRNAs [59–62]. This redundancy in miRNA-mRNA interaction is a particularly critical characteristic of miRNA function as it enables a single miRNA to regulate a many unique transcripts, eliminating the need for excessively large numbers of very specific miRNA.

3.2. miRNA regulation of gene expression

3.2.1. 5′ to 3′ exonucleic decay

The initial stages of cap-dependent mRNA translation are primed by interaction between 5′ bound eukaryotic initiation factors (eIF) and 3′ poly(A)-binding proteins (PABP), which both circularise mRNA for efficient translation and promote assembly of a translation initiation complex in the 5′ UTR [63]. The mRNA 5′ methylguanosine cap and 3′ poly(A) tail are therefore considered as two critical *cis*-acting factors in translation initiation and are thus ideal targets for translational repression and degradation by miRNA and the RISC [64].

An extensive body of research has since revealed that the RISC induces activation of the 5′ to 3′ mRNA decay pathway to facilitate degradation of target mRNAs. The first step of this pathway is characterised by recruitment of the PAN2-PAN3 and CCR4-NOT deadenylation complexes to target mRNA, which trigger sequential cleavage of the 3′ poly(A) tail [65, 66]. Co-immunoprecipitation and structural analysis suggest that the RISC indirectly recruits these deadenylation factors through the action of GW182 proteins, which bind both AGO family members in addition to the PAN3 and NOT1/9 deadenylase subunits [67–70]. Erosion of the poly(A) tail subsequently stimulates the removal of the 5′ methylguanosine cap via DCP2 and associated decapping factors, recruited to the target mRNA via CCR4-NOT [71]. The exposed mRNA is then subject to 5′ to 3′ digestion by XRN1 exonuclease [71].

3.2.2. Inhibition of active translation

RISC-mediated degradation of mRNA has long been recognised as the canonical mechanism through which miRNAs specifically modulate the transcriptome and therefore translation. Emerging evidence suggests the RISC may also function to repress translation through a number of mechanisms (**Figure 3**), foremost of which is inhibition of active translation. This form of translational repression arose as a potential facet of RISC function following the initial discovery of miRNA in association with polysomes [72]; however, no evidence was uncovered regarding a link between miRNA binding and arrest of active translation. A similar discovery has also been observed for the dendrite-abundant translational repressor FMRP, which has been shown to form translationally active complexes with ribosomes in mouse cortical preparations [73]. Further studies have identified CDS-bound phosphorylated FMRP is associated with stalled ribosomes, leading to the current hypothesis that FMRP halts active protein synthesis through binding actively translating ribosomes [74–76]. This holds significance for neuronal miRNA function since FMRP has been shown to interact with AGO1 [77], AGO2 [78], MOV10 (RISC RNA helicase) [79] and specific microRNAs [80], raising the possibility that miRNA and the RISC may act as a targeting mechanism for FMRP. Considering these interactions together in conjunction with the dendritic enrichment of FMRP, miRNA- and FMRP-mediated stalling of actively translating ribosomes could constitute an exciting dimension to miRNA function particularly relevant to synaptic translation.

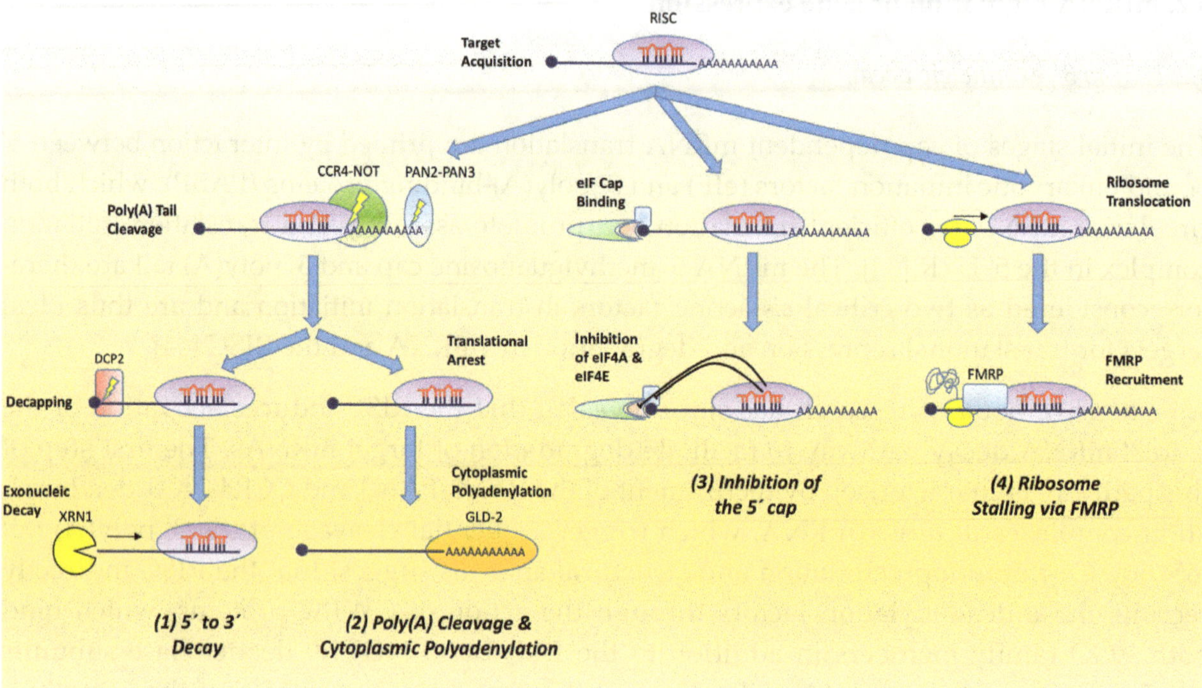

Figure 3. Mechanisms of miRNA-mediated translational repression. The RISC acquires target mRNAs through complementary base pairing, triggering one of a number of repressive pathways. (1) Transcript degradation is stimulated through RISC recruitment of deadenylase complexes to cleave the mRNA poly(A) tail, followed by decapping and exonuclease decay. (2) Cleavage of the poly(A) tail reduces the capacity for target mRNA to act as a substrate for protein synthesis, leading to translational repression likely reversible by cytoplasmic poly(A) polymerases. (3) The RISC may additionally stimulate dissociation of eIFs from the mRNA 5′ cap, or alternatively, (4) recruit FMRP to halt active synthesis through ribosome stalling.

3.2.3. Poly(A) tail erosion and cytoplasmic polyadenylation

While RISC induction of mRNA decay constitutes an effective mechanism through which translation may be fine-tuned for cellular needs, in the neuronal context, this mechanism relies heavily on both transcriptional activity and mRNA trafficking to maintain transcriptomic supply at dendrites. Consequently, a system by which the translational competency of mRNAs could be modulated during periods of quiescence and in response to plasticity-inducing stimuli would significantly relieve pressure applied by RISC degradation of transcripts. A major candidate mechanism through which this may be achieved is modulation of mRNA poly(A) tail length, since this structure and associated PABPs facilitate 5′–3′ interactions required for translation initiation [63]. The manipulation of reporter mRNA in HeLa cultures [81] and cell-free systems [82] has indeed revealed let-7 translational arrest of reporter luciferase depends on the expression of a poly(A) tail, emphasising the role of the poly(A) tail as a conduit through which translational competency may be altered by miRNA. A requirement for such a system to exist, however, is the functional decoupling of poly(A) tail erosion and mRNA decay. Recent studies illustrate that this occurs in embryonic culture systems such that deadenylated targets of miRNA, including miR-35-42, miR-51-56 and miR-155, have been shown to accumulate in a stable manner [83, 84], suggesting miRNA-mediated poly(A) tail cleavage does not necessarily instigate mRNA decay.

This potential dimension to miRNA function becomes particularly interesting in the neural context, as cytoplasmic polyadenylation has the potential to reinstate the translational activity of poly(A) deficient mRNAs. Poly(A) polymerase GLD-2 is a promising contender for this function due to its neuronal enrichment, cytoplasmic localisation and participation in translational enhancement via poly(A) tail extension [85, 86]. In addition to these features, GLD-2 function increases the abundance and stability of poorly translated mRNAs and is also required for the induction of LTP, suggesting that cytoplasmic polyadenylation could play a significant role in synaptic plasticity [85, 87, 88]. Regardless, the role of GLD-2 and deadenylase counterpart PARN (poly(A)-specific ribonuclease) in bidirectional regulation of poly(A) tail length and neuronal translation as part of the cytoplasmic polyadenylation complex illustrates the significance of cytoplasmic polyadenylation in neuronal translational control [85].

3.2.4. *Inhibition of translation initiation*

Further emerging evidence implicates miRNA and the RISC in direct inhibition of translation initiation through interaction with 5′ cap-bound eIFs responsible for mediating ribosomal assembly in the mRNA 5′ UTR [63]. At present, AGO1-RISC has been shown to indirectly stimulate disassociation of eIF4E via GW182, and eIF4A through a mechanism independent of GW182, inhibiting the assembly of an eIF4F translation initiation complex [89, 90]. While it is clear that this interaction acts to prevent translation of target mRNAs, there is uncertainty regarding whether this is another mechanism of translationally arresting mRNA or simply a precursor to mRNA degradation. The recent discovery of an RNA-independent association between CCR4-NOT subunit NOT1 and eIF4A2 RNA helicase involved in RISC degradation of target mRNA [91] suggests the latter is likely but does not rule out the possibility of eIF interference as a means of transcript repression.

3.3. microRNAs in synaptic function

Considering the array of confirmed and emerging miRNA functions, miRNA degradation and/or repression of transcripts constitutes an effective mechanism for fine-tuning highly dynamic translation at the post-synaptic compartment. While miRNAs are thought to be largely stable mRNA species, new evidence suggests that miRNAs are subject to activity-dependent synthesis and rapid turnover in dendritic spines [42]. Dendritic synthesis of miRNA became particularly apparent following the discovery of pre-miRs [92] and their inactive processing enzyme Dicer at the post-synaptic density (PSD) whereby activity-dependent stimulation of Calpain I was sufficient to induce Dicer function [93]. These data were supported by the detection of mature miRNA species enriched in mouse forebrain synaptoneurosomes [92]. Activity-dependent degradation of miRNA has also recently been observed in mouse retinal neurons; however, the exact mechanism of degradation remains elusive [94]. Interestingly, exosome release may act as a means of post-synaptic miRNA clearance, as MAP1B-enriched neuronal exosomes released in response to depolarisation have recently been shown to contain miRNA (miR-638, miR-149*, miR-4281 and let-7e) normally downregulated by depolarisation in the dendritic compartment [95].

Supporting the critical role of miRNA in synaptic function, microarray analysis and deep-sequencing have revealed that subsets of miRNA are subject to differential expression up to 24-h post-induction of hippocampal synaptic plasticity [96, 97]. These data have since been extended through the development of a conditional *Dicer 1* knockout in the adult mouse forebrain shown to result in enhanced LTP, learning and memory [98]. Reflecting on these discoveries, it is perhaps not surprising that a number of neuron-enriched miRNA have been described in terms of the regulation of synaptic function.

Arguably the most studied miRNA in the context of synaptic function, miR-132 is widely regarded for its role in the regulation of synaptic plasticity in brain regions such as the visual cortex [99] and hippocampus [100]. Following neuronal activity, miR-132 is subject to a rapid increase in CREB-mediated (cAMP response element-binding protein) transcription, resulting in stimulation of dendritic growth and branching through suppression of p250GAP (p250 GTPase activating protein) [101, 102]. These modifications to dendritic morphology are characterised by expression of stubby, mushroom-like dendritic spines which act to potentiate synaptic transmission [80]. miR-132 expression additionally directs the upregulation of NR2A, NR2B and GluR1 glutamate receptor subunits following BDNF stimulation [103], revealing this miRNA may direct synaptic plasticity through guiding both morphological and physiological change. A particularly interesting aspect of miR-132 function, however, is its relationship with FMRP, which provides novel insight regarding potential interplay between miRNA and FMRP homologues. Specifically, miR-132 effects on dendritic morphology are abolished following FMRP knockdown, uncovering a functional relationship between these molecules likely to be responsible for miR-132-associated regulation of plasticity-relevant transcripts [80]. A similar relationship has been observed for miR-125b whereby FMRP deficits inhibit miR-125b negative regulation of both dendritic spine morphology and NR2A [80], further supporting the role of FMRP in neuronal miRNA function.

Aside from miR-132, several recent studies have implicated a variety of other neuron-enriched or specific miRNAs in the modification of synaptic function. miR-134 is a key example which modulates dendritic spine volume through the regulation of *Limk1* expression, resulting in dendritic spine volume deficits when miR-134 is overexpressed [104, 105]. This function of miR-134 in the negative regulation of dendritic spine morphology is reflected in the impairment of mouse contextual fear learning following miR-134 overexpression in the CA1 hippocampus; however, post-transcriptional miR-134 regulation of the CREB transcription factor appears to significantly contribute to this deficiency [106]. Another miRNA involved in the inhibition of synaptic plasticity is miR-137 which decreases dendritic complexity and length through downregulation of mind bomb-1 ubiquitin ligase while additionally inhibiting pre-synaptic vesicle release [107, 108]. miR-137 also directly influences AMPA receptor expression through the regulation of GluA1, leading to synaptic silencing and deficits in hippocampal learning when overexpressed in mice [109].

Considering these examples alone, it is evident that miRNAs modulate a variety of synaptic characteristics through post-transcriptional regulation of a number of unique mRNA species, emphasising the importance of miRNA in coordinating a number of gene expression networks to fine-tune synaptic plasticity. Moreover, miRNA species appear to provide the basis through which the induction of plastic alterations to the synapse may be bidirectionally regulated. This not only implicates specific miRNA species such as miR-132 in the enhancement of synaptic plasticity, but also additionally implies miRNA including miR-134 and miR-137 act as a breaking mechanism to prevent excessive potentiation or depression of individual synapses. Despite this extensive understanding of miRNA function, many are yet to be fully characterised in relation to synaptic and indeed neuronal function.

4. P-bodies and mRNP granules: linking mRNA transport, translation and repression

miRNA regulation of gene expression is sequestered within subcellular granules known as processing bodies (P-bodies), proposed to form through aggregation of translationally arrested mRNA and mRNA degradation machinery [110]. These granules were initially described as cytoplasmic "speckles" termed GW-bodies, observed as aggregates of GW182 complexed with mRNA [111]. P-bodies have since been characterised as foci of mRNA degradation due to their enrichment of translationally repressive RBPs such as Argonaute proteins, DCP1 & DCP2 decapping enzymes, Pat1 & edc3 decapping factors and XRN1 exonuclease [110]. Considering these granules are both enriched at the post-synaptic density and actively migrate to post-synaptic compartments following neuronal activity [112–114], P-bodies are currently heavily implicated in post-synaptic translational regulation.

Neuronal mRNP granules similarly form by the aggregation of messenger RNPs to provide a vehicle for mRNA distal transport while maintaining mRNAs in a translationally arrested state [18]. Interestingly, *Drosophila* Staufen and FMRP mRNP granules are enriched with homologues of mRNA decay machinery including DCP1, XRN1 and AGO2 [24], demonstrating these granules bear similarity to P-bodies. In conjunction with this observation, an exciting interaction between these granules has recently been reported whereby 50% of dendritic P-bodies have been shown to dock with neuronal mRNPs [113], raising the prospect that these granules exchange their contents.

Drawing from these observations, a fascinating scenario is the potential for neuronal RNP granules to unload their mRNA and mRNA degradation cargo to P-bodies for repression until translation is appropriate, thereby acting as a means of mRNA storage with the potential for degradation if specific transcripts are not required. In support of this possibility, mapping of mRNA localisation during yeast glucose starvation and tetracycline transcriptional suppression indicates mRNA can associate with polysomes from P-bodies [115], revealing mRNA may be subjected to translation following sequestration in P-bodies. Adding to this evidence, cationic amino acid transporter–1 mRNA has recently been observed undergoing release from miR-122 repression and subsequently associating with polysomes from P-bodies during cellular stress [116], further implicating miRNA in repressing translation without necessarily instigating mRNA decay. While the potential underlying mechanisms driving mRNA de-repression in P-bodies remains unclear, *Drosophila* GLD-2 poly(A) polymerase has been observed to co-localise with FMR1 in neuronal mRNP granules [87] and may therefore be delivered to P-bodies, lending to the possibility of cytoplasmic poly(A) tail lengthening in de-repressing mRNA.

In addition to their mRNA, P-bodies themselves respond to cellular stimuli as synaptic input induces as much as a 60% decrease in dendritic P-body abundance [113], while artificial stimulation of cap-dependent translation decreases P-body biogenesis in PNS sensory neurons [117]. Overall, these observations imply that these repressive granules could dissociate in a pro-translational environment to release a collection of mRNAs for novel protein synthesis. A subset of dendritic P-body-like granules containing miRNAs repressed mRNAs and lacking XRN1, which respond to synaptic activation may represent a subcategory of P-bodies specifically designed for such a purpose [112]. Stress granules, which contain translationally stalled mRNAs, translational enhancers (such as eIFs and PABPs) and interact with P-bodies, are another key candidate for mRNA storage; however, their functional relevance is limited to periods of exposure to stressful cellular stimuli [118].

5. Emerging non-coding RNAs in post-transcriptional regulation of synaptic translation

5.1. Long non-coding RNA

Long non-coding RNA (lncRNA) is a broad category of >200nt non-coding transcripts characterised by widespread genomic distribution and involvement in a variety of regulatory functions [119]. Like miRNA, lncRNAs inhabit a range of genomic regions including intergenic, telomeric and gene regulatory sequences [119]. Protein-coding genes have also been identified as a source of lncRNA expression wherein these RNA may reside in antisense, overlapping, intronic or bidirectional configurations relative to protein-coding sequences [120]. From these genes, lncRNAs are transcribed by RNA polymerase II following which many are subject to posttranscriptional modifications including alternative splicing, 5′ capping and polyadenylation [121]. Despite this similarity to mRNA, recent studies have revealed the genomic origin of lncRNA dictates the functional role of individual lncRNA species, which may serve as regulators of translation, transcription and epigenetic modifications, or act as miRNA precursors or sponges [120, 122]. Translational regulation is a particularly interesting aspect of lncRNA function due to the range of emerging post-transcriptional mechanisms through which this may be achieved. This holds significance in the context of neuronal function as the adult brain has recently been identified as a source of substantial lncRNA enrichment, reflected in the discovery of 849 (of 1328 examined) lncRNAs subject to specific patterns of expression in mice [123]. Accordingly, a number of lncRNAs have exhibited roles in the regulation of synaptic translation and synaptic function, adding further complexity to the nature of neuronal translation.

The rodent lncRNA *Bc1* and its primate orthologue *BC200* are prime examples of neuronal lncRNAs, which modulate post-synaptic translation of plasticity-associated mRNA, including Arc, CaMKII and MAP1B [124]. Current studies indicate that *Bc1/BC200* instigates translational repression at somatodendritic compartments through inhibition of eIF4A and eIF4B activity at the mRNA 5′ cap, thereby suppressing translation initiation [125]. In conjunction with this observation, *BC200* alone has been shown to contain *cis*-acting adenine-rich elements which potentially facilitate interaction with PABPs [126], indicating this lncRNA may additionally interfere with 5′ to 3′ mRNA interactions required for translation initiation. FMRP may further contribute to the multidimensional nature of *Bc1/BC200* lncRNA function as oligonucleotide masking of an mRNA recognition motif within the *Bc1* lncRNA primary sequence inhibits FMRP interaction with MAP1B mRNA [124]. This suggests that *Bcl* lncRNA may potentially act as a guide in FMRP association with plasticity-associated mRNA analogous to miRNA and the RISC; however, the exact functional mechanism of these relationships is yet to be elucidated.

In addition to *Bc1/BC200*, other emerging lncRNAs have been implicated in synaptic regulation through multiple post-transcriptional mechanisms. lncRNA Malat1 is one such example, which modulates synaptic density through positive regulation of neuroligin 1 and SynCAM1 mRNA expression and alternative splicing of CaMKIIB [127]. Interestingly, this occurs within nuclear speckles, known for their role as sites of mRNA storage and processing, revealing this lncRNA modulates synaptic properties from the nucleus via a post-transcriptional mechanism [127]. lncRNA Tsx has additionally been shown to enhance short-term hippocampal memory in mice through an elusive mechanism, suggesting a role for this lncRNA in the regulation of synaptic plasticity [128].

Considering these examples together, it is evident that current understanding of the exact mechanisms through which various lncRNAs post-transcriptionally modulate synaptic properties is limited. Despite this gap in the literature, lncRNAs appear to bidirectionally regulate post-synaptic translation, suggesting lncRNAs may act to fine-tune protein synthesis rather than strongly influence gene expression networks. Supporting this theory, mRNAs with roles in synaptogenesis including *CamkIIa* and *Dag1* have been observed in complex with their antisense lncRNA counterparts in synaptoneurosomes of the adult mouse forebrain [129]. This further raises the possibility that lncRNAs could block translation via binding target mRNAs while additionally inhibiting miRNA-mediated mRNA decay through masking miRNA recognition elements. This distinct prospect further underscores the complex and multidimensional nature of post-transcriptional lncRNA function in the regulation of synaptic properties and emphasises the need for extensive characterisation of individual lncRNA species.

5.2. Circular RNA

Circular RNAs (circRNAs), as their name implies, are a class of circular long non-coding RNAs produced by exonic or intronic splicing which lack 5′ cap and 3′ poly(A) tail structures and exhibit exonuclease-resistance [130]. Unlike miRNA and RBPs which generally serve to regulate translation through direct modulation of mRNA characteristics, emerging evidence implicates circRNA as miRNA sponges, serving as a regulatory mechanism by which miRNA translational regulation may be dampened. A well-characterised example is the brain-enriched circRNA ciRS-7 (also known as CDR1as) which contains as many as 74 conventional seed-binding sites for miR-7 that allow this circRNA to function as a more potent miRNA sponge than traditional anti-miRs used for miRNA knockdown [131, 132]. While this circRNA demonstrates highly specific miRNA sponging, it is unclear whether this is a unique example or common among other species. For comparison, circHIPK3 and circRNA mlb, respectively, knockdown 9 and 2 unique miRNA [133, 134].

circHIPK3 is a particularly interesting example as overexpression of this species triggers a reduction of midbrain size in developing zebrafish [133], indicating circRNA may exert substantial influence over neuronal structure and function. Considering this, the function of this RNA class bears significant implications in the neuronal context since circRNAs exhibit substantial brain enrichment and accumulate during nervous system development and with age [135, 136]. circRNA may also act to fine-tune plasticity-associated translation as evidenced through their subcellular enrichment within dendritic compartments of cortical pyramidal neurons and interneurons, and differential expression of at least 42 distinct species during bicuculline-induced synaptic plasticity [134]. Together, these studies therefore implicate circRNA in both neuronal development and plasticity and provide an exciting added dimension to neuronal translational control. Further characterisation of individual circRNA will no doubt be integral in both determining the status of miRNA sponging as a primary circRNA function and the functional significance of these RNA in neuronal structure and function.

6. Towards a unified model of neuronal post-transcriptional regulation of translation

Since the initial discovery of extrasomatic neuronal translation, it has become evident that a number of regulatory systems fine-tune neuronal protein synthesis in an exquisitely coordinated manner to control structural and physiological characteristics associated with synaptic plasticity. Since these regulatory systems are continually exhibiting varying degrees of overlap, deciphering the mechanisms through which these systems both function in isolation and interact is of critical importance in revealing the intricate details of neuronal post-transcriptional regulation of translation.

A key example is the interplay between neuronal transport mRNP granules and P-bodies at the post-synaptic compartment [113]. The possibility of mRNP granules delivering cargo to P-bodies is an enticing prospect further exemplified by the potential for P-bodies to isolate and store repressed mRNAs for translation under suitable conditions [115]. What remains to be considered is the potential for P-bodies to export cargo to neuronal mRNP granules, perhaps acting as a means of mRNA recycling especially interesting in the context of the proposed "Sushi Belt" theory of neuronal mRNA transport [18]. As P-bodies, neuronal mRNP granules, polysomes and stress granules display multiple degrees of functional interaction, an overlying mechanism of mRNA transport, storage, repression and translation is likely at play to exert considerable influence over the available pool of translatable mRNA at the post-synaptic compartment.

With regard to miRNA function in the neuronal context, an increasing body of evidence underscores the fact that miRNAs are not simply mediators of mRNA decay. For neurons in particular, the existence of reversible systems of translational repression would present an energetically favourable mechanism of translational control capable of reducing total reliance on novel transcription and extra-somatic mRNA trafficking to dendrites. Indeed, the role of cytoplasmic poly(A) polymerases such as GLD-2 in enhancing activity-dependent translation [85] shows potential for cytoplasmic poly(A) tail modulation as a reversible mechanism of neuronal translational control, warranting investigation of the theoretical decoupling of miRNA repression and degradation of mRNA in the neuronal context. Furthermore, uncovering the functional relevance of FMRP in mediating miRNA ribosome stalling will likely reveal a neuron-specific aspect to miRNA function which may prove critical in characterising the role of FMRP in the biogenesis of neuronal disease. Further miRNA studies in conjunction with high-throughput ribosome profiling [137], poly(A) tail sequencing [138] and co-immunoprecipitation sequencing will prove critical in revealing the existence and functional significance of these repressive systems in coordinating post-synaptic neuronal translation.

From the presented examples miR-132, miR-134 and miR-137, plasticity-relevant miRNA species clearly regulate dynamic morphological and physiological changes at the post-synaptic compartment through interaction with a variety of targets. However, it is important to note that these miRNA constitute well-described examples subject to intensive research. Additional miRNAs, such as miR-9, miR-22, miR-124 and miR-188, among others [139], have all displayed an association with synaptic plasticity and therefore stress the need for further characterisation of specific miRNA and how together they exquisitely coordinate gene expression networks in regulation of synaptic plasticity. This holds true for lncRNAs, which appear to regulate synaptic plasticity via an assortment of posttranscriptional mechanisms [119], stressing the need for further investigation of individual lncRNA species and the mechanisms through which they act. Considering the potential role of circRNA in regulating miRNA [131–134] and their post-synaptic enrichment, emphasis should no doubt be additionally placed on characterising these non-coding RNA in the context of neuronal translational control. Expression of circRNA is likely to partially account for the distinct complexity of neuronal translation and could act as novel therapeutic target or biomarker in neurological disease.

Continual advancement in high-throughput technology and analysis will substantially further our ability to characterise and integrate these regulatory systems into a unified model of neuronal posttranscriptional regulation of neuronal translation. Increasing our knowledge of this aspect of the central dogma of molecular biology in the neuronal context will subsequently facilitate characterisation of the molecular events underlying synaptic plasticity, fuelling our understanding of learning and memory.

Author details

Dylan Kiltschewskij[1,2] and Murray J. Cairns[1,2,3*]

*Address all correspondence to: murray.cairns@newcastle.edu.au

1 School of Biomedical Sciences and Pharmacy, Faculty of Health, The University of Newcastle, Callaghan, Australia

2 Priority Research Centre for Brain and Mental Health Research, Hunter Medical Research Institute, New Lambton, Australia

3 Schizophrenia Research Institute, Sydney, Australia

References

[1] Huganir, R.L. and R.A. Nicoll, AMPARs and synaptic plasticity: the last 25 years. Neuron, 2013. **80**(3): pp. 704–17.

[2] Sutton, M.A. and E.M. Schuman, Dendritic protein synthesis, synaptic plasticity, and memory. Cell, 2006. **127**(1): pp. 49–58.

[3] Steward, O., et al., Protein synthesis and processing in cytoplasmic microdomains beneath postsynaptic sites on CNS neurons. A mechanism for establishing and maintaining a mosaic postsynaptic receptive surface. Mol Neurobiol, 1988. **2**(4): pp. 227–61.

[4] Torre, E.R. and O. Steward, Demonstration of local protein synthesis within dendrites using a new cell culture system that permits the isolation of living axons and dendrites from their cell bodies. J Neurosci, 1992. **12**(3): pp. 762–72.

[5] Cajigas, I.J., et al., The local transcriptome in the synaptic neuropil revealed by deep sequencing and high-resolution imaging. Neuron, 2012. **74**(3): pp. 453–66.

[6] Kislauskis, E.H., et al., Isoform-specific 3′-untranslated sequences sort alpha-cardiac and beta-cytoplasmic actin messenger RNAs to different cytoplasmic compartments. J Cell Biol, 1993. **123**(1): pp. 165–72.

[7] La Via, L., et al., Modulation of dendritic AMPA receptor mRNA trafficking by RNA splicing and editing. Nucleic Acids Res, 2013. **41**(1): pp. 617–31.

[8] An, J.J., et al., Distinct role of long 3′ UTR BDNF mRNA in spine morphology and synaptic plasticity in hippocampal neurons. Cell, 2008. **134**(1): pp. 175–87.

[9] Blichenberg, A., et al., Identification of a cis-acting dendritic targeting element in MAP2 mRNAs. J Neurosci, 1999. **19**(20): pp. 8818–29.

[10] Mayford, M., et al., The 3′-untranslated region of CaMKII alpha is a cis-acting signal for the localization and translation of mRNA in dendrites. Proc Natl Acad Sci U S A, 1996. **93**(23): pp. 13250–5.

[11] Martin, K.C. and A. Ephrussi, mRNA localization: gene expression in the spatial dimension. Cell, 2009. **136**(4): pp. 719–30.

[12] Chartrand, P., et al., Structural elements required for the localization of ASH1 mRNA and of a green fluorescent protein reporter particle in vivo. Curr Biol, 1999. **9**(6): pp. 333–6.

[13] Serano, T.L. and R.S. Cohen, A small predicted stem-loop structure mediates oocyte localization of Drosophila K10 mRNA. Development, 1995. **121**(11): pp. 3809–18.

[14] Jambor, H., et al., A stem-loop structure directs oskar mRNA to microtubule minus ends. RNA, 2014. **20**(4): pp. 429–39.

[15] Meer, E.J., et al., Identification of a cis-acting element that localizes mRNA to synapses. Proc Natl Acad Sci U S A, 2012. **109**(12): pp. 4639–44.

[16] Knowles, R.B., et al., Translocation of RNA granules in living neurons. J Neurosci, 1996. **16**(24): pp. 7812–20.

[17] Shan, J., et al., A molecular mechanism for mRNA trafficking in neuronal dendrites. J Neurosci, 2003. **23**(26): pp. 8859–66.

[18] Doyle, M. and M.A. Kiebler, Mechanisms of dendritic mRNA transport and its role in synaptic tagging. EMBO J, 2011. **30**(17): pp. 3540–52.

[19] Hutten, S., T. Sharangdhar, and M. Kiebler, Unmasking the messenger. RNA Biol, 2014. **11**(8): pp. 992–7.

[20] Li, Z., et al., The fragile X mental retardation protein inhibits translation via interacting with mRNA. Nucleic Acids Res, 2001. **29**(11): pp. 2276–83.

[21] Antar, L.N., et al., Localization of FMRP-associated mRNA granules and requirement of microtubules for activity-dependent trafficking in hippocampal neurons. Genes Brain Behav, 2005. **4**(6): pp. 350–9.

[22] Dictenberg, J.B., et al., A direct role for FMRP in activity-dependent dendritic mRNA transport links filopodial-spine morphogenesis to fragile X syndrome. Dev Cell, 2008. **14**(6): pp. 926–39.

[23] Price, T.J., et al., The RNA binding and transport proteins staufen and fragile X mental retardation protein are expressed by rat primary afferent neurons and localize to peripheral and central axons. Neuroscience, 2006. **141**(4): pp. 2107–16.

[24] Barbee, S.A., et al., Staufen- and FMRP-containing neuronal RNPs are structurally and functionally related to somatic P bodies. Neuron, 2006. **52**(6): pp. 997–1009.

[25] Laver, J.D., et al., Genome-wide analysis of Staufen-associated mRNAs identifies secondary structures that confer target specificity. Nucleic Acids Res, 2013. **41**(20): pp. 9438–60.

[26] Farina, K.L., et al., Two ZBP1 KH domains facilitate beta-actin mRNA localization, granule formation, and cytoskeletal attachment. J Cell Biol, 2003. **160**(1): pp. 77–87.

[27] Tiruchinapalli, D.M., et al., Activity-dependent trafficking and dynamic localization of zipcode binding protein 1 and beta-actin mRNA in dendrites and spines of hippocampal neurons. J Neurosci, 2003. **23**(8): pp. 3251–61.

[28] Donnelly, C.J., et al., Axonally synthesized beta-actin and GAP-43 proteins support distinct modes of axonal growth. J Neurosci, 2013. **33**(8): pp. 3311–22.

[29] Davidovic, L., et al., The fragile X mental retardation protein is a molecular adaptor between the neurospecific KIF3C kinesin and dendritic RNA granules. Hum Mol Genet, 2007. **16**(24): pp. 3047–58.

[30] Song, T., et al., Specific interaction of KIF11 with ZBP1 regulates the transport of beta-actin mRNA and cell motility. J Cell Sci, 2015. **128**(5): pp. 1001–10.

[31] Kohrmann, M., et al., Microtubule-dependent recruitment of Staufen-green fluorescent protein into large RNA-containing granules and subsequent dendritic transport in living hippocampal neurons. Mol Biol Cell, 1999. **10**(9): pp. 2945–53.

[32] Dienstbier, M., et al., Egalitarian is a selective RNA-binding protein linking mRNA localization signals to the dynein motor. Genes Dev, 2009. **23**(13): pp. 1546–58.

[33] Rook, M.S., M. Lu, and K.S. Kosik, CaMKIIalpha 3′ untranslated region-directed mRNA translocation in living neurons: visualization by GFP linkage. J Neurosci, 2000. **20**(17): pp. 6385–93.

[34] Frey, U. and R.G. Morris, Synaptic tagging and long-term potentiation. Nature, 1997. **385**(6616): pp. 533–6.

[35] Morris, R.G. and U. Frey, Hippocampal synaptic plasticity: role in spatial learning or the automatic recording of attended experience? Philos Trans R Soc Lond B Biol Sci, 1997. **352**(1360): pp. 1489–503.

[36] Wang, S.H., R.L. Redondo, and R.G. Morris, Relevance of synaptic tagging and capture to the persistence of long-term potentiation and everyday spatial memory. Proc Natl Acad Sci U S A, 2010. **107**(45): pp. 19537–42.

[37] Barco, A., M. Lopez de Armentia, and J.M. Alarcon, Synapse-specific stabilization of plasticity processes: the synaptic tagging and capture hypothesis revisited 10 years later. Neurosci Biobehav Rev, 2008. **32**(4): pp. 831–51.

[38] Redondo, R.L. and R.G. Morris, Making memories last: the synaptic tagging and capture hypothesis. Nat Rev Neurosci, 2011. **12**(1): pp. 17–30.

[39] Lee, R.C., R.L. Feinbaum, and V. Ambros, The *C. elegans* heterochronic gene lin-4 encodes small RNAs with antisense complementarity to lin-14. Cell, 1993. **75**(5): pp. 843–54.

[40] Wightman, B., I. Ha, and G. Ruvkun, Posttranscriptional regulation of the heterochronic gene lin-14 by lin-4 mediates temporal pattern formation in *C. elegans*. Cell, 1993. **75**(5): pp. 855–62.

[41] Chou, C.H., et al., miRTarBase 2016: updates to the experimentally validated miRNA-target interactions database. Nucleic Acids Res, 2016. **44**(D1): pp. D239–47.

[42] Krol, J., I. Loedige, and W. Filipowicz, The widespread regulation of microRNA biogenesis, function and decay. Nat Rev Genet, 2010. **11**(9): pp. 597–610.

[43] Wang, W., E.J. Kwon, and L.H. Tsai, MicroRNAs in learning, memory, and neurological diseases. Learn Mem, 2012. **19**(9): pp. 359–68.

[44] Rodriguez, A., et al., Identification of mammalian microRNA host genes and transcription units. Genome Res, 2004. **14**(10A): pp. 1902–10.

[45] Bortolin-Cavaille, M.L., et al., C19MC microRNAs are processed from introns of large Pol-II, non-protein-coding transcripts. Nucleic Acids Res, 2009. **37**(10): pp. 3464–73.

[46] Cai, X., C.H. Hagedorn, and B.R. Cullen, Human microRNAs are processed from capped, polyadenylated transcripts that can also function as mRNAs. RNA, 2004. **10**(12): pp. 1957–66.

[47] Lee, Y., et al., MicroRNA genes are transcribed by RNA polymerase II. EMBO J, 2004. **23**(20): pp. 4051–60.

[48] Baskerville, S. and D.P. Bartel, Microarray profiling of microRNAs reveals frequent coexpression with neighboring miRNAs and host genes. RNA, 2005. **11**(3): pp. 241–7.

[49] Han, J., et al., Molecular basis for the recognition of primary microRNAs by the Drosha-DGCR8 complex. Cell, 2006. **125**(5): pp. 887–901.

[50] Bohnsack, M.T., K. Czaplinski, and D. Gorlich, Exportin 5 is a RanGTP-dependent dsRNA-binding protein that mediates nuclear export of pre-miRNAs. RNA, 2004. **10**(2): pp. 185–91.

[51] Yi, R., et al., Exportin-5 mediates the nuclear export of pre-microRNAs and short hairpin RNAs. Genes Dev, 2003. **17**(24): pp. 3011–6.

[52] Macrae, I.J., et al., Structural basis for double-stranded RNA processing by Dicer. Science, 2006. **311**(5758): pp. 195–8.

[53] Hutvagner, G., et al., A cellular function for the RNA-interference enzyme Dicer in the maturation of the let-7 small temporal RNA. Science, 2001. **293**(5531): pp. 834–8.

[54] Ender, C. and G. Meister, Argonaute proteins at a glance. J Cell Sci, 2010. **123**(Pt 11): pp. 1819–23.

[55] Takeda, A., et al., The mechanism selecting the guide strand from small RNA duplexes is different among argonaute proteins. Plant Cell Physiol, 2008. **49**(4): pp. 493–500.

[56] Sasaki, T., et al., Identification of eight members of the Argonaute family in the human genome. Genomics, 2003. **82**(3): pp. 323–30.

[57] Janowski, B.A., et al., Involvement of AGO1 and AGO2 in mammalian transcriptional silencing. Nat Struct Mol Biol, 2006. **13**(9): pp. 787–92.

[58] Khvorova, A., A. Reynolds, and S.D. Jayasena, Functional siRNAs and miRNAs exhibit strand bias. Cell, 2003. **115**(2): pp. 209–16.

[59] Lewis, B.P., et al., Prediction of mammalian microRNA targets. Cell, 2003. **115**(7): pp. 787–98.

[60] Lytle, J.R., T.A. Yario, and J.A. Steitz, Target mRNAs are repressed as efficiently by microRNA-binding sites in the 5′ UTR as in the 3′ UTR. Proc Natl Acad Sci U S A, 2007. **104**(23): pp. 9667–72.

[61] Lewis, B.P., C.B. Burge, and D.P. Bartel, Conserved seed pairing, often flanked by adenosines, indicates that thousands of human genes are microRNA targets. Cell, 2005. **120**(1): pp. 15–20.

[62] Hausser, J., et al., Analysis of CDS-located miRNA target sites suggests that they can effectively inhibit translation. Genome Res, 2013. **23**(4): pp. 604–15.

[63] Dobrikov, M., et al., Phosphorylation of eukaryotic translation initiation factor 4G1 (eIF4G1) by protein kinase C{alpha} regulates eIF4G1 binding to Mnk1. Mol Cell Biol, 2011. **31**(14): pp. 2947–59.

[64] Guo, H., et al., Mammalian microRNAs predominantly act to decrease target mRNA levels. Nature, 2010. **466**(7308): pp. 835–40.

[65] Fabian, M.R., et al., miRNA-mediated deadenylation is orchestrated by GW182 through two conserved motifs that interact with CCR4-NOT. Nat Struct Mol Biol, 2011. **18**(11): pp. 1211–7.

[66] Chen, C.Y., et al., Ago-TNRC6 triggers microRNA-mediated decay by promoting two deadenylation steps. Nat Struct Mol Biol, 2009. **16**(11): pp. 1160–6.

[67] Braun, J.E., et al., GW182 proteins directly recruit cytoplasmic deadenylase complexes to miRNA targets. Mol Cell, 2011. **44**(1): pp. 120–33.

[68] Kuzuoglu-Ozturk, D., et al., The *Caenorhabditis elegans* GW182 protein AIN-1 interacts with PAB-1 and subunits of the PAN2-PAN3 and CCR4-NOT deadenylase complexes. Nucleic Acids Res, 2012. **40**(12): pp. 5651–65.

[69] Chen, Y., et al., A DDX6-CNOT1 complex and W-binding pockets in CNOT9 reveal direct links between miRNA target recognition and silencing. Mol Cell, 2014. **54**(5): pp. 737–50.

[70] Huntzinger, E., et al., The interactions of GW182 proteins with PABP and deadenylases are required for both translational repression and degradation of miRNA targets. Nucleic Acids Res, 2013. **41**(2): pp. 978–94.

[71] Behm-Ansmant, I., et al., mRNA degradation by miRNAs and GW182 requires both CCR4:NOT deadenylase and DCP1:DCP2 decapping complexes. Genes Dev, 2006. **20**(14): pp. 1885–98.

[72] Maroney, P.A., et al., Evidence that microRNAs are associated with translating messenger RNAs in human cells. Nat Struct Mol Biol, 2006. **13**(12): pp. 1102–7.

[73] Stefani, G., et al., Fragile X mental retardation protein is associated with translating polyribosomes in neuronal cells. J Neurosci, 2004. **24**(33): pp. 7272–6.

[74] Chen, E., et al., Fragile X mental retardation protein regulates translation by binding directly to the ribosome. Mol Cell, 2014. **54**(3): pp. 407–17.

[75] Darnell, J.C., et al., FMRP stalls ribosomal translocation on mRNAs linked to synaptic function and autism. Cell, 2011. **146**(2): pp. 247–61.

[76] Ceman, S., et al., Phosphorylation influences the translation state of FMRP-associated polyribosomes. Hum Mol Genet, 2003. **12**(24): pp. 3295–305.

[77] Bolduc, F.V., et al., Excess protein synthesis in Drosophila fragile X mutants impairs long-term memory. Nat Neurosci, 2008. **11**(10): pp. 1143–5.

[78] Muddashetty, R.S., et al., Reversible inhibition of PSD-95 mRNA translation by miR-125a, FMRP phosphorylation, and mGluR signaling. Mol Cell, 2011. **42**(5): pp. 673–88.

[79] Kenny, P.J., et al., MOV10 and FMRP regulate AGO2 association with microRNA recognition elements. Cell Rep, 2014. **9**(5): pp. 1729–41.

[80] Edbauer, D., et al., Regulation of synaptic structure and function by FMRP-associated microRNAs miR-125b and miR-132. Neuron, 2010. **65**(3): pp. 373–84.

[81] Beilharz, T.H., et al., microRNA-mediated messenger RNA deadenylation contributes to translational repression in mammalian cells. PLoS One, 2009. **4**(8): p. e6783.

[82] Wakiyama, M., et al., Let-7 microRNA-mediated mRNA deadenylation and translational repression in a mammalian cell-free system. Genes Dev, 2007. **21**(15): pp. 1857–62.

[83] Subtelny, A.O., et al., Poly(A)-tail profiling reveals an embryonic switch in translational control. Nature, 2014. **508**(7494): pp. 66–71.

[84] Wu, E., et al., Pervasive and cooperative deadenylation of 3′UTRs by embryonic microRNA families. Mol Cell, 2010. **40**(4): pp. 558–70.

[85] Udagawa, T., et al., Bidirectional control of mRNA translation and synaptic plasticity by the cytoplasmic polyadenylation complex. Mol Cell, 2012. **47**(2): pp. 253–66.

[86] Rouhana, L., et al., Vertebrate GLD2 poly(A) polymerases in the germline and the brain. RNA, 2005. **11**(7): pp. 1117–30.

[87] Kwak, J.E., et al., GLD2 poly(A) polymerase is required for long-term memory. Proc Natl Acad Sci U S A, 2008. **105**(38): pp. 14644–9.

[88] Nousch, M., et al., The cytoplasmic poly(A) polymerases GLD-2 and GLD-4 promote general gene expression via distinct mechanisms. Nucleic Acids Res, 2014. **42**(18): pp. 11622–33.

[89] Fukaya, T., H.O. Iwakawa, and Y. Tomari, MicroRNAs block assembly of eIF4F translation initiation complex in Drosophila. Mol Cell, 2014. **56**(1): pp. 67–78.

[90] Mathonnet, G., et al., MicroRNA inhibition of translation initiation in vitro by targeting the cap-binding complex eIF4F. Science, 2007. **317**(5845): pp. 1764–7.

[91] Meijer, H.A., et al., Translational repression and eIF4A2 activity are critical for microRNA-mediated gene regulation. Science, 2013. **340**(6128): pp. 82–5.

[92] Lugli, G., et al., Expression of microRNAs and their precursors in synaptic fractions of adult mouse forebrain. J Neurochem, 2008. **106**(2): pp. 650–61.

[93] Lugli, G., et al., Dicer and eIF2c are enriched at postsynaptic densities in adult mouse brain and are modified by neuronal activity in a calpain-dependent manner. J Neurochem, 2005. **94**(4): pp. 896–905.

[94] Krol, J., et al., Characterizing light-regulated retinal microRNAs reveals rapid turnover as a common property of neuronal microRNAs. Cell, 2010. **141**(4): pp. 618–31.

[95] Goldie, B.J., et al., Activity-associated miRNA are packaged in Map1b-enriched exosomes released from depolarized neurons. Nucleic Acids Res, 2014. **42**(14): pp. 9195–208.

[96] Park, C.S. and S.J. Tang, Regulation of microRNA expression by induction of bidirectional synaptic plasticity. J Mol Neurosci, 2009. **38**(1): pp. 50–6.

[97] Eacker, S.M., et al., Neuronal activity regulates hippocampal miRNA expression. PLoS One, 2011. **6**(10): p. e25068.

[98] Konopka, W., et al., MicroRNA loss enhances learning and memory in mice. J Neurosci, 2010. **30**(44): pp. 14835–42.

[99] Mellios, N., et al., miR-132, an experience-dependent microRNA, is essential for visual cortex plasticity. Nat Neurosci, 2011. **14**(10): pp. 1240–2.

[100] Wang, R.Y., et al., In vivo knockdown of hippocampal miR-132 expression impairs memory acquisition of trace fear conditioning. Hippocampus, 2013. **23**(7): pp. 625–33.

[101] Impey, S., et al., Defining the CREB regulon: a genome-wide analysis of transcription factor regulatory regions. Cell, 2004. **119**(7): pp. 1041–54.

[102] Wayman, G.A., et al., An activity-regulated microRNA controls dendritic plasticity by down-regulating p250GAP. Proc Natl Acad Sci U S A, 2008. **105**(26): pp. 9093–8.

[103] Kawashima, H., et al., Glucocorticoid attenuates brain-derived neurotrophic factor-dependent upregulation of glutamate receptors via the suppression of microRNA-132 expression. Neuroscience, 2010. **165**(4): pp. 1301–11.

[104] Schratt, G.M., et al., A brain-specific microRNA regulates dendritic spine development. Nature, 2006. **439**(7074): pp. 283–9.

[105] Christensen, M., et al., Recombinant adeno-associated virus-mediated microRNA delivery into the postnatal mouse brain reveals a role for miR-134 in dendritogenesis in vivo. Front Neural Circuits, 2010. **3**: p. 16.

[106] Gao, J., et al., A novel pathway regulates memory and plasticity via SIRT1 and miR-134. Nature, 2010. **466**(7310): pp. 1105–9.

[107] Smrt, R.D., et al., MicroRNA miR-137 regulates neuronal maturation by targeting ubiquitin ligase mind bomb-1. Stem Cells, 2010. **28**(6): pp. 1060–70.

[108] Siegert, S., et al., The schizophrenia risk gene product miR-137 alters presynaptic plasticity. Nat Neurosci, 2015. **18**(7): pp. 1008–16.

[109] Olde Loohuis, N.F., et al., MicroRNA-137 Controls AMPA-Receptor-Mediated Transmission and mGluR-Dependent LTD. Cell Rep, 2015. **11**(12): pp. 1876–84.

[110] Decker, C.J. and R. Parker, P-bodies and stress granules: possible roles in the control of translation and mRNA degradation. Cold Spring Harb Perspect Biol, 2012. **4**(9): p. a012286.

[111] Eystathioy, T., et al., A phosphorylated cytoplasmic autoantigen, GW182, associates with a unique population of human mRNAs within novel cytoplasmic speckles. Mol Biol Cell, 2002. **13**(4): pp. 1338–51.

[112] Cougot, N., et al., Dendrites of mammalian neurons contain specialized P-body-like structures that respond to neuronal activation. J Neurosci, 2008. **28**(51): pp. 13793–804.

[113] Zeitelhofer, M., et al., Dynamic interaction between P-bodies and transport ribonucleoprotein particles in dendrites of mature hippocampal neurons. J Neurosci, 2008. **28**(30): pp. 7555–62.

[114] Oh, J.Y., et al., Activity-dependent synaptic localization of processing bodies and their role in dendritic structural plasticity. J Cell Sci, 2013. **126**(Pt 9): pp. 2114–23.

[115] Brengues, M., D. Teixeira, and R. Parker, Movement of eukaryotic mRNAs between polysomes and cytoplasmic processing bodies. Science, 2005. **310**(5747): pp. 486–9.

[116] Bhattacharyya, S.N., et al., Relief of microRNA-mediated translational repression in human cells subjected to stress. Cell, 2006. **125**(6): pp. 1111–24.

[117] Melemedjian, O.K., et al., Bidirectional regulation of P body formation mediated by eIF4F complex formation in sensory neurons. Neurosci Lett, 2014. **563**: pp. 169–74.

[118] Kedersha, N., et al., Stress granules and processing bodies are dynamically linked sites of mRNP remodeling. J Cell Biol, 2005. **169**(6): pp. 871–84.

[119] Qureshi, I.A. and M.F. Mehler, Emerging roles of non-coding RNAs in brain evolution, development, plasticity and disease. Nat Rev Neurosci, 2012. **13**(8): pp. 528–41.

[120] Qureshi, I.A., J.S. Mattick, and M.F. Mehler, Long non-coding RNAs in nervous system function and disease. Brain Res, 2010. **1338**: pp. 20–35.

[121] Kapranov, P., et al., RNA maps reveal new RNA classes and a possible function for pervasive transcription. Science, 2007. **316**(5830): pp. 1484–8.

[122] Shi, X., et al., Long non-coding RNAs: a new frontier in the study of human diseases. Cancer Lett, 2013. **339**(2): pp. 159–66.

[123] Mercer, T.R., et al., Specific expression of long noncoding RNAs in the mouse brain. Proc Natl Acad Sci U S A, 2008. **105**(2): pp. 716–21.

[124] Zalfa, F., et al., The fragile X syndrome protein FMRP associates with BC1 RNA and regulates the translation of specific mRNAs at synapses. Cell, 2003. **112**(3): pp. 317–27.

[125] Eom, T., et al., Dual nature of translational control by regulatory BC RNAs. Mol Cell Biol, 2011. **31**(22): pp. 4538–49.

[126] Duning, K., et al., SYNCRIP, a component of dendritically localized mRNPs, binds to the translation regulator BC200 RNA. J Neurochem, 2008. **105**(2): pp. 351–9.

[127] Bernard, D., et al., A long nuclear-retained non-coding RNA regulates synaptogenesis by modulating gene expression. EMBO J, 2010. **29**(18): pp. 3082–93.

[128] Anguera, M.C., et al., Tsx produces a long noncoding RNA and has general functions in the germline, stem cells, and brain. PLoS Genet, 2011. **7**(9): p. e1002248.

[129] Smalheiser, N.R., et al., Natural antisense transcripts are co-expressed with sense mRNAs in synaptoneurosomes of adult mouse forebrain. Neurosci Res, 2008. **62**(4): pp. 236–9.

[130] Vicens, Q. and E. Westhof, Biogenesis of Circular RNAs. Cell, 2014. **159**(1): pp. 13–4.

[131] Hansen, T.B., et al., Natural RNA circles function as efficient microRNA sponges. Nature, 2013. **495**(7441): pp. 384–8.

[132] Memczak, S., et al., Circular RNAs are a large class of animal RNAs with regulatory potency. Nature, 2013. **495**(7441): pp. 333–8.

[133] Zheng, Q., et al., Circular RNA profiling reveals an abundant circHIPK3 that regulates cell growth by sponging multiple miRNAs. Nat Commun, 2016. **7**: p. 11215.

[134] Westholm, J.O., et al., Genome-wide analysis of drosophila circular RNAs reveals their structural and sequence properties and age-dependent neural accumulation. Cell Rep, 2014. **9**(5): pp. 1966–80.

[135] You, X., et al., Neural circular RNAs are derived from synaptic genes and regulated by development and plasticity. Nat Neurosci, 2015. **18**(4): pp. 603–10.

[136] Szabo, L., et al., Statistically based splicing detection reveals neural enrichment and tissue-specific induction of circular RNA during human fetal development. Genome Biol, 2015. **16**: pp. 126.

[137] Ingolia, N.T., et al., The ribosome profiling strategy for monitoring translation in vivo by deep sequencing of ribosome-protected mRNA fragments. Nat Protoc, 2012. **7**(8): pp. 1534–50.

[138] Harrison, P.F., et al., PAT-seq: a method to study the integration of 3′-UTR dynamics with gene expression in the eukaryotic transcriptome. RNA, 2015. **21**(8): pp. 1502–10.

[139] Ye, Y., et al., Role of MicroRNA in Governing Synaptic Plasticity. Neural Plast, 2016. **2016**: p. 4959523.

5

The Ghrelin Receptor Regulates Dendritic Spines and the NMDA Receptor–Mediated Synaptic Transmission in the Hippocampus

Masako Isokawa

Abstract

Increasing evidence suggests the involvement of ghrelin (an orexigenic hormone) and its cognate receptor growth hormone secretagogue receptor (GHSR1a, also known as the ghrelin receptor) in extra-hypothalamic functions such as hippocampal learning and memory. However, cellular and molecular mechanisms underlying the ghrelin-regulated hippocampal neuron activity are poorly understood. In this chapter, we show the following: (1) ghrelin promoted phosphorylation of the *N*-methyl-D-aspartate receptor (NMDAR) subunit 1 (GluN1) in a PKC/PKA-dependent manner and amplified NMDAR-mediated excitatory postsynaptic currents, (2) ghrelin stimulated phosphorylation of CREB (cAMP response-element-binding protein), and (3) ghrelin increased phalloidin binding to F-actin, suggesting possible reorganization of dendritic spines; all occurred through the activation of GHSR1a in the CA1 pyramidal cell of the hippocampus in cultured slice preparations. Interestingly, the ghrelin's effects on GluN1 and CREB phosphorylation were negatively modulated by exogenous application of endocannabinoids, 2-arachidonoylglycerol (2-AG), and anandamide (ANE), in type 1 cannabinoid receptor (CB1R)-dependent and -independent manners, respectively. It is suggested that ghrelin and the ghrelin receptor regulate synaptic transmission and plasticity in the hippocampus, interacting with the endogenous cannabinoid system, which may be essential and necessary for successful acquisition of metabolic state–dependent learning and adaptive appetitive behavior.

Keywords: GluN1 phosphorylation, NMDAR-EPSC, ghrelin binding, GHSR1a KO mice, Phalloidin, CREB, endocannabinoid, CB1R

1. Introduction

We empirically know that we can learn things more easily, accurately, and quickly when we are interested, motivated, and reward-driven. Numerous animal models of learning have placed experimental subjects under fasted conditions in order for successful acquisition of specific tasks by using food as a reward [1]. This suggests the possibility that a molecule, which plays a critical role in appetitive behavior and/or reward-related feeling, may also be involved in the acquisition of learning.

1.1. Hippocampus in reward-related learning

Although the mesolimbic dopaminergic system is central to the study of motivational and reward-related learning, the neurobiological basis of reward-related learning cannot be explained completely without the participation of the hippocampus. The hippocampus is a primary site of activity-dependent plasticity and neuromodulation that have been hypothesized to be the neuronal substrate for learning and memory. The hippocampus lies upstream of the dopaminergic reward circuit and sends a major output to the reward system. More specifically, the hippocampal glutamatergic outputs regulate reward responses in the nucleus accumbens [2]. Therefore, cellular and synaptic plasticity within the hippocampus alters the transfer of information throughout the brain's reward system.

1.2. Ghrelin in reward-related learning

Ghrelin is a unique acylated 28 amino acid peptide hormone that is released from the stomach when it is empty. Ghrelin was originally identified as an endogenous ligand for the growth hormone secretagogue receptor (GHSR1a, now known as the ghrelin receptor) [3]. Activation of GHSR1a initiates a release of growth hormone from pituitary glands. Activation of GHSR1a also stimulates feeding center in the hypothalamus [4]. Indeed, the hypothalamus shows the highest localization of GHSR1a [4]. However, increasing evidence suggests that ghrelin may have numerous physiological functions in the brain outside the hypothalamus. For example, ghrelin stimulates the brain's reward center [5]. Ghrelin improves memory retention [6]. Thus, the accelerated acquisition of learning under fasted conditions suggests the potential importance of ghrelin as a key molecule for cellular and molecular mechanisms of reward-related learning and memory [7–9].

1.3. Source of ghrelin: brain or stomach?

Systemic ghrelin can cross the blood-brain barrier and enter the hippocampus [10]. Thus, peripheral ghrelin could be a source to be utilized by hippocampal neurons. On the other hand, in the mouse model, acylated ghrelin was readily transported across the blood-brain barrier in the brain-to-blood direction, but the quantity of its transport in the blood-to-brain direction appeared negligible [11]. Furthermore, vagotomy prevented peripheral ghrelin's effect on the hypothalamus [12], suggesting that ghrelin's direct effect on the brain may be of intrinsic origin [13, 14]. Neurons in the hypothalamus and septum are reported to be immunopositive to ghrelin [4] and likely to release ghrelin [15]. The septal neurons project directly to the hippocampus making monosynaptic connections [16]. Thus, centrally produced ghrelin in the septal neuron could be a source of ghrelin for hippocampal synapses, independently of systemic ghrelin, and contributes to neuron plasticity leading to contextual learning.

1.4. Investigating hippocampal GHSR1a in isolation

The hippocampus receives hypothalamic and arcuate projections directly from the fornix, while being situated centrally for functional interactions with other limbic cortexes by exchanging reciprocal synaptic connections. Thus, GHSR1a in the hippocampus is likely a direct target of hypothalamic and limbic cortical inputs including those from the septum. Each of these inputs may provide ghrelin independently or collectively to the hippocampal GHSR1a. Identifying the source(s) of ghrelin that affects hippocampal neuron function is an important scientific issue. Unfortunately, it is beyond the scope of this chapter because our goal is to first identify cellular and molecular mechanisms underlying the GHSR1a-involved process of hippocampal learning. Here, we review our progress in determining direct effects of ghrelin and GHSR1a-mediated cellular signaling in the hippocampal neuron synapse transmission and plasticity in isolation, without secondary modulation originating in the extra-hippocampal network activity, by using the hippocampal slice culture model and exogenous application of ghrelin.

2. Localization of GHSR1a in the hippocampus of cultured slices

2.1. Fluorescent ghrelin binding

We demonstrate the localization of GHSR1a in the cultured hippocampal slices with the use of three different methods. First of all, an octanoylated form of FITC-conjugated ghrelin (1 μM) was used in the rat hippocampal slice culture. Ghrelin can bind to GHSR1a only when it is octanoylated [17]. Thus, FITC-conjugated octanoylated ghrelin is a useful and reliable molecule that specifically binds to the receptor [18]. Non-octanoylated form of FITC-conjugated ghrelin was used as a control in order to confirm the specificity of octanoylated ghrelin binding. After 1 h of incubation followed by fixation (with 4% paraformaldehyde), intense binding was detected in the pyramidal cell layer of all CA fields with the given focal plane shown in **Figure 1a** [19]. However, by imaging FITC signals in many different focal planes in the same specimen using a confocal microscope (Fluoview 1000, Olympus), we learned that the actual binding ranged from dentate gyrus granule cell layer to CA1, CA2, and CA3 pyramidal cell layers, suggesting that GHSR1a has ample expression in the cultured hippocampus and is widely distributed throughout the dentate gyrus and Ammons horn.

2.2. eGFP-tagged GHSR1a expression in transgenic mouse hippocampus in slice culture

According to the eGFP-tagged reporter gene mapping of the whole mouse brain, GHSR1a is reported to be highly localized in the hippocampus [20]. However, it is not determined whether transgenic mouse hippocampus retains the expression of functional GHSR1a in the

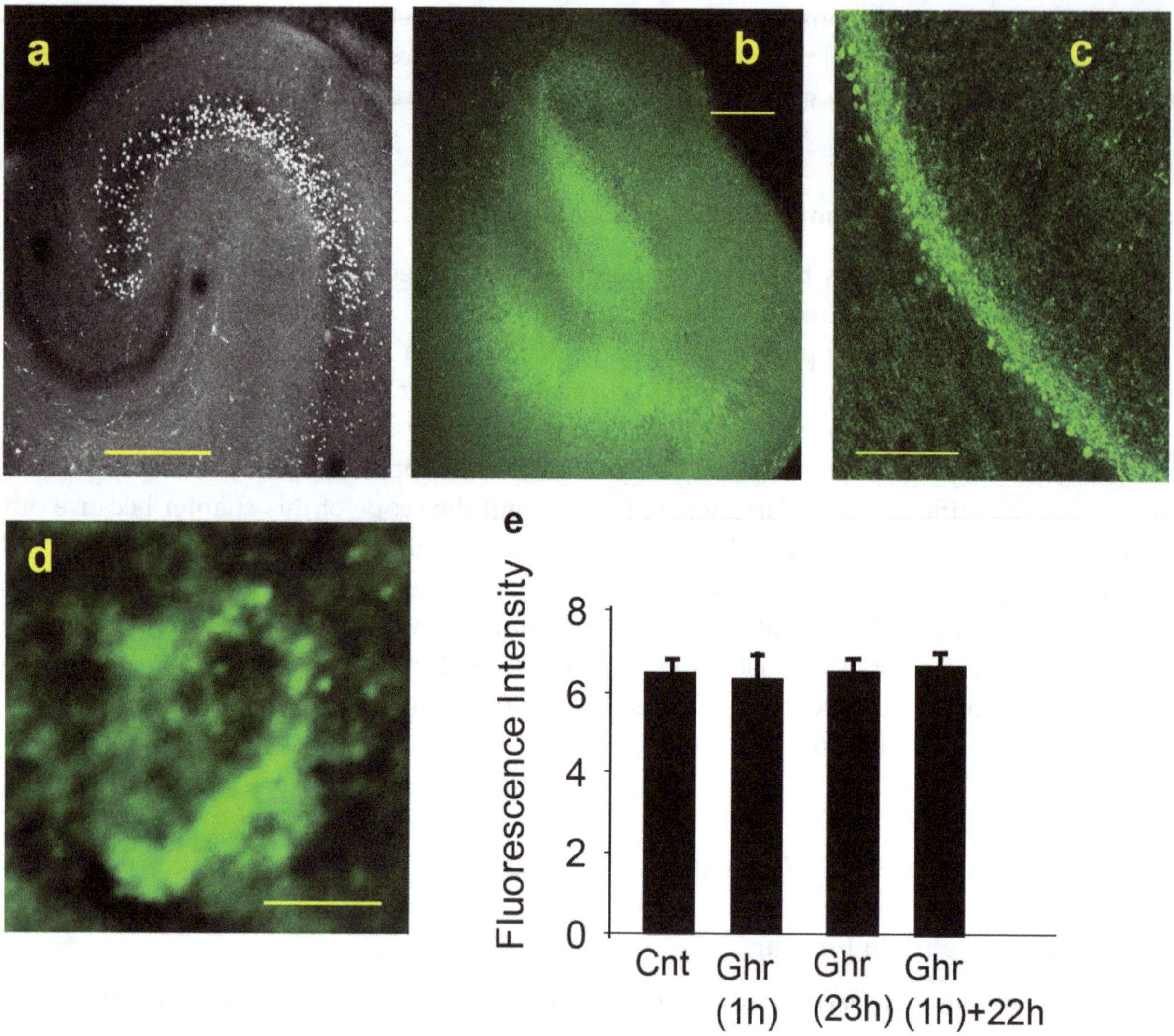

Figure 1. Localization of GHSR1a in cultured hippocampus in slices. **a**. Binding of the octanoylated form of FITC-conjugated ghrelin. **b**. eGFP signals from GHSR1a-expressing cells in mouse hippocampal slices. **c**. eGFP signals from CA1 pyramidal cell layer. **d**. GHSR1a immunoreactivity. **e**. GHSR1a expression was quantified in an arbitrary scale in control, 1-h incubation in ghrelin, 23-h incubation in ghrelin, and 1-h incubation in ghrelin followed by 22-h incubation in control media without ghrelin. Calibrations: (a) and (b) 500 μm, (c) 200 μm, and (d) 5 μm. (Modified with permission from Muniz and Isokawa [19]).

in vitro culture. Hippocampal slices were prepared from eGFP-tagged GHSR1a-expressing transgenic mouse brains, where the eGFP gene was inserted downstream of the GHSR1a promoter (Jackson Lab, B6;129S7-Ghsr<tm2Rgs</J/Stock# 019908). Up to 3 weeks in culture, the localization of GHSR1a was identified by live-imaging eGFP fluorescence. **Figure 1b** shows eGFP signals that are visible in the infra-pyramidal blade of the dentate gyrus and the pyramidal cell layer of the CA1 region. With higher magnification, the CA1 pyramidal cell layer became clearly detectable with resolution that is sufficient to identify individual neurons (**Figure 1c**). Under different focal planes, eGFP signals were detected in other CA fields (i.e., CA2 and CA3) in the pyramidal cell layer and from the supra-pyramidal blade of the dentate gyrus granule cell layer.

2.3. Immunohistochemistry of GHSR1a

In addition to receptor binding and eGFP tagging, we investigated the localization of GHSR1a immunohistochemically in the cultured rat hippocampal slices using two different antibodies raised against GHSR1a (rabbit polyclonal anti-GHSR1a from Phoenix Pharmaceutical, Burlingame, CA, and from Santa Cruz Biotechnology Lab, Santa Cruz, CA). With both antibodies, GHSR1a immunoreactivity was successfully detected in the dentate gyrus and the Ammons horn of our rat hippocampal slice culture. More specifically, fluorescent signals collected from secondary antibody (Alexa 488, Life Technologies, Grand Island, NY) by confocal imaging revealed that GHSR1a was localized primarily as numerous aggregates surrounding the soma (**Figure 1d**). Together, these observations provide cellular and molecular evidence that the ghrelin receptor, GHSR1a, is expressed and localized in the cultured rat and mouse hippocampus in slices in a similar manner to what was reported in the in vivo whole brain specimen.

2.4. Receptor internalization in the hippocampal slice culture

GHSR1a exhibits an unusually high constitutive activity, which is the ability to propagate the intracellular signal in the absence of agonist [21, 22]. Thus, it may be possible that the downstream-signaling level, determined by constitutive activity, could reflect membrane expression of the receptor. In addition, agonist-induced internalization is a widely acknowledged process among all G-protein–coupled receptors including GHSR1a [23]. Thus, we were concerned whether GHSR1a in our hippocampal slice culture might have undergone such a process during the application of ghrelin in our experiments. Live slice cultures were incubated in ghrelin (100 nM) for either 1 or 23 h. At the end of the incubation, the specimens were fixed and processed for immunohistochemistry. GHSR1a immunoreactivity was imaged with a confocal microscope and quantified using image analysis software (IPLab, BD Bioscience, San Jose, CA). We did not find any difference in the magnitude of GHSR1a immunoreactivity between 1-h incubation and 23-h incubation, when compared with control (**Figure 1e**) [24]. We also conducted a "second" control, which was to incubate the slices in ghrelin for 1 h and the additional 22 h in control media (without ghrelin). At the end of the experiment, slices were fixed and processed for immunohistochemistry. There were no differences in the GHSR1a immunoreactivity between control and the "second" control. This finding suggested that GHSR1a did not appear to be internalized by the exogenous application of agonist to a significant extent even if a long-term incubation of 23 h was employed. There was a report that GHSR1a hardly desensitized with the nM range of concentrations of ghrelin [25], which is in agreement with our observation and supports the present finding.

3. Phosphorylation of GluN1 by ghrelin

Subunit phosphorylation is a critical step to facilitate the NMDAR channel function and to induce plasticity in excitatory synapses [26]. Among various phosphorylation sites in the NMDAR , we focused on the phosphorylation of Ser 896 and Ser 897 in the GluN1 subunit. The phosphorylation of Ser 896 is dependent on protein kinase C, and the phosphorylation of Ser 897 is dependent on protein kinase A [27]. The reason for investigating these two phosphorylation sites are as follows: (1) GHSR1a is a Gq-coupled receptor, so that the activation of GHSR1a initiates inositol trisphosphate-mediated-signaling pathways leading to the activation of protein kinase C [28]; and (2) GHSR1a can cause a robust activation of cAMP/PKA-signaling cascade, which has been reported in the process of procuring sufficient energy [29].

3.1. Dose-dependent increase of pGluN1

Phosphorylation of GluN1 was studied using a goat polyclonal anti-pGluN1 at Ser 896/897 (Santa Cruz Biotechnology, Santa Cruz, CA) and Alexa 488 secondary antibody. Phosphorylated GluN1 (pGluN1) was quantified based on the fluorescent signal, captured by a confocal microscope. Representative pGluN1 signals were manually selected as a strongly fluorescing small puncta (examples are shown by yellow arrows in **Figure 2a**). A total of 236 representative puncta were manually selected from 30 confocal images, and the area and intensities of these puncta were measured using IPLab (BD Bioscience, San Jose, CA). Based on the measurement, selection criteria were established and applied to 2024 confocal images taken from 157 hippocampal slices. Among them, 35513 pGluN1 immunoreactive puncta, taken from 1714 confocal images, satisfied the selection criteria, and were used for data analysis.

Exogenous application of ghrelin (1–1000 nM) increased the magnitude of phosphorylation in GluN1 in a dose-dependent manner. The ghrelin-induced increase in pGluN1 immunoreactivity peaked at a concentration of 10 nM ($r^2 = 0.899$, $p < 0.0001$, $n = 56$; analysis of variance (ANOVA)) (**Figure 2b**). The ghrelin-induced changes in pGluN1 immunoreactivity were sensitive to and inhibited by the GHSR1a antagonist, D-Lys3-GHRP6 (1 μM), and an inverse agonist, substance *P*-analog (10 μM), when they were applied with ghrelin (100 nM). However, the application of D-Lys3-GHRP6 or substance *P*-analog alone (without ghrelin) did not have any effect as compared with control ($p < 0.001$, $n = 47$, unpaired *t*-test) (**Figure 2c** and **d**). This suggested the possibility that (1) there were few endogenous ghrelin molecules present in our cultured hippocampal slices, or (2) constitutive activation of GHSR1a (if any) did not appear to affect the phosphorylation state of GluN1 in cultured hippocampus in slices.

3.2. Effect of ghrelin on pGluN1 in GHSR1a knockout mouse

In cultured hippocampal slices prepared from homozygous GHSR1a knockout (-/-) mice, exogenous application of ghrelin (100 nM) failed to cause any change in pGluN1 immunoreactivity (**Figure 2e** and **f**) when compared with the wild-type GHSR1a (+/+) mouse hippocampus ($p < 0.005$, $n = 31$, unpaired *t*-test) (**Figure 2e** and **f**). Slices prepared from heterozygous GHSR1a knockout (+/-) mouse hippocampus also failed to show any change in pGluN1 immunoreactivity in response to ghrelin (100 nM) (**Figure 2e** and **f**). This suggested that a small reduction in the expression of GHSR1a could negate the ghrelin's effect on the GluN1 subunit phosphorylation at Ser 896/897. Furthermore, we found that the baseline pGluN1 was elevated in homozygous GHSR1a knockout (-/-) mice as compared with wild-type GHSR1a (+/+) mice in both control and ghrelin. This suggested that the NMDAR channel may be hyperactive in the hippocampus of homozygous GHSR1a knockout (-/-) mouse. It might be

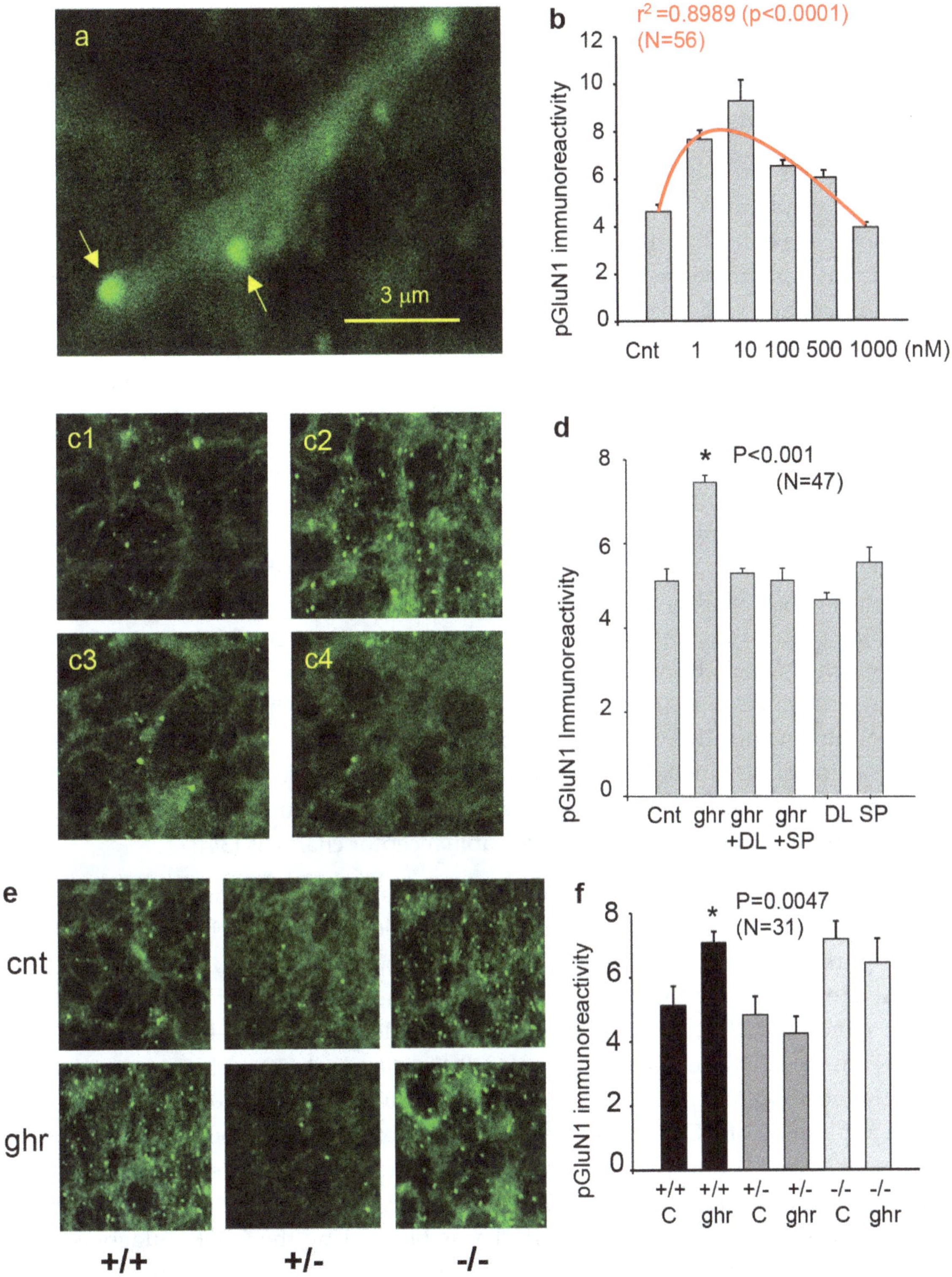

Figure 2. pGluN1 immunoreactivity in cultured rat hippocampal slices. **a.** Representative pGluN1 signals are indicated by yellow arrows. **b.** Dose-dependent changes in pGluN1. **c1–c4.** pGluN1 in control (c1), ghrelin (c2), ghrelin and D-Lys3-GHRP6 (c3), and ghrelin and substance *P*-analogue (c4). **d.** Quantification of pGluN1 in control (c), ghrelin (ghr), ghrelin and D-Lys3-GHRP6 (ghr + DL), ghrelin and substance *P*-analogue (ghr+SP), D-Lys3-GHRP6 alone (DL), and substance *P*-analogue alone (SP). **e.** pGluN1 in control (cnt) and ghrelin (ghr) in wild type (+/+), heterozygous GHSR1a knockout mice (+/-), and homozygous GHSR1a knockout mice (-/-). **f.** Quantification of pGluN1 in wild-type and GHSR1a knockout mice. (Modified with permission from Muniz and Isokawa [19]).

possible that some compensatory mechanisms had switched on under the total absence of GHSR1a, in order to readjust homeostatic balance in the NMDAR channel activity.

3.3. Endocannabinoids negatively modulate ghrelin's effect on pGluN1

Endocannabinoids (eCB) and the type 1 cannabinoid receptor (CB1R) have been implicated essentially in regulating a feeding behavior. They stimulate hypothalamic orexigenic neurons, enhance appetite, and initiate food consumption [30]. Interestingly, there is a report to suggest that ghrelin may exert its orexigenic effect through the endogenous cannabinoid system by producing eCBs in the hypothalamus [31]. However, to date, there is no evidence in the hippocampus that a similar interaction might occur between ghrelin and the endocannabinoid system. We tested if eCBs such as 2-AG (2-arachidonoylglycerol) and anandamide might modulate the effect of ghrelin on the phosphorylation of GluN1 [32].

Hippocampal slices were incubated in 20 nM of R(+)-methanandamide (non-hydrolyzing form of anandamide) together with 100 nM of ghrelin. The magnitude of pGluN1 immunoreactivity remained unchanged when compared to the control ($p = 0.939$) (**Figure 3a**), suggesting that the effect of ghrelin on pGluN1 was negated by R(+)-methanandamide. Interestingly, the inhibitory effect of R(+)-methanandamide was not blocked by the CB1R antagonist, AM251 (5 μM), which suggested that R(+)-methanandamide exerted its effect independently of CB1R. We then tested the antagonist of TRPV1 (transient receptor potential vanilloid type 1), since anandamide is also an agonist of this receptor [33]. Neither capsazepine (caps, 5 μM) nor iodoresiniferatoxin (IRTX, 10 nM), antagonists of TRPV1, was effective of blocking the inhibitory action of R(+)-methanandamide (**Figure 3a**). It may be possible that R(+)-methanandamide directly inhibited the NMDAR channel, since anandamide was reported to directly interact and inhibit nonspecific cation-permeable receptor channels [34].

Next, we tested the effect of 2-AG. Similar to the result of R(+)-anandamide, the application of 2-AG (10 μM) negated the stimulatory effect of ghrelin on the phosphorylation of GluN1 (**Figure 3b**). A negative effect of 2-AG was blocked by the CB1R antagonist, AM251 (5 μM), suggesting that the effect of 2-AG was exerted through the activation of CB1R. A synthetic agonist of CB1R, WIN 55,212 (4 μM), also blocked the ghrelin's stimulatory effect on pGluN1 in the CB1R-dependent manner. We then applied 150 mM KCl in the attempt of depolarizing neurons and mobilizing endogenous 2-AG (instead of exogenously applying 2-AG). The application of KCl mimicked the inhibitory effect of 2-AG on the ghrelin-mediated enhancement of GluN1 phosphorylation. The magnitude of pGluN1 remained unchanged in the presence of ghrelin during KCl application and was comparable to control. KCl-mediated inhibition of the ghrelin's stimulatory effect was blocked by the CB1R antagonist, AM251 (5 μM), suggesting that the application of KCl successfully mobilized endogenous 2-AG. Finally, we used an inhibitor of MAGL (monoacylglycerol lipase), JZL184 (100 nM). MAGL is the degradation enzyme for 2-AG. Thus, JZL184 slows down the rate of 2-AG degradation while maintaining an elevated concentration of ambient 2-AG and making the effect of endogenous 2-AG longer and more intense. As shown in **Figure 3b**, JZL184 was effective of negating the ghrelin's action on the phosphorylation of pGluN1 ($p < 0.0001$), and this effect was reversed by the CB1R antagonist, AM251 ($p < 0.05$). Although we cannot estimate the

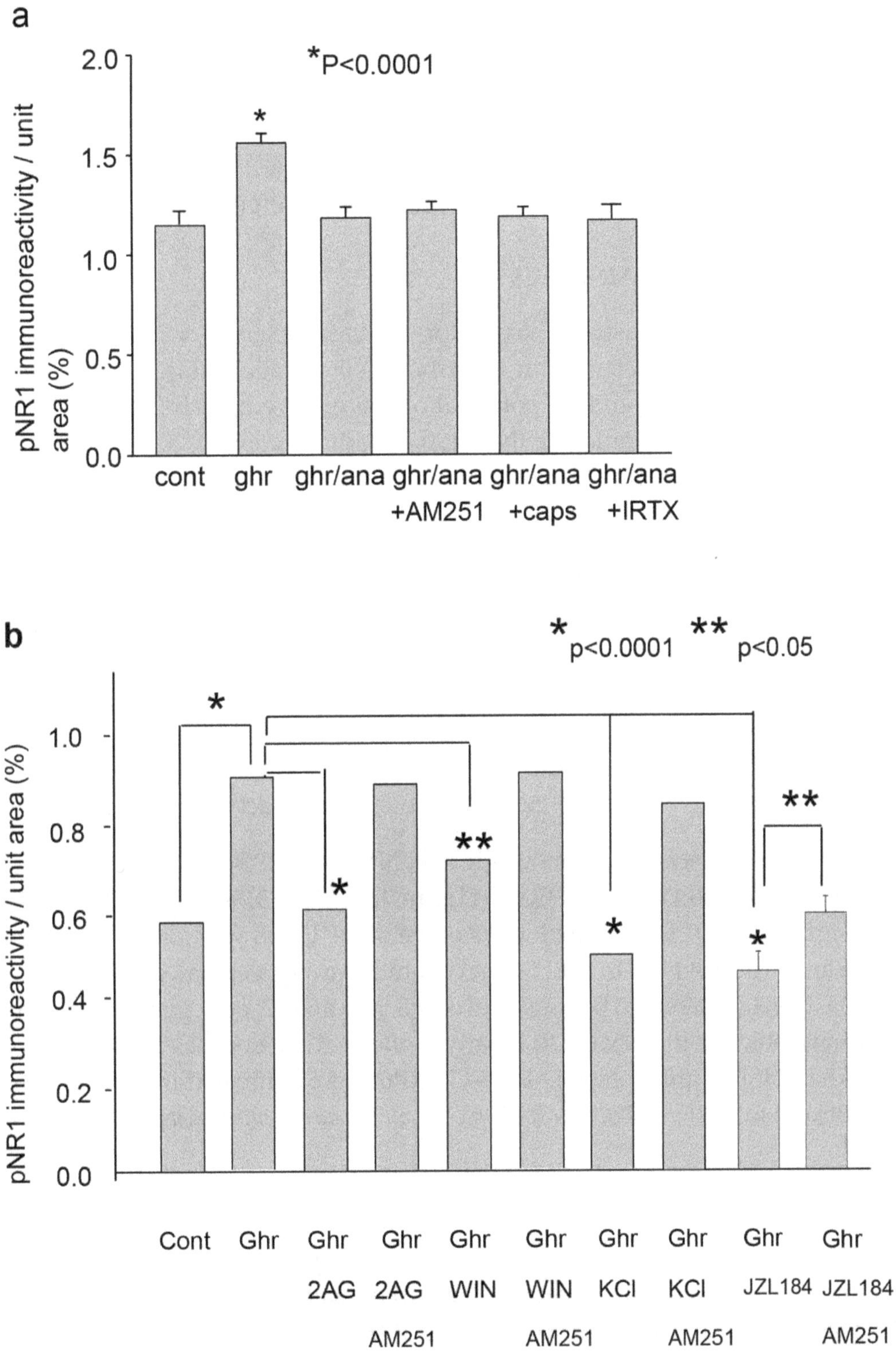

Figure 3. Effects of endocannabinoids on ghrelin-induced increase in pGluN1. **a**. Co-application of ghrelin (200 nM) and R(+)-methanandamide (20 nM) blocked the stimulatory effect of ghrelin on the phosphorylation of GluN1. This inhibitory effect of R(+)-methanandamide was independent of CB1R and TRPV1. **b**. Co-application of ghrelin (200 nM) with 2-AG (10 μM), WIN55,212 (4 μM), KCl (150 mM), and JZL 184 (100 nM), all negated the stimulatory effect of ghrelin on the phosphorylation of GluN1. The CB1R antagonist, AM251 (5 μM), blocked the inhibitory effect of 2-AG, WIN55212, KCl, and JZL 184 on the phosphorylation of GluN1, indicating that these compounds exerted their effects through the activation of CB1R. (Modified with permission from Cuellar and Isokawa [32]).

intrinsic concentration of 2-AG and the rate of increase by JZL184 in our hippocampal slice culture, a physiological range of fluctuation in the concentration of eCBs appears to be sufficient to interact and modulate the ghrelin-signaling cascade on the GluN1 subunit.

4. Ghrelin amplifies NMDAR-mediated synaptic currents

4.1. Ghrelin on evoked NMDAR-EPSCs

NMDAR-EPSCs (*N*-methyl-D-aspartate receptor–mediated excitatory postsynaptic currents) were isolated with a patch electrode in the whole-cell voltage-clamp configuration in single CA1 pyramidal cells at a holding potential of +40 mV (Axopatch 200A and pClamp 10, Molecular Devices), while stimulating the stratum radiatum every 20 s. Extracellular solution (ACSF: artificial cerebrospinal fluid) contained 50 μM picrotoxin and 10 μM NBQX (2,3-dihydroxy-6-nitro-7-sulfamoyl-benzo[F] quinoxaline) in order to block GABAergic induced pluripotent stem cells (IPSCs) and AMPA (α-amino-3-hydroxy-5-methyl-4-isoxazolepropionic acid) receptor–mediated EPSC component. A brief local application of ghrelin (100 nM) enhanced NMDAR-EPSCs (*$*F = 29.12, p < 0.001$, $**F = 28.39, p < 0.005$, $n = 30$, one-way repeated measure ANOVA*) (**Figure 4a**). This increase was sensitive to D-Lys3-GHRP-6 (GHSR1a antagonist, 100 μM). Subsequent bath application of D-Lys3-GHRP6 reduced the amplitude of NMDAR-EPSCs (*$*t = 10.18, p < 0.0006$, $**t = 14.96, p < 0.0002$, $n = 41$, unpaired t-test*). Complete blockade of EPSCs by APV (100 μM, the antagonist of NMDAR) supported our interpretation that the recorded EPSCs were indeed generated solely by the activation of the NMDAR.

Interestingly, in the absence of exogenous ghrelin, NMDAR-EPSCs were reduced in the peak amplitude in response to D-Lys3-GHRP6 (**Figure 4c**) (*$*F = 63.58, p < 0.001$, $n = 37$, one-way repeated measure ANOVA*). This reduction was reversible. Upon washout of the antagonist of GHSR1a, the amplitude of NMDAR-EPSCs recovered. We suggest that, in cultured hippocampal slices, (1) GHSR1a is likely to be constitutively active and (2) endogenous ghrelin might be present and available for the NMDAR. Finally, none of the responses presented above with ghrelin and the GHSR1a antagonist, D-Lys3-GHRP6, were generated in slices prepared from GHSR1a knockout mice (*$F = 0.772, p > 0.77$, $n = 18$, one-way repeated measure ANOVA*).

4.2. Ghrelin on spontaneous NMDAR-EPSCs

Spontaneously occurring NMDAR-EPSCs (sEPSCs) responded to exogenous application of ghrelin and the GHSR1a antagonist similarly to evoked NMDAR-EPSCs. The amplitude of sEPSCs was 100 pA in average in control ACSF (**Figure 4d1**). However, it was increased by twofolds in response to exogenous application of ghrelin (**Figure 4d2**). The increase was recovered to the control level following the bath application of D-Lys3-GHRP6 (100 μM) (**Figure 4d3**). Although the amplitude of sEPSCs changed in response to the application of agonist and antagonist of GHSR1a, the frequency of sEPSCs did not change significantly, suggesting that the effect of ghrelin and GHSR1a signaling was likely postsynaptic.

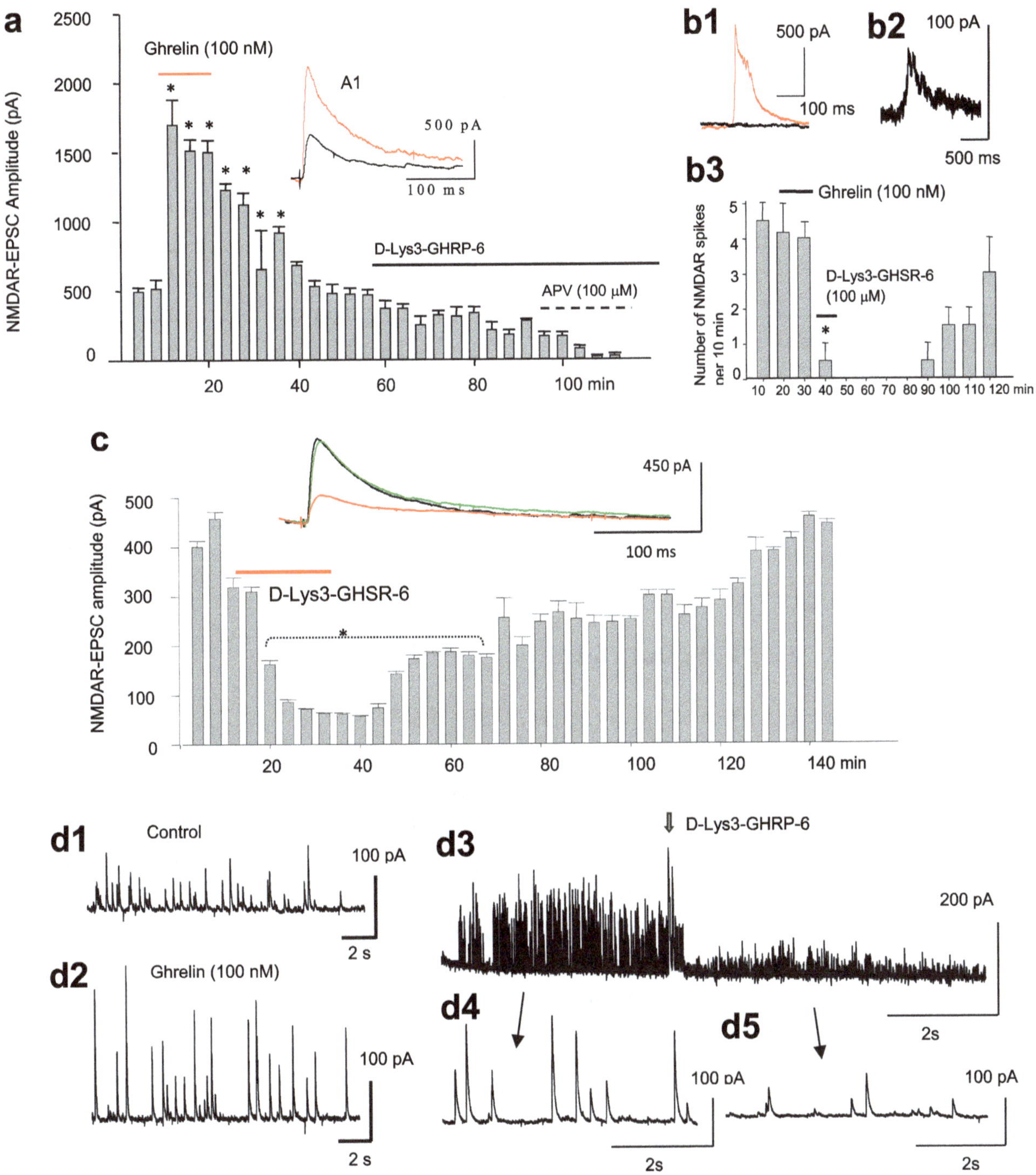

Figure 4. Effect of ghrelin on the NMDA receptor–mediated EPSCs. **a.** Single pyramidal neurons in the CA1 of cultured rat hippocampal slices were voltage clamped at +40 mV in the presence of picrotoxin and NBQX. Stratum radiatum was stimulated every 20 s in order to avoid a rundown. Recording pipette contained cesium-based solution with QX-314 and MgATP. Local brief puff application of ghrelin (100 nM) increased the EPSC amplitude transiently, which was blocked by the GHSR1a antagonist, D-Lys3-GHRP6 (100 μM), and was totally eliminated by the NMDAR antagonist, APV (100 μM). **b.** NMDA spike currents in control (red trace in **b1**), in the presence of D-Lys3-GHRP6 (black trace in **b1**), and in wash (**b2**). Bar graph in b3 represents the occurrence of NMDA spikes per 10 min for a total of 120 min of gap-free recording. **c.** Reversible inhibition of NMDAR-EPSCs by D-Lys3-GHRP6 in the absence of ghrelin. **d1–4.** Spontaneous NMDAR-EPSCs. (Modified with permission from Muniz and Isokawa [19]).

4.3. Ghrelin on NMDA spike currents

NMDA spikes are spontaneously generated local electrical signals at dendritic branches [35] where NMDARs are highly localized [36]. The generation of NMDA spikes is promoted by glutamate spillover at any single point in the entire dendritic tree [37] that may involve extra-synaptic receptors [38]. In our rat hippocampal slice culture, NMDA spike currents were insensitive to exogenous application of ghrelin. However, the generation of NMDA spike currents was blocked by the bath application of GHSR1a antagonist, D-Lys3-GHRP6, in the absence of ghrelin (**Figure 4d**) (*chi-square* = 20.135, $p < 0.045$, $n = 12$, *Friedman one-way repeated measure ANOVA*). The blockade of NMDA spike currents by the GHSR1a antagonist was reversible, and upon washout of D-Lys3-GHRP6, NMDA spike currents recovered. Although we cannot rule out the possibility that D-Lys3-GHRP6 interacted with the NMDAR directly, inhibiting its function independently of GHSR1a [39], our finding of the inhibitory effect of D-Lys3-GHRP6 on the NMDA spike suggests that GHSR1a-mediated intracellular signaling modulates the activity of extra-synaptic NMDARs and supports our interpretation that GHSR1a is likely present on pyramidal cell dendrites with physical proximity to the NMDA receptor.

5. Ghrelin-induced phosphorylation of CREB

The family of CREB (cAMP response element-binding protein) transcription factors is involved in a variety of biological processes including the plasticity of the nervous system [40]. In order for CREB to be active, it needs to be phosphorylated before being translocated to the nucleus. Thus, the identification of a phosphorylated CREB is a reliable assay for predicting the occurrence of plasticity, learning, and memory in neurons. We previously reported in the in vivo-fasting model in rats that metabolic demand stimulated and upregulated the phosphorylation of CREB by twofolds in the hippocampus together with other limbic cortexes such as piriform cortex, the entorhinal cortex, and the cortico-amygdala transitional zone [41]. Here, we discuss the NMDA receptor–mediated and ghrelin-enhanced phosphorylation of CREB in our cultured hippocampal slices.

5.1. Ghrelin-stimulated phosphorylation of CREB

CREB activity was assayed immunohistochemically using a rabbit polyclonal antibody against phosphorylated CREB (pCREB at Ser 133) (Cell Signaling, Danvers, MA) (**Figure 5a–c**). pCREB immunoreactivity was quantified using an auto-segmentation tool provided by IPLab imaging software. Low concentrations of ghrelin in 50 and 100 nM did not have any effect on pCREB expression. However, 200 nM and above concentrations of ghrelin increased the expression of pCREB by fourfolds compared to control ($p < 0.01$) (**Figure 5d**). The magnitude of pCREB expression was not different among 200, 500, and 1000 nM. A steep change in response to differing concentrations of ghrelin may be explained by the unique process of ghrelin des-octanoylation [42]. Finally, the effect of ghrelin was mediated by GHSR1a, since the antagonist of GHSR1a, D-Lys3-GHRP6 (100 μM), blocked the ghrelin-mediated increase in the expression of pCREB (**Figure 5e**).

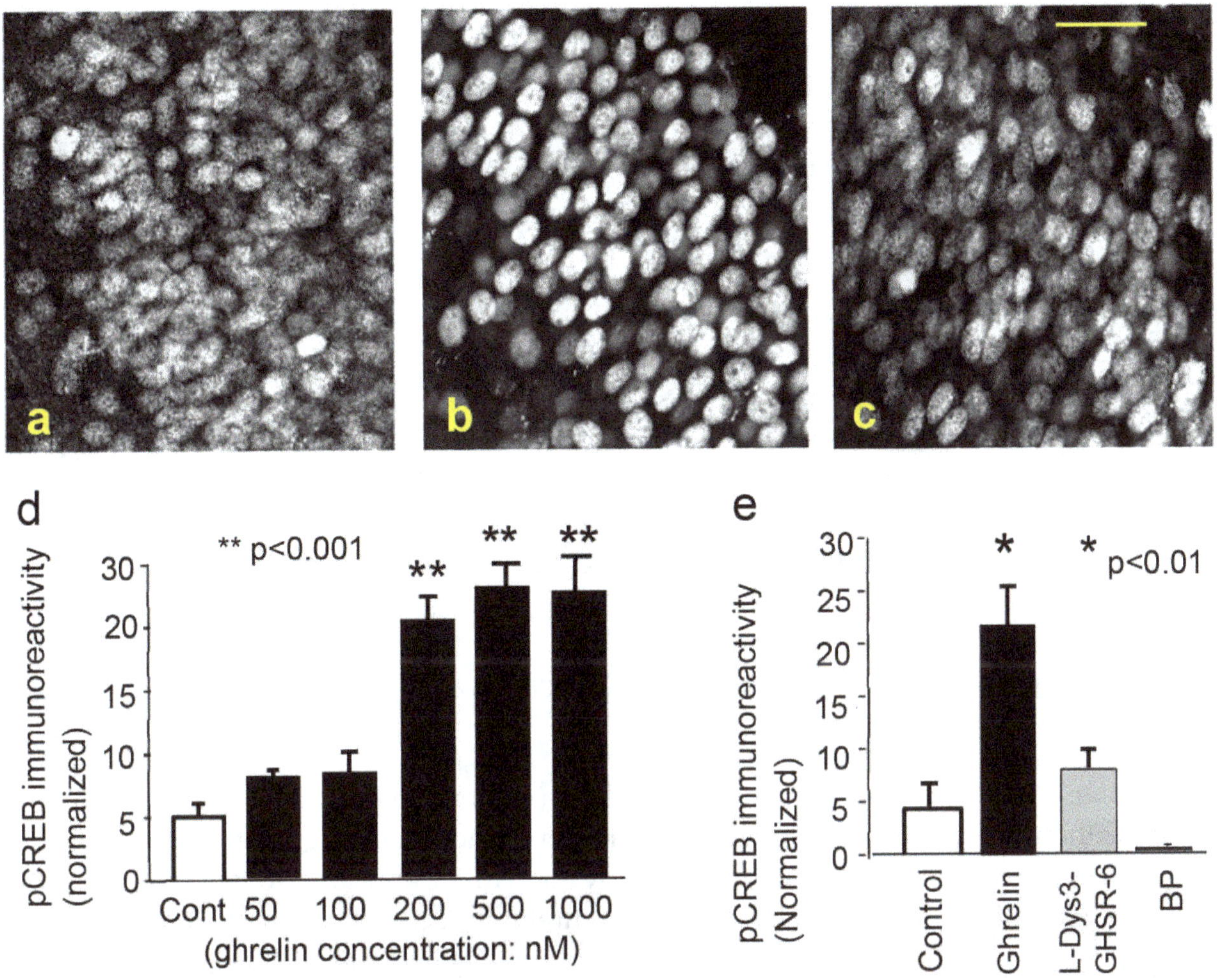

Figure 5. Effects of ghrelin on pCREB. **a–c.** pCREB immunoreactivity in control (**a**), ghrelin (**b**, 200 nM), and in D-Lys3-GHRP6 (**c**, 100 μM). **d.** pCREB in response to ghrelin doses. **e.** Summary graph of pCREB in control, ghrelin, and D-Lys3-GHRP6. Calibration: 30 μm. (Modified with permission from Cuellar and Isokawa [32]).

5.2. Effect of endocannabinoids on ghrelin-mediated upregulation of pCREB

Synergistic involvement of the endogenous cannabinoid system is suggested in the ghrelin-mediated CREB phosphorylation in the hypothalamus [31]. However, in the hippocampus, the contribution of endocannabinoids and the cannabinoid receptor in short- and long-term plasticity has been explained independently of ghrelin and GHSR1a. Furthermore, in Section 3.3, we discussed that ghrelin-mediated enhancement of GluN1 subunit phosphorylation appeared to be negatively modulated, instead of synergistically amplified, by eCBs. Here, we examined potential interactions of the endogenous cannabinoid system to ghrelin-induced hippocampal plasticity at the level of CREB phosphorylation.

A low concentration (20 nM) of R(+)-methanandamide, a nonhydrolyzing form of anandamide, inhibited ghrelin-induced increase of pCREB (**Figure 6**). This inhibitory effect of R(+)-methanandamide was not blocked by the CB1R antagonist AM251 (5 μM) or the TRPV1 antagonist capsazepine (5 μM), suggesting that the action of R(+)-methanandamide on the ghrelin-mediated phosphorylation of CREB may be independent of the CB1R or TRPV1.

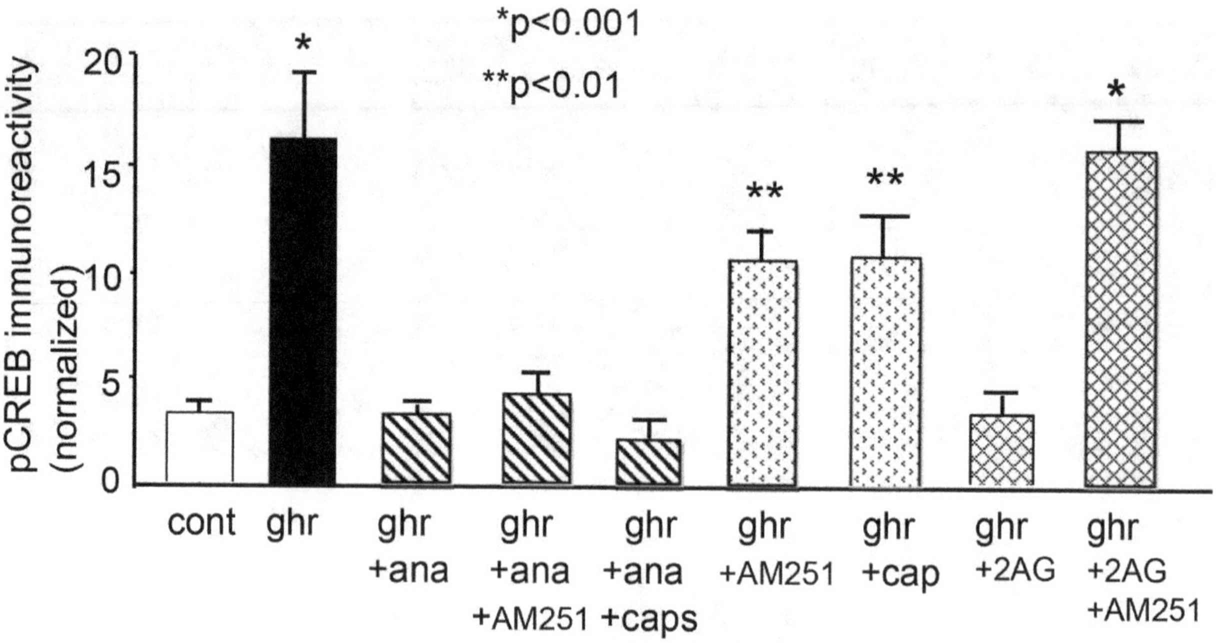

Figure 6. Effects of eCBs on ghrelin-mediated phosphorylation of CREB in the hippocampus. (Modified with permission from Cuellar and Isokawa [32]).

Furthermore, incubation of slices in AM251 alone (without anandamide) or in capsazepine alone (without anandamide) did not block a ghrelin-induced increase in CREB phosphorylation. These results suggested that neither CB1R nor TRPV1 appeared to be involved in the negative effect of R(+)-methanandamide on the ghrelin-induced phosphorylation of CREB.

We next examined the effect of 2-AG on the ghrelin-induced upregulation of pCREB. Similar to R(+)-methanandamide, 2-AG (10 μM) inhibited ghrelin-induced increase in pCREB (**Figure 6**). However, in contrast to R(+)-methanandamide, the inhibitory effect of 2-AG was blocked by CB1R antagonist AM251, suggesting that the action of 2-AG was mediated through the activation of CB1R.

Although we cannot rule out the possibility that eCBs negatively modulated the ghrelin's stimulatory effect on CREB phosphorylation independently of the phosphorylation of the NMDAR GluN1 subunit, our interpretation is that the target of the negative effect of eCBs is the NMDAR, because (1) GluN1 phosphorylation by ghrelin was negated by both 2-AG and anandamide in the identical manner to CREB phosphorylation and (2) the NMDAR is situated upstream of the signaling cascade of CREB activation, having the NMDAR as a necessary molecule in the induction of hippocampal synaptic plasticity.

6. Ghrelin and dendritic spines

CREB-induced gene expression includes reorganization of cytoskeletal proteins. Diano et al. [10] reported that ghrelin upregulated the number of spine synapses in the hippocampus. However, it is elusive whether the increase in synapse occurred on existing spines or on newly generated spines. We examined changes in the number of dendritic spines with a hypothesis that ghrelin might stimulate the generation of dendritic spines. Polymerized actin (F-actin) is highly localized in dendritic spines. Thus, we used phalloidin, a mushroom toxin that has a high affinity to F-actin, as a marker for the identification of dendritic spines. Alexa 488-conjugated phalloidin was visualized and relative changes in fluorescence puncta were quantified using confocal microscope and imaging software (IPLab) (**Figure 7a**).

6.1. Short-term effect of ghrelin on dendritic spines

Ghrelin was applied for 60 min with a concentration of 200 nM to cultured rat hippocampal slices. At the end of the incubation, the slices were fixed with 4% paraformaldehyde and treated with fluorescent phalloidin for confocal visualization of dendritic spines. In control, the average spine density, measured as phalloidin fluorescence was 0.302/unit area ± 0.039 standard error of mean (SEM) ($n = 30$ images taken from 10 slices). Ghrelin increased the average spine density to 0.499/unit area ± 0.058 SEM ($n = 30$, $p < 0.001$) (**Figure 7b**). The antagonist of GHSR1a, D-Lys3-GHRP6 (100 μM), blocked the ghrelin's stimulatory effect on spine generation, and the average spine density returned to the control level (0.333/unit area + 0.041 SEM, $n = 30$). These results suggested that ghrelin may increase the number (or the size) of spines by activating GHSR1a and the downstream-signaling molecules, and that 60 min of incubation in ghrelin is sufficient to induce the generation of "new" spines.

6.2. Long-term effect of ghrelin on dendritic spines

Ghrelin was applied for 23 h at a concentration of 200 nM to cultured rat hippocampal slices. At the end of the incubation, the slices were fixed and treated with fluorescent phalloidin for confocal visualization. Similar to the 60-min application, ghrelin-treated slices expressed a higher density of dendritic spines compared with the control (0.618/unit area ± 0.043 SEM, 30 images from 10 slices, $p < 0.001$) (**Figure 7c**). Spine density remained elevated at the end of the 23-h application. Pre-application of slices with D-Lys3-GHRP6 for 2 h before the application of ghrelin blocked the increase of phalloidin fluorescence, and the spine density stayed at a control level (0.322/unit area ± 0.024 SEM, $n = 30$).

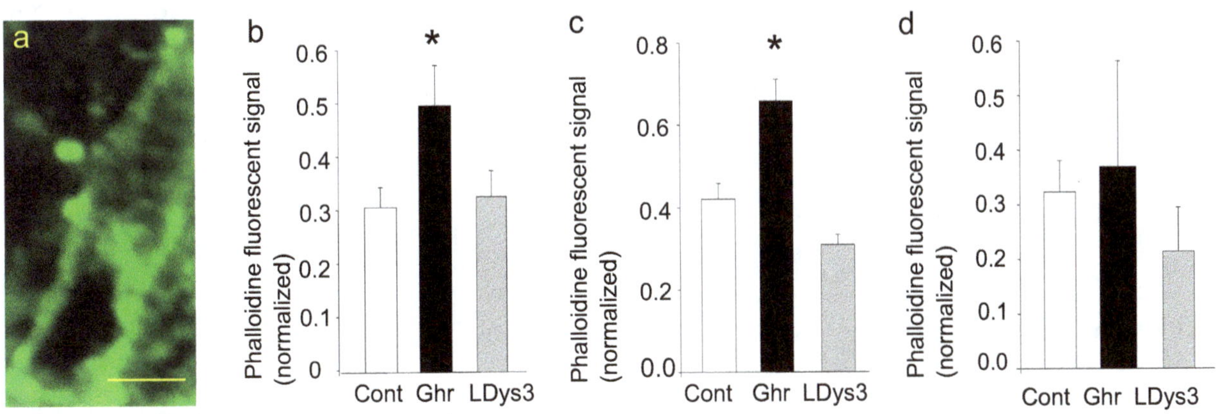

Figure 7. Dendritic spines visualized with Alexa 488-conjugated phalloidin. **a.** Representative phalloidin image. **b.** Phalloidin signals in response to 60-min incubation in ghrelin. **c.** Phalloidin signals in response to 23-h incubation in ghrelin. **d.** Phalloidin signals in response to 22-h incubation in control media after 60-min application of ghrelin. (Modified with permission from Berrout and Isokawa [24]).

6.3. Ghrelin is required to maintain "newly added" spines

Our results indicated that a 60-min application of ghrelin was sufficient to increase spine density. Our results also showed that spine density remained elevated after 23-h application of ghrelin. A question raised from this result is whether the maintenance of elevated spine density in 23 h of incubation with ghrelin really required 23 h of continual availability of ghrelin (since 60-min application was sufficient to increase spine density). In order to answer the question, we incubated hippocampal slices in ghrelin-containing culture media for 60 min, then removed the slices from ghrelin-containing media and incubated in control media for additional 22 h without ghrelin. At the end of the incubation period (of 1 h with ghrelin and the subsequent 22 h without ghrelin), the slices were fixed and treated with fluorescent phalloidin for confocal visualization of dendritic spines. At the end of this combined treatment, spine density was 0.370/unit area ± 0.193 SEM, which was comparable to a control level (0.314/unit area ± 0.057 SEM) (**Figure 7d**). It appears that spine density can increase in response to ghrelin within 60 min and remain elevated for up to 23 h as long as ghrelin is present. However, once ghrelin is removed and no longer available to activate GHSR1a, "newly added" spines retract and the spine density recovers to a control level. In conclusion, ghrelin can add "new" spines to hippocampal neuron dendrites, and that continual availability of ghrelin is a prerequisite together with non-desensitizing activity of GHSR1a for this form of spine plasticity.

7. Concluding remarks

The hippocampus plays a critical role in employing food-searching strategies. Ghrelin is thought to be essential in order to retain memories regarding the spatial localization of food sources [43]. Food search is typically initiated when metabolic demand increases, and the search typically does not end until the metabolic demand is fulfilled. During fasting, a serum ghrelin level increases and stays increased until fasting ends. The rate of ghrelin crossing the blood–brain barrier also increases in a ghrelin concentration-dependent manner [10]. Although it is not known whether the concentration of intrinsic ghrelin in the hippocampus (if any) may fluctuate with metabolic demand, ghrelin can be a key molecule for metabolic demand–induced neuron plasticity in the hippocampus, which serves as a cellular and molecular substratum for food-related memories and learning. Ghrelin-dependent maintenance of plasticity and the loss of plasticity in the absence of ghrelin may nicely explain when and how long such plasticity is required in order for organisms to successfully exercise adaptive appetitive behavior for survival.

Acknowledgements

This work was supported by the NIH (2R15DA021683). The author thanks Dr. Len Luyt at the University of Western Ontario for providing FITC-conjugated ghrelin, and N. Estrada, JN Cuellar, L Berrout, and BG Muniz for their assistance in immunohistochemistry and data analysis.

Author details

Masako Isokawa

*Address all correspondence to: masako.isokawa@utrgv.edu

Department of Health and Biomedical Sciences, The University of Texas Rio Grande Valley, One West University Boulevard, Brownsville, TX, USA

References

[1] Purves D, Augustine GJ, Fitzpatrick D, Hall WC (2012) Neuroscience 5e, Sinauer Associates, Inc., MA, USA, ISBN: 978-0-87893-695-3.

[2] Grace AA, Floresco SB, Goto Y, Lodge DJ (2007) Regulation of firing of dopaminergic neurons and control of goal-directed behaviors. Trends Neurosci. 30:220–227.

[3] Kojima M (1999). Ghrelin is a growth-hormone-releasing acylated peptide from stomach. Nature 402:656–660.

[4] Cowley MA, Smith RG, Diano S, Tschop M, Pronchuk N, Grove KL, Strasburger CJ, Bidlingmaier M, Esterman M, Heiman ML, Garcia-Segura LM, Nillni EA, Mendez P, Low MJ, Sotonyi P, Friedman JM, Liu H, Pinto S, Colmers WF, Cone D, Horvath TL (2003) The distribution and mechanism of action of ghrelin in the CNS demonstrates a novel hypothalamic circuit regulating energy homeostasis. Neuron 37:649–661.

[5] Malik S, McGlone F, Bedrossian D, Dagher A (2008) Ghrelin modulates brain activity in areas that control appetitive behavior. Cell Metab. 7:400–409.

[6] Carlini VP, Ghersi M, Schiöth HB, de Barioglio SR (2010) Ghrelin and memory: differential effects on acquisition and retrieval. Peptides 31:1190–1193.

[7] Ferrini F, Salio C, Lossi L, Merighi A (2009) Ghrelin in central neurons. Curr. Neuropharmacol. 7:37–49.

[8] Andrews ZB (2010) The extra-hypothalamic actions of ghrelin on neuronal function. Cell 34:31–40.

[9] Albarran-Zeckler RG, Sun Y, Smith RG (2011) Physiological roles revealed by ghrelin and ghrelin receptor deficient mice. Peptides 32:2229–2235.

[10] Diano S, Farr SA, Benoit SC, McNay WC, da Silvo I, Horvath B, Gaskin FS, Nonaka N, Jaeger LB, Banks WA, Morley JE, Pinto S, Sherwin RS, Xu L, Yamada KA, Sleeman MW, Tschöp MH, Horvath TL (2006) Ghrelin controls hippocampal spine synapse density and memory performance. Nat. Neurosci. 9:381–388.

[11] Banks WA, Tschop M, Heiman ML (2002) Extent and direction of ghrelin transport across the blood brain barrier is determined by its unique primary structure. J. Pharmacol. Exp. Ther. 302:822–827.

[12] Date Y, Murakami N, Toshinai K, Matsukura S, Niijima A, Matsuo H, Kangawa K, Nakazato M (2002) The role of the gastric afferent vagal nerve in ghrelin-induced feeding and growth hormone secretion in rats. Gastroenterology 123:1120–1128.

[13] Nakazato M, Murakami N, Date Y, Kojima M, Matsuo H, Kangawa K, Matsukura S (2001) A role for ghrelin in the central regulation of feeding. Nature 409:194–198.

[14] Tschop M, Smiley DL, Heiman ML (2000) Ghrelin induces adiposity in rodents. Nature 407:908–913.

[15] Gong Y, Xu L, Wang H, Guo F, Sun X, Gao S. (2013) Involvements of the lateral hypothalamic area in gastric motility and its regulation by the lateral septum. Gen. Comp. Endocrinol. 194:275–285.

[16] Huh CY, Goutagny R, Williams S (2010) Glutamatergic neurons of the mouse medial septum and diagonal band of broca synaptically drive hippocampal pyramidal cells: relevance for hippocampal theta rhythm. J. Neurosci. 30:15951–15961. Doi: 10.1523/JNEUROSCI.3663-10.2010.

[17] Hosoda H, Kojima M, Matsuo H, Kangawa K (2000) Ghrelin and des-acyl ghrelin: two major forms of rat ghrelin peptide in gastrointestinal tissue. Biochem. Biophys. Res. Commun. 279:909–913.

[18] McGirr R, McFarland MS, McTavish J, Luyt LG, Dhanvantari S (2011) Design and characterization of a fluorescent ghrelin analog for imaging the growth hormone secretagogue receptor 1a. Regulatory Peptides 172:69–76.

[19] Muniz BG, Isokawa M (2015) Ghrelin receptor activity amplifies hippocampal N-methyl-D-aspartate receptor-mediated postsynaptic currents and increases phosphorylation of the GluN1 subunit at Ser896 and Ser 897. Eur. J. Neurosci. 42:3045–3053. Doi:10.1111/ejn.13107.

[20] Mani BK, Walker AK, Lopez-Soto EJ, Raingo J, Lee CE, Perello M, Andrews ZB & Zigman JM (2014) Neuroanatomical characterization of a growth hormone secretagogue receptor-green fluorescent protein reporter mouse. J. Comp. Neurol. 522:3644–3666.

[21] Holst B, Cygankiewicz A, Jensen TH, Schwartz, TW (2003) High constitutive signaling of the ghrelin receptor – identification of a potent inverse agonist. Mol. Endocrinol. 17:2201–2210.

[22] Mear Y, Enjalbert A, Thirion S (2013) GHSR1a constitutive activity and its physiological relevance. Front. Neurosci. 7, Article 87. DOI: 10.3389/fnins.2013.00087.

[23] Holliday ND, Host B, Rodionova EA, Schwartz TQ, Cox HM (2007) Importance of constitutive activity and arrestin-independent mechanisms for intracellular trafficking of the ghrelin receptor. Mol. Endocrinol. 21:3100–3112.

[24] Berrout L, Isokawa M (2012) Ghrelin promotes reorganization of dendritic spines in cultured rat hippocampal slices. Neurosci. Lett. 516:280–284.

[25] Camina JP, Carreura NC, Messari SE, Llorens-Cortes C, Smith RG, Casanuev FF (2004) Desensitization and endocytosis mechanisms of ghrelin-activated growth hormone secretagogue receptor 1a. Endocrinology 145:930–940.

[26] Skeberdis VA, Chevaleyre V, Lau CG, Goldberg JH, Pettit DL, Suadicani SO, Lin Y, Bennett MV, Yuste R, Castillo PE, Zukin RS (2006) Protein kinase A regulates calcium permeability of NMDA receptors. Nat. Neurosci. 9:501–510.

[27] Leonard AS, Hell JW (1997) Cyclic AMP-dependent protein kinase and protein kinase C phosphorylate N-methyl-D-aspartate receptors at different sites. J. Biol. Chem. 272:12107–12115.

[28] Camina JP (2006) Cell biology of the ghrelin receptor. J. Neuroendocrinol. 18:65–76.

[29] Kohno D, Gao HZ, Muroya S, Kikuyama S, Yada T (2003) Ghrelin directly interacts with neuropeptide-Y-containing neurons in the rat arcuate nucleus: Ca2+ signaling via protein kinase A and *N*-type channel-dependent mechanisms and cross-talk with leptin and orexin. Diabetes 52:948–956.

[30] Jo Y-H, Chen Y-JJ, Chua SC, Jr., Talmage DA, Role LW (2005) Integration of endocannabinoid and leptin signaling in an appetite-related neural circuit. Neuron 48:1055–1066.

[31] Kola B, Farkas I, Christ-Crain M, Wittmann G, Lolli F, Amin F, Harvey-White J, Liposits Z, Kunos G, Grossman AB, Fekete C, Korbonits M (2008) The orexigenic effect of ghrelin is mediated through central activation of the endogenous cannabinoid system. PLoS One 3(3):e1979. doi:10.1371/journal.pone.0001797.

[32] Cuellar JN, Isokawa M (2011) Ghrelin-induced activation of cAMP signal transduction and its negative regulation by endocannabinoids in the hippocampus. Neuropharmacology 60:842–851.

[33] Al-Hayani A, Wease KN, Ross RA, Pertwee RG, Davies SN (2001) The endogenous cannabinoid anadamide activates vanilloid receptors in the rat hippocampal slice. Neuropharmacology 41:1000–1005.

[34] Spivak CE, Lupica CR, Oz M (2007) The endocannabinoid anandamide inhibits the function of $\alpha 4\beta 2$ nicotinic acetylcholine receptors. Mol. Pharmacol. 72:1024–1032.

[35] Antic SD, Zhou W-L, Moore AR, Hort SM, Ikonomu KD (2010) The decade of the dendritic NMDA spike. J. Neurosci. Res. 88:2991–3001.

[36] Ding JD, Kennedy MB, Weinberg RJ (2013) Subcellular organization of CaMKII in rat hippocampal pyramidal neurons. J. Comp. Neurol. 521:3570–3583.

[37] Chalifoux JR, Carter AG (2011) Glutamate spillover promotes the generation of NMDA spikes. J. Neurosci. 31:16435–16446.

[38] Petralia RS (2012) Distribution of extrasynaptic NMDA receptors on neurons. Scientific World Journal. 2012;2012:267120. doi: 10.1100/2012/267120. Epub 2012 Apr 30.

[39] Pinilla L, Barreiro ML, Tena-Sempere M, Aguilar E (2003) Role of ghrelin in the control of growth hormone secretion in prepubertal rats: interactions with excitatory amino acids. Neuroendocrinology 77:83–90.

[40] Pittenger C, Huyang YY, Paletzki RF, Bourtchouladze R, Canlin H, Vronskaya S, Kandel ER (2002) Reversible inhibition of CREB/ATF transcription factors in region CA1 of the dorsal hippocampus disrupts hippocampus dependent spatial memory. Neuron 34:447–462.

[41] Estrada NM, Isokawa M (2009) Metabolic demand stimulates CREB signaling in the limbic cortex: Implication for the induction of hippocampal synaptic plasticity by intrinsic stimulus for survival. Front. Syst. Neurosci. 10.3389/neuro.06.005.2009.

[42] De Vriese C, Gregoire F, Lema-Kisoka R, Waelbroeck M, Robberecht P, Delporte C (2004) Ghrelin degradation by serum and tissue homogenates: identification of the cleavage sites. Endocrinology 145:4997–5005.

[43] Cong W-N, Golden E, Pantaleo N, White CM, Maudsley S, Martin B (2010) Ghrelin receptor signaling: a promising therapeutic target for metabolic syndrome and cognitive dysfunction. CNS Neurol. Dis. Drug Target 9:557–563.

6

Neuroplasticity in Bipolar Disorder: Insights from Neuroimaging

Marlos Vasconcelos Rocha, Fabiana Nery,
Amanda Galvão-de-Almeida,
Lucas de Castro Quarantini and
Ângela Miranda-Scippa

Abstract

Background: Advances in neuroimaging techniques have produced evidence about disrupted frontolimbic circuits related to emotional regulation. These neuroimaging studies may suggest impairments in cellular plasticity in bipolar disorder (BD) patients. However, the long-term use of mood stabilizers may restore these dysfunctions by neurotrophic effects

Objectives: Review the major structures of the brain that underpin this disorder, synthesize the main findings in neuroimaging in BD, and debate neuroplastic effects of psychopharmacological treatment on findings from the neuroimaging studies.

Methods: We undertook a review from neuroimaging in BD. Search words entered were "bipolar disorder", "mania", "depression", "mixed states", "suicide", "psychosis" "lithium", "mood stabilizers", "neuroplasticity", magnetic resonance imaging", "functional magnetic resonance", "FDG-PET","SPECT".

Results: The literature highlighted specific brain areas that support emotional regulation and processing. Moreover, there is heterogeneity across studies and some findings are controversial, but some results suggest neuroplastic effects from the long-term psychopharmacological treatment (particularly mood stabilizers) in bipolar disorder.

Conclusion: The findings in neuroimaging studies suggest there is fronto-limbic circuitry dysregulation in BD; changes in specific brain areas have been replicated in several studies, which may reflect impairments in neuroplastic phenomena. Evidence from neuroimaging studies have been also show that long-term treatment may be associated with metabolic/functional compensation or structural restoration in bipolar responders.

Keywords: bipolar disorder, neuroimaging, treatment, neuroplasticity

1. Introduction

Bipolar disorder (BD) affects around 3% of the population [1] and is a serious multifactorial disease, caused by combination of genetic vulnerability and environmental stressors with abnormalities in neurotransmitter and neuroendocrine systems, and intracellular signaling pathways as well. Clinically, BD is characterized by recurrent changes of thought, behavior, cognition, mood, and desynchronization of circadian rhythm, which imply in affective phases—mania, hypomania, depression, and mixed states. As a result, BD is a condition often difficult to diagnose, since at least 50% of patients with BD have an initial episode of depression and 35% may have a delay in their diagnosis in up to 10 years [2]. In this context, samples more homogeneous in neuroimaging studies in BD may allow better understanding of BD pathophysiology, through the establishment of putative associations between areas and neuronal circuits and clinical phenotypes, and also to clarify the utility of the various neuroimaging methods for determining potential neurobiological markers of BD.

In this sense, some authors propose concepts in neuroimaging biomarkers for mood disorders, such as *prognostic biomarkers* that characterize the risk for onset or progression of the disease, *predictive biomarkers* associated with the likelihood of therapeutic response, and *pharmacodynamic biomarkers*, which show biological response related to drug treatment [3].

The majority of neuroimaging studies in BD have been demonstrated abnormalities in different cortical and subcortical areas involved in emotional processing and regulation, while *postmortem* histopathological studies of these regions have shown abnormal reductions of synaptic markers and glial cells in prefrontal cortex and hippocampus and point to a dysfunction of the complex intracellular mechanisms, which involve second messengers systems, regulation of the genic expression and synthesis of trophic factors [4]. Overall, these neuropathological and neuroimaging studies may suggest impairments in cellular plasticity and resilience in patients who suffer from mood disorders.

Conversely, a substantial body of evidence suggests that long-term psychopharmacological treatment with antidepressants and mood stabilizers—in particular lithium and valproate—may compensate for this dysfunction by reducing the pathological limbic activity subjacent to affective symptoms and by regulating gene expression of neurotrophic factors that exert neuroplastic effects within the pathways modulating emotional expression. Such effects may be associated with structural restoration or enlargement of specific brain areas in chronically treated BD patients evaluated in multiple neuroimaging studies, when compared to healthy controls [5–7].

Keeping these issues in mind, the purpose of this chapter is to review the major cortical and subcortical structures of the brain that underpin this disorder, describe the main findings in structural and functional neuroimaging in BD, and synthesize impaired major cellular plasticity mechanisms and potential neuroplastic effects of mood stabilizers on structural and functional findings from the neuroimaging studies.

2. Circuits and neuronal models of emotion regulation

- Ventrolateral prefrontal circuit: Constituted by the ventrolateral prefrontal cortex (VLPFC)—Brodmann areas (BA) 10 and 47—which sends fibers to the ventromedial striatum (ventromedial caudate nucleus, ventral putamen, nucleus accumbens, and olfactory tubercle) and which projects to the globus pallidus (GP); pallidal fibers follow for ventral anterior and dorsomedial nuclei of the thalamus, which connects again to VLPFC. The anterior temporal cortex (areas comprising BA 20 and BA 38) maintains reciprocal connections with VLPFC and amygdala [8, 9].
- Ventromedial prefrontal circuit: Formed by the ventromedial prefrontal cortex (VMPFC), defined by BA 11 and 12, of which depart fibers to follow to the ventromedial striatum and ventral caudate nucleus. From these regions, projections run for ventral anterior, dorsomedial and ventrolateral nuclei of the thalamus, closing the circuit with thalamic pathways to the ventromedial cortex. It should be mentioned projections of these cortical areas also to the entorhinal cortex and amygdala—lesion in these areas produces impairment in the allocation of emotional valence of information, a process that facilitates storage of information—as well as reciprocal connections between the insula with the amygdala and the VMPFC [9].
- Anterior cingulate circuit: The ACC is the most part of BA 24, 25, and 32. These cortical areas maintain connections with the ventral medial striatum, of which follow fibers to the rostral lateral and ventral GP, which in turn sends projections for dorsomedial nucleus of the thalamus; fibers depart from this topography and return to the ACC, closing this circuit [8, 9].

The ACC is divided functionally into ventral or "affective" region (more anterior portions of BA 25 [paragenual] and BA 24 [subgenual]) and dorsal or "cognitive" region (posterior prelimbic area [BA 32] and more posterior portions of BA 24).

The affective division of the ACC has connections with the amygdala, the periaqueductal gray matter, the anterior thalamic nuclei, the ventral striatum, and the insula; it contributes to the regulation of endocrine and autonomic functions, generation of appropriate social behavior, and part of the global emotional response by activation of somatic and visceral states relevant to emotional experience; cognitive division includes the posterior portions of BA 24 and 32 and connects to the periaqueductal gray matter and primary and associative cortical motor areas; it is associated with inhibition responses [10] and monitoring conflicts [11, 12].

- Dorsolateral prefrontal circuit (DLPFC) includes BA 10, 45, and 9/46 Brodmann, which covers part of the lateral surface of the frontal lobes. These regions depart fibers to the dorsolateral caudate nucleus, which in turn sends fibers to the GP and then to ventroanterior, dorsomedial, and ventrolateral nuclei of the thalamus; thalamic pathways from these nuclei return to DLPFC [8, 9].

Compounding these circuits, the cerebellum receives cortical projections from nuclei located in the base of the pons; the fibers of the pontine nuclei decussate and follow the middle cerebellar peduncle to specific cerebellar targets: while the motor cortex projects to the cerebellum (paravermian region) through lateral pontine nuclei, associative cortical areas of the prefrontal, parietal, and temporal regions as well as ACC reach the cerebellum through pontine nuclei medial [13].

The amygdala is divided into three major sections: basolateral, corticomedial, and central. The basolateral nucleus participates in the sensory information integration from external and internal environments, which are linked to learned information and are processed by associative cortical areas, with subsequent planning, selection, and implementation of the action; corticomedial nucleus contributes to the presence of emotional attributes related to sensory and nociceptive stimuli; and the central nucleus is the convergence site of all signs of the amygdala. The amygdala regulates the fight, flight, or freeze behaviors together with the periaqueductal gray matter and contributes to motor and autonomic responses to emotional stimuli [14].

Among several neural circuit models related to processes of emotional perception and regulation proposed in the literature, the Mary Phillips and coworkers' model highlights over others [15, 16]. This model proposes the existence of two neuronal systems: a ventral system comprising subcortical (the amygdala, the insula, the ventral striatum) and cortical structures (the hippocampus, the anterior cingulate, and prefrontal cortex) and would be linked to identification of the emotional meaning of a stimulus associated with generation of affective states and autonomic regulation; the dorsal system would be represented by dorsal regions of the anterior cingulate and PFC as well as the hippocampus and would support cognitive processes such as selective attention, planning, performance monitoring, and voluntary regulation of emotional states.

The assessment of neuroimaging findings in BD allows to corroborate the relevance of this model, from the identification of dysfunction in different cortical and subcortical areas—as already stated, structures involved in processing and emotion regulation—abnormal increase in activity of the amygdala during performance of emotional and non-emotional tasks; abnormal decrease in activity of the VLPFC and orbital frontal cortex (OFC); and abnormal decrease in functional connectivity between the amygdala and the prefrontal cortex during emotional regulation tasks. Moreover, in studies involving reward paradigms (anticipation of reward), there is abnormal increase in activity of the ventral striatum, the VLPFC and OFC [17, 18].

3. Main findings of neuroimaging in BD

3.1. White matter

The white matter (WM) hyperintensity is a change often described in BD patients, both in adult [19] and pediatric [20] samples. Among the WM association bundles, the corpus callosum (CC) is one of the structures of great interest in BD research. In this region, studies using diffusion tensor technique (DTI) often show loss of structural integrity of the CC in its various segments (genu, body, or splenius) [21, 22]. Moreover, a recent study conducted by our group evaluated bipolar patients type I euthymic and showed reduction of CC in the areas of the genu and isthmus when compared to healthy controls, confirming data from other studies [23, 24], but with no significant difference between suicide and non-suicidal [25]; a meta-analysis documented the volume reduction of this structure in bipolar patients [26]. Finally, another study found that bipolar patients without suicide attempt had lower values of fractional anisotropy (FA) in the genu and body of the CC when compared to unipolar depressed and healthy controls, and bipolar suicide patients had reduction of FA in all regions of the CC when compared to healthy controls [27]. In addition, more recent studies have shown that in euthymic and non-euthymic bipolar patients with a history of psychotic symptoms was observed higher area of the rostrum of the CC [28] and lower FA in the body of the CC in bipolar euthymic or depressed patients [29]; importantly, changes of the CC have also been described in children and adolescents with BD [30] and in groups of risk for BD, such as first-degree relatives [31].

Furthermore, loss of functional integrity was verified in other associative bundles of white matter, for instance, uncinate fasciculus (which connects the orbital frontal cortex and areas of the ventromedial prefrontal cortex to the amygdala and hippocampus) was studied in some works, in which the results are inconsistent, with bilateral reduction of AF [32, 33] or increased AF to the left in this region [34]. Finally, lower FA in the left orbital frontal WM among patients with attempted suicide, a finding that correlated with higher impulsivity score [35].

Taken together, these findings suggest that WM abnormalities in BD may compromise the interhemispheric neuronal transmission and subsequent emotional processing/regulation—which may represent a potential anatomical biomarker of the disease—and precede the onset of bipolar disorder and predispose to brain development changes during the neurodevelopmental process of the central nervous system (CNS) in children and adolescents.

3.2. Frontal lobe

The anterior cingulate cortex (ACC), dorsolateral prefrontal cortex (DLPFC), and orbital frontal cortex (OFC) represent the most widely studied frontal lobe areas in BD research.

Studies assessed the ACC through MRI showed volumetric reduction of the subgenual AC (sgACC) (areas 24 and 25 Brodmann), a finding confirmed in a meta-analysis [36]. In studies with proton magnetic resonance spectroscopy (H^{+}MRS), reduction of the N-acetyl-aspartate (NAA) and increase of the choline in the ACC are the most consistent results [37]. Interestingly, some studies showed that long-term treatment with lithium increased the sgACC volume [6] and was associated to higher levels of NAA in this region [38, 39]. Additionally, Functional changes on PET studies were observed both in patients at resting state as in those undergoing activation tasks in the CC: most of them show hyperactivity ACC, notably the sgACC in patients in depressive [40] and manic [41] states.

Studies that evaluated the pregenual ACC (pgACC) also reported abnormalities, with reduction of the left pgACC volume, both in adults [42, 43] and in adolescents [44].

Another H⁺MRS study of this region detected in patients with mania increased relationship glutamine/glutamate, a finding that may be related to impairment of glial-neuronal cell interaction in the interpretation of the authors [45].

Some studies have demonstrated reduction in DLPFC volume in adults [46, 47] and pediatric samples [48], whereas other studies using H⁺MRS reported reduction of NAA in this region [49, 50]. At last, hypometabolism of the DLPFC with ^{18}FDG-PET and functional magnetic resonance imaging (fMRI) in patients with BD was found, both in mania [51] and in depression [52–54].

Other studies evaluating the OFC showed reduction of its volume both in adults [46, 55–57] and in pediatric patients [58, 59], but the heterogeneity of their samples may limit the interpretation of results. A H⁺MRS study of this region demonstrated the decrease of the NAA and the choline in hospitalized non-euthymic bipolar patients (mixed or manic episode), but a minority was in use of lithium [60], whereas our group reported normal metabolic levels in medial orbital frontal cortex in BD I euthymic outpatients with and without suicidal behavior [7]. In fact, in our sample, 30.2% of the subjects were prescribed the first mood stabilizer in the year after the first affective episode, 22% after the first year before the fifth year, and 47.8% 5 years after the first affective episode, and it was demonstrated a higher prevalence of suicide attempts in the latter group [61]. These results support the protective clinical effect of the use of mood stabilizers on the suicidal behavior.

Finally, in patients with mania, hypoactivation of the VLPFC and the OFC in fMRI studies was documented [62, 63].

3.3. Amygdala

Volumetric abnormalities of amygdala are among the most common findings, especially in adolescent samples, in which smaller volumes were reported, but with controversial results among adults. While the reduction of the amygdala among adolescents may represent an anatomical characteristic finding of this clinical subgroup, inconsistent results in adults may result from clinical course, the proportion of adult patients with early BD compounding the sample or neuroplastic effects associated with treatment [15].

The studies of fMRI suggest abnormality of the amygdala in response to a variety of experimental paradigms (resting state, processing of emotional stimuli, and cognitive tasks with or without emotional valence) in the context of the various affective states [11]. On the other hand, some authors reported the absence of hyperactivity of the amygdala during euthymia, which may reflect normalization of the amygdala function induced by long-term treatment, possible evidence of neuroplasticity [64].

3.4. Cerebellum

Most structural neuroimaging studies of the cerebellum showed a reduction in the volume of sub-regions of the cerebellar vermis [65–68], and reduction of the cerebellar volume may be associated with genetic predisposition to BD [69]. Additionally, reduction of the density of the gray matter of the cerebellar vermis has been reported in untreated BD patients, but not in patients under treatment, which may suggest possible neuroprotective effects associated with psychopharmacological drug use [70].

3.5. Hippocampus

Data from a meta-analysis that summarized the results of 25 studies of hippocampal structure have found reduced hippocampal volume, especially in bipolar adolescent samples and reported apparent relationship between increased hippocampal volume and lithium therapy, which may explain the non-significant difference in hippocampal volume in most studies with samples of adult patients when compared to healthy controls [71].

4. Evidence of impairment of cellular resilience and plasticity in BD

There is growing evidence in literature of changes of neuroprotective processes and cellular plasticity and resilience pathways in BD from morphometric and neuropathological studies. Particularly, several mechanisms have founded to be involved as putative etiologic theories that underlie the neurobiological basis of BD, including proinflammatory cytokines, intracellular signaling cascades, and disrupted neurotrophic factor pathways.

More specifically, inflammatory mediators, such as interleukins, tumor necrosis factor alpha (TNF-a), and C-reactive protein, may influence several aspects of the pathophysiology of BD through changes in regulation of neuronal excitability, neuronal survival, synaptic transmission, and plasticity [72, 73]. Several studies have demonstrated a low-grade proinflammatory state in BD during euthymia [74–77], whereas both mania and depression seem to be associated with even more increased circulating cytokines [78, 79]. In addition, it has been suggested that proinflammatory cytokines may be one of the mechanisms of progression of BD, according to some studies [77, 80].

In terms of dysfunction of intracellular signaling cascades, there is a solid evidence of impaired regulation of calcium signaling and increased intracellular calcium levels, with subsequent loss of modulation of neuronal and glial activity, increased oxidative stress, and shortened survival cell [81–83]. Besides, Bcl-2, a protein with both antiapoptotic and neuroprotective properties highly expressed in the limbic system [84, 85], is associated with calcium regulation, reducing its release; Bcl-2 polymorphism AA was associated with both higher cytosolic calcium levels in lymphoblasts [86] and age-related decreases in brain gray matter volume [87].

Additional important signaling cascades involved in BD pathophysiology are those associated with members of the neurotrophin family, especially brain-derived neurotrophic factor (BDNF), which exerts its biological effects through activation of intracellular systems, including the extracellular signal-regulated kinase (ERK)/mitogen-activated protein kinase (MAPK) pathway [88].

BDNF is essential for neuroplastic phenomena, such as neurogenesis, neuronal survival, normal maturation of neural development pathways, and synaptic plasticity and dendritic growth in adulthood as well [89], and it has been demonstrated circulating BDNF is reduced during manic and depressive states [90, 91], while ERK/MAPK pathway is an important intracellular mediator of biological effects of neurotrophic factors, acting on several proteins involved in cellular plasticity, such as glycogen synthase K-3 (GSK-3)—a major regulator of apoptosis—and cAMP response element-binding protein (CREB), which is a facilitator of the expression of neurotrophic/neuroprotective proteins such as Bcl-2 and BDNF [92, 93].

Information about histopathological abnormalities of neuronal and glial cells from *postmortem* studies in mental illness is scarce and its interpretation may be limited due to employment of different techniques and presence of confounding factors such as illicit-drugs and alcohol abuse [94]. However, particularly in BD patients, these abnormalities seem to be concentrated on frontolimbic regions associated with emotional regulation, including the DLPFC and ACC [95].

Although histopathological findings vary among regions and layers of the prefrontal cortex in BD patients, the majority of *postmortem* studies points up reductions in the neuronal density and size, glial cell density and changes in protein expression (implicated in the regulation of synaptic plasticity), which likely result from a combination of dendritic atrophy and/or cell loss in the DLPFC and ACC [95].

In this context, it is possible to hypothesize a link among the neuropathological, neuroimaging, and clinical findings, which dendritic atrophy and cell loss may result in reductions of volume in prefrontal areas, as abnormal synaptic interactions among cortical and subcortical brain structures may result in structural and functional intra- and interhemispheric disconnections and culminate in more vulnerability to stressful stimuli from environment, emotional dysregulation, and BD-related affective, cognitive, and behavioral symptoms [96].

However, lithium and valproic acid, respectively, through inhibition of glycogen synthase kinase-3 (GSK-3) and the histone deacetylases (HDACs), regulate the transcription and expression of neurotrophic, angiogenic, and neuroprotective proteins, such as BDNF, glial cell line-derived neurotrophic factor (GDNF), and angiogenic vascular endothelial growth factor (VEGF). Also, lithium in particular acts on factors that affect apoptotic signaling, such as Bcl-2, p53, Bax, caspase, and heat shock proteins (HSP); both lithium and valproate activate ERK/MAPK pathway. Finally, lithium contributes to induction of the ubiquitin-proteasome system and autophagy, two major intracellular quality control mechanisms for protein clearance that prevent abnormal protein accumulation. Overall, these findings highlight the properties of lithium and probably other mood stabilizers to suppress cell death, attenuate neuroinflammation, and promote angiogenesis and cellular plasticity in BD patients, which contribute to the reduction of neuronal loss [5].

However, not all neuroimaging studies show benefits from long-term use of mood stabilizers. For instance, in a study that evaluated both medicated with antipsychotics or lithium manic (most hospitalized) and outpatient euthymic patients and healthy controls using fMRI demonstrated loss of functional connectivity between amygdala and ACC in manic, but not in euthymic patients;

according to its authors, these findings may suggest a state-dependent neuronal dysfunction [97], but these results may be a marker of treatment non-response, since all patients were medicated.

This latter hypothesis has been brought up a longitudinal study in which bipolar I patients were assigned to euthymic, responders, and non-responders to lithium therapy. When baseline and after treatment volumes of the hippocampus, amygdala, PFC, DLPFC, and ACC volumes were compared, there was a significant enlargement in the left PFC and DLPF in bipolar I patients who responded to treatment, and the left hippocampus and right ACC volumes were decreased in non-responders [98].

5. Conclusion

In summary, the main findings in structural and functional neuroimaging studies suggest that there is frontolimbic circuitry dysregulation in BD, characterized by impairment of control of subcortical regions by cortical ones; changes in specific brain areas have been replicated in several studies, which may reflect impairments in physiological neuroplastic phenomena in the central nervous system. However, growing body of evidence from neuroimaging studies also shows that long-term treatment with mood stabilizers may be associated with metabolic/functional compensation or structural restoration, at least in bipolar responders, and neuroimaging techniques may be considered as a potential tool for establishing prognostic, predictive, or pharmacodynamic biomarkers in BD in the future.

Author details

Marlos Vasconcelos Rocha[1, 2*], Fabiana Nery[2, 3], Amanda Galvão-de-Almeida[2, 3], Lucas de Castro Quarantini[2, 3] and Ângela Miranda-Scippa[2, 3]

*Address all correspondence to: mfvrocha@gmail.com

1 Department of Cognitive Neurology, University Hospital Professor Edgard Santos, Salvador, Bahia, Brazil

2 Program of Mood and Anxiety Disorders (CETHA), Federal University of Bahia, Bahia, Brazil

3 Department of Neuroscience and Mental Health, Federal University of Bahia, Salvador, Bahia, Brazil

References

[1] Kessler RC, Demler O, Frank RG, Olfson M, Pincus HA, Walters EE, et al. Prevalence and treatment of mental disorders, 1990 to 2003. N Engl J Med. 2005 Jun 16; 352(24):2515-2523.

[2] Hirschfeld RM, Lewis L, Vornik LA. Perceptions and impact of bipolar disorder: how far have we really come? Results of the national depressive and manic-depressive association 2000 survey of individuals with bipolar disorder. J Clin Psychiatry. 2003 Feb; 64(2):161-174.

[3] Savitz JB, Rauch SL, Drevets WC. Clinical application of brain imaging for the diagnosis of mood disorders: the current state of play. Mol Psychiatry. 2013 May; 18(5):528-539.

[4] Rajkowska G, Halaris A, Selemon LD. Reductions in neuronal and glial density characterize the dorsolateral prefrontal cortex in bipolar disorder. Biol Psychiatry. 2001 May 1; 49(9):741-752.

[5] Chiu TC, Wang Z, Hunsberger JG, Chuang DM. Therapeutic potential of mood stabilizers lithium and valproic acid: beyond bipolar disorder. Pharmacol Rev. 2013 Jan 8; 65(1):105-142.

[6] Moore GJ, Cortese BM, Glitz DA, Zajac-Benitez C, Quiroz JA, Uhde TW, Drevets WC, Manji HK: A longitudinal study of the effects of lithium treatment on prefrontal and subgenual prefrontal gray matter volume in treatment-responsive bipolar disorder patients. J Clin Psychiatry. 2009 May; 70(5):699-705.

[7] Rocha MV, Nery-Fernandes F, Guimarães JL, Quarantini L de C, de Oliveira IR, Ladeia-Rocha GG, Jackowski AP, de Araujo Neto C, Miranda-Scippa Â. Normal metabolic levels in prefrontal córtex in euthymic bipolar I patients with and without suicide attempts. Neural Plast. 2015; 2015:165180.

[8] Tekin S, Cummings JL. Frontal-subcortical neuronal circuits and clinical psychiatry: an update. J Psychosom Res. 2002 Aug; 53(2):647-654.

[9] Strakowski SM, Adler CM, Almeida J, Altshuler LL, Blumberg HP, Chang KD, et al. The functional neuroanatomy of bipolar disorder: a consensus model. Bipolar Disord. 2012 Jun; 14(4):313-325

[10] Zald DH, Kim SW. Anatomy and function of the orbital frontal cortex, I: anatomy, neurocircuitry, and obsessive-compulsive disorder. J Neuropsychiatry Clin Neurosci. 1996 Spring; 8(2):125-138.

[11] MacDonald AW 3rd, Cohen JD, Stenger VA, Carter CS. Dissociating the role of the dorsolateral prefrontal and anterior cingulate cortex in cognitive control. Science. 2000 Jun 9; 288(5472):1835-1838.

[12] Kerns JG, Cohen JD, MacDonald AW 3rd, Cho RY, Stenger VA, Carter CS. Anterior cingulate conflict monitoring and adjustments in control. Science. 2004 Feb 13; 303(5660): 1023-1026.

[13] Parvizi J, Anderson SW, Martin CO, Damasio H, Damasio AR. Pathological laughter and crying: a link to the cerebellum. Brain. 2001 Sep; 124(Pt 9):1708-1719.

[14] LeDoux J. The amygdala. Curr Biol. 2007 Oct; 17(20):R868-R874.

[15] Phillips ML, Drevets WC, Rauch SL, Lane R. Neurobiology of emotion perception I: the neural basis of normal emotion perception. Biol Psychiatry. 2003 Sep 1; 54(5):504-514.

[16] Phillips ML, Ladoucer CD, Drevets WC. A neural model of voluntary and automatic emotional regulation: implications for understanding the pathophysiology and neurodevelopment of bipolar disorder. Mol Psychiatry. 2008 Sep; 13(9):829, 833-857.

[17] Blond BN, Fredericks CA, Blumberg HP. Functional neuroanatomy of bipolar disorder: structure, function, and connectivity in an amygdala-anterior paralimbic neural system. Bipolar Disord. 2012 Jun; 14(4):340-355.

[18] Phillips ML, Swartz HA. A critical appraisal of neuroimaging studies of bipolar disorder: toward a new conceptualization of underlying neural circuitry and a road map for future research. Am J Psychiatry. 2014 Aug; 171(8):829-843.

[19] Soares JC, Mann JJ. The anatomy of mood disorders – review of structural neuroimaging studies. Biol Psychiatry. 1997 Jan 1; 41(1):86-106.

[20] Lyoo IK, Lee HK, Jung JH, Noam GG, Renshaw PF. White matter hyperintensities on magnetic resonance imaging of the brain in children with psychiatric disorders. Compr Psychiatry. 2002 Sep-Oct; 43(5):361-368.

[21] Wang F, Kalmar JH, Edmiston E, Chepenik LG, Bhagwagar Z, Spencer L, et al. Abnormal corpus callosum integrity in bipolar disorder: a diffusion tensor imaging study. Biol Psychiatry. 2008 Oct 15; 64(8):730-733.

[22] Bruno S, Cercignani M, Ron MA. White matter abnormalities in bipolar disorder: a voxel-based diffusion tensor imaging study. Bipolar Disord. 2008; 10(4):460-468.

[23] Brambilla P, Nicoletti MA, Sassi RB, Mallinger AG, Frank E, Kupfer DJ, et al. Magnetic resonance imaging study of corpus callosum abnormalities in patients with bipolar disorder. Biol. Psychiatry. 2003; 54(11):1294-1297.

[24] Atmaca M, Ozdemir H, Yildirim H. Corpus callosum areas in first-episode patients with bipolar disorder. Psychol Med. 2007 May; 37(5):699-704.

[25] Nery-Fernandes F, Rocha MV, Jackowski A, Ladeia G, Guimarães JL, Quarantini L de C, et al. Reduced posterior corpus callosum area in suicidal and non-suicidal patients with bipolar disorder. J Affect Disord. 2012 Dec 15; 142(1-3):150-155.

[26] Arnone D, McIntosh AM, Chandra P, Ebmeier KP. Meta-analysis of magnetic resonance imaging studies of the corpus callosum in bipolar disorder. Acta Psychiatr Scand. 2008; 118(5):357-362.

[27] Cyprien F, de Champfleur NM, Deverdun J, Olié E, Le Bars E, Bonafé A, et al. Corpus callosum integrity is affected by mood disorders and also by the suicide attempt history: a diffusion tensor imaging study. J Affect Disord. 2016 Jul 19; 206:115-124.

[28] Sarrazin S, Poupon C, Linke J, Wessa M, Phillips M, Delavest M, et al. A multicenter tractography study of deep white matter tracts in bipolar I disorder: psychotic peatures and interhemispheric disconnectivity. JAMA Psychiatry. 2014 Apr; 71(4):388-396.

[29] Sarrazin S, d'Albis MA, McDonald C, Linke J, Wessa M, Phillips M, et al. Corpus callosum area in patients with bipolar disorder with and without psychotic features: an international multicenter study. J Psychiatry Neurosci. 2015 Sep; 40(5):352-359.

[30] Caetano SC, Silveira CM, Kaur S, Nicoletti M, Hatch JP, Brambilla P, et al. Abnormal corpus callosum myelination in pediatric bipolar patients. J Affect Disord. 2008; 108:297-301.

[31] Versace A, Ladouceur CD, Romero S, Birmaher B, Axelson DA, Kupfer DJ, et al. Altered development of white matter in youth at high familial risk for bipolar disorder: a diffusion tensor imaging study. J Am Acad Child Adolesc Psychiatry. 2010; 49:1249-1259.

[32] Mcintosh AM, Muñoz-Maniega S, Lymer GK, Mckirdy J, Hall J, Sussmann JE, et al. White matter tractography in bipolar disorder and schizophrenia. Biol Psychiatry. 2008 Dec 15; 64(12):1088-1092.

[33] Sussmann JE, Lymer GK, McKirdy J, Moorhead TW, Muñoz-Maniega S, Job D, et al. White matter abnormalities in bipolar disorder and schizophrenia detected using diffusion tensor magnetic resonance imaging. Bipolar Disord. 2009 Feb; 11(1):11-18.

[34] Houenou J, Wessa M, Douaud G, Leboyer M, Chanraud S, Perrin M. Increased white matter connectivity in euthymic bipolar patients: diffusion tensor tractography between the subgenual cingulate and the amygdalo-hippocampal complex. Mol Psychiatry. 2007 Nov; 12(11):1001-1010.

[35] Mahon K, Burdick KE, Ardekani BA, Szeszko PR. Relationship between suicidality and impulsivity in bipolar I disorder: a diffusion tensor imaging study. Bipolar Disord. 2012 Feb; 14(1):80-89.

[36] Heng S, Song AW, Sim K. White matter abnormalities in bipolar disorder: insight from diffusion tensor imaging studies. J Neural Transm. 2010 May; 117(5):639-654.

[37] Yildiz-Yesiloglu A, Ankerst DP. Neurochemical alterations of the brain in bipolar disorder and their implications for pathophysiology: a systematic review of the in vivo proton magnetic resonance spectroscopy findings. Prog Neuropsychopharmacol Biol Psychiatry. 2006 Aug 30; 30(6):969-995.

[38] Moore GJ, Galloway MP. Magnetic resonance spectroscopy: neurochemistry and treatment effects in affective disorders. Psychopharmacol Bull. 2002 Spring; 36(2):5-23.

[39] Forester BP, Finn CT, Berlow YA, Wardrop M, Renshaw PF, Moore CM. Brain lithium, N-acetyl aspartate and myo-inositol levels in older adults with bipolar disorder treated with lithium: a lithium-7 and proton magnetic resonance spectroscopy study. Bipolar Disord. 2008 Sep; 10(6):691-700.

[40] Drevets WC. Neuroimaging studies of mood disorders. Biol Psychiatry. 2000 Oct 15; 48(8):813-829.

[41] Blumberg HP, Stern E, Martinez D, Ricketts S, de Asis J, White T, et al. Increased anterior cingulate and caudate activity in bipolar mania. Biol Psychiatry. 2000 Dec 1; 48(11):1045-1052.

[42] Fornito A, Malhi GS, Lagopoulos J, Ivanovski B, Wood SJ, Saling MM, et al. Anatomical abnormalities of the anterior cingulate and paracingulate cortex in patients with bipolar I patients. Psychiatry Res. 2008 Feb 28; 162(2):123-132.

[43] Matsuo K, Nicoletti MA, Peluso MA, Hatch JP, Nemoto K, Watanabe Y, et al. Anterior cingulate volumes associated with trait impulsivity in individuals with bipolar disorder. Bipolar Disord. 2009 Sep; 11(6):628-636.

[44] Kalmar JH, Wang F, Spencer L, Edmiston E, Lacadie CM, Martin A, et al. Preliminary evidence for progressive prefrontal abnormalities in adolescents and young adults with bipolar disorder. J Int Neuropsychol Soc. 2009 May; 15(3):476-481

[45] Ongur D, Jensen JE, Prescot AP, Stork C, Lundy M, Cohen BM, et al. Abnormal glutamatergic neurotransmission and neuronal-glial interactions in acute mania. Biol Psychiatry. 2008 Oct 15; 64(8):718-726.

[46] Frangou S. The Maudsley Bipolar Disorder Project. Epilepsia. 2005; 46(Suppl 4):19-25.

[47] Brooks JO 3rd, Bonner JC, Rosen AC, Wang PW, Hoblyn JC, Hill SJ, et al. Dorsolateral and dorsomedial prefrontal gray matter density changes associated with bipolar depression. Psychiatry Res. 2009 Jun 30; 172(3):200-204.

[48] Dickstein DP, Miham MP, Nugent AC, Drevets WC, Charney DS, Pine DS, et al. Frontotemporal alterations in pediatric bipolar disorder: results of a voxel-based morphometry study. Arch Gen Psychiatry. 2005 Jul; 62(7):734-741.

[49] Molina V, Sánchez J, Sanz J, Reig S, Benito C, Leal I, et al. Dorsolateral prefrontal N-acetyl-aspartate concentration in male patients with chronic schizophrenia and with chronic bipolar disorder. Eur Psychiatry. 2007 Nov; 22(8):505-512.

[50] Kalayci D, Ozdel O, Sözeri-Varma G, Kiroglu Y, Tümkaya S. A proton magnetic resonance spectroscopy study in schizoaffective disorder: comparison of bipolar disorder and schizophrenia. Prog Neuropsychopharmacol Biol Psychiatry. 2012 Apr 27; 37(1):176-181.

[51] Brooks JO 3rd, Hoblyn JC, Ketter TA. Metabolic evidence of corticolimbic dysregulation in bipolar mania. Psychiatry Res. 2010 Feb 28; 181(2):136-140.

[52] Altshuler L, Bookheimer S, Townsend J, Proenza MA, Sabb F, Mintz J, et al. Regional brain changes in bipolar I depression: a functional magnetic resonance imaging study. Bipolar Disord. 2008 Sep; 10(6):708-717.

[53] Brooks JO 3rd, Wang PW, Bonner JC, Rosen AC, Hoblyn JC, Hill SJ, et al. Decreased prefrontal, anterior cingulate, insula, and ventral striatal metabolism in medication-free depressed outpatients with bipolar disorder. J Psychiatry Res. 2009 Jan; 43(3):181-188.

[54] Hosokawa T, Momose T, Kasai K. Brain glucose metabolism difference between bipolar and unipolar mood disorders in depressed and euthymic states. Prog Neuropsychopharmacol Biol Psychiatry. 2009 Mar 17; 33(2):243-250.

[55] Lyoo IK, Sung YH, Dager Sr, Friedman SD, Lee JY, Kim SJ, et al. Regional cerebral cortical thinning in bipolar disorder. Bipolar Disord. 2006 Feb; 8(1):65-74.

[56] Nugent AC, Miham MP, Bain EE, Mah L, Cannon DM, Marret S, et al. Cortical abnormalities in bipolar disorder investigated with MRI and voxel-based morphometry. Neuroimage. 2006 Apr 1; 30(2):485-497.

[57] Narita K, Suda M, Takei Y, Aoyama Y, Majima T, Kameyama M, et al. Volume reduction of ventromedial prefrontal cortex in bipolar II patients with rapid cycling: a voxel-based morphometric study. Prog Neuropsychopharmacol Biol Psychiatry. 2011 Mar 30; 35(2):439-445.

[58] Wilke M, Kowatch RA, DelBello MP, Mills NP, Holland SK. Voxel-based morphometry in adolescents with bipolar disorder: first results. Psychiatry Res. 2004 May 30; 131(1):57-69.

[59] James A, Hough M, James S, Burge L, Winmill L, Nijhawan S, et al. Structural brain and neuropsychometric changes associated with pediatric bipolar disorder with psychosis. Bipolar Disord. 2011 Feb; 13(1):16-27.

[60] Cecil KM, DelBello MP, Morey R, Strakowski SM. Frontal lobe differences in bipolar disorder as determined by proton MR spectroscopy. Bipolar Disord. 2002 Dec; 4(6):357-365.

[61] Nery-Fernandes F, Quarantini L de C, Galvão-de-Almeida A, Rocha MV, Kapczinski F, Miranda-Scippa A. Lower rates of comorbidities in euthymic bipolar patients. World J Biol Psychiatry. 2009; 10(4 Pt 2):474-479.

[62] Altshuler LL, Bookheimer SY, Townsend J, Proenza MA, Eisenberger N, Sabb F, et al. Blunted activation in orbitofrontal cortex during mania: a functional magnetic resonance imaging study. Biol Psychiatry. 2005 Nov 15; 58(10):763-769.

[63] Mazzola-Pomietto P, Kaladjian A, Azorin JM, Anton JL, Jeanningros R. Bilateral decrease in ventrolateral prefrontal cortex activation during motor response inhibition in mania. J Psychiatr Res. 2009 Jan; 43(4):432-441.

[64] Blumberg HP, Donegan NH, Sanislow CA, Collins S, Lacadie C, Skudlarski P, et al. Preliminary evidence for medication effects on functional abnormalities in the amygdala and anterior cingulate in bipolar disorder. Psychopharmacology (Berl). 2005 Dec; 183(3):308-313.

[65] DelBello MP, Strakowski SM, Zimmerman ME, Hawkins JM, Sax KW. MRI analysis of the cerebellum in bipolar disorder: a pilot study. Neuropsychopharmacology. 1999 Jul; 21(1):63-68.

[66] Mills NP, DelBello MP, Adler CM, Strakowski SM. MRI analysis of cerebellar vermal abnormalities in bipolar disorder. Am J Psychiatry. 2005 Aug; 162(8):1530-1532.

[67] Monkul ES, Hatch JP, Sassi RB, Axelson D, Brambilla P, Nicoletti MA, et al. MRI study of the cerebellum in young bipolar patients. Prog Neuropsychopharmacol Biol Psychiatry. 2008 Apr 1; 32(3):613-619.

[68] Baldaçara L, Nery-Fernandes F, Rocha M, Quarantini L de C, Rocha GG, Guimarães JL, et al. Is cerebellar volume related to bipolar disorder? J Affect Disord. 2011 Dec; 135(1-3):305-309.

[69] Sariçiçek A, Yalin N, Hidiroglu C, Çavusoglu B, Tas C, Ceylan D, et al. Neuroanatomical correlates of genetic risk for bipolar disorder: a voxel-based morphometry study in bipolar type I patients and healthy first degree relatives. J Affect Disord. 2015 Nov 1; 186:110-118.

[70] Kim D, Cho HB, Dager S, Yurgelun-Todd DA, Yoon S, Lee JH, et al. Posterior cerebellar vermal deficits in bipolar disorder. J Affect Disord. 2013 Sep 5; 150(2):499-506.

[71] Danzer R, Kelley K. Twenty years of research in cytocine-induced sickness behavior. Brain Behav Immun. 2007 Feb; 21(2):153-160.

[72] Yirmiya R, Goshen I. Immune modulation of learning, memory, neural plasticity and neurogenesis. Brain Behav Immun. 2011 Feb; 25(2):181-213.

[73] Kapcsinski F, Dal-Pizzol A, Teixeira AL, Magalhães PV, Kauer-Sant'Anna M, Klamt F, et al. Peripheral biomarkers and illness activity in bipolar disorder. J Psychiatr Res. 2011 Feb; 45(2):156-161.

[74] Hope S, Dieset I, Agaitz I, Steen N, Ueland T, Melle I, et al. Affective Symtoms are associated with markers of inflammation and immune activation in bipolar disorder but not schizophrenia. J Psychiatr Res. 2011 Dec; 45(12):1608-1616.

[75] Kim YK, Jung HG, Mint AM, Kim H, Park SH. Imbalance between proinflammatory and anti-inflammatory cytokines in bipolar disorder. J Affect Disord. 2007 Dec; 104(1-3):91-95.

[76] Doganavsargill-Baysal O, Cinemre B, Aksoy UM, Akbas H, Metin O, Fettahoglu C, et al. Levels of TNF-α, Soluble receptors (sTNFR1, sTNFR2), and cognition in bipolar disorder. Hum Psychopharmacol. 2013 Mar; 28(2):160-167.

[77] Maes M, Bosmaus E, Calabrese J, Smith R, Meltzer HY, et al. Interleukin-2 and interleukin-6 in schizophrenia and mania: effects of neuroleptics and mood stabilizers. J Psychiatr Res. 1995; 29(2):141-152.

[78] Kauer Sant'Anna M, Kapczinski F, Andreazza AC, et al. Brain-derived neurotrophic factor and inflammatory markers in patients with early- vs. late-stage bipolar disorder. Int J Neuropsychopharmacol. 2009; 12(4):447-458.

[79] Grande I, Magalhães PV, Chendo I, et al. Staging bipolar disorder: clinical, biochemical and functional correlates. Acta Psychiatr Scand. 2014; 129(6):557-567.

[80] Kato T, Ishiwata M, Mori K, Washizuka S, Tajima O, Akyiama T, et al. Mechanisms of altered Ca^{2+} signalling in transformed lymphoblastoid cells from patients with bipolar disorder. Int J Neuropsychopharmacol. 2003 Dec; 6(4):379-389.

[81] Akimoto T, Kusumi I, Suzuki K, Koyama T. Effects of calmodulin and protein kinase C on transient Ca^{2+} increase and capacitative Ca^{2+} entry in human platelets: relevant to pathophysiology of bipolar disorder. Prog Neuropsychopharmacol Biol Psychiatry. 2007 Jan; 31(1):136-141.

[82] Andreazza AC, Kauer-Sant'Anna M, Frey BN, Bond DJ, Kapczinski F, Young LT, et al. Oxidative Stress markers in bipolar disorder: a meta-analysis. J Affect Disord. 2008 Dec; 111(2-3):135-144.

[83] Bernier PJ, Parent A. The anti-apoptosis bcl-2 proto-oncogene is preferentially expressed in limbic structures of the primate brain. Neuroscience. 1998 Feb; 82(3):635-640.

[84] Liu L, Schulz S, Lee S, Reutiman TJ, Fatemi SH. Hippocampal CA1 pyramidal cell size is reduced in bipolar disorder. Cell Mol Neurobiol. 2007 May; 27(3):351-358.

[85] Machado-Vieira R, Pivovarova N, Stanika R, Yuan P, Wang Y, Zhou R, et al. The bcl-2 gene polymorphism rs956572AA increases inositol 1,4,5-triphosphate receptor mediated endoplasmic reticulum calcium release in subjects with bipolar disorder. Biol Psychiatry. 2011 Feb; 69(4):344-352.

[86] Liu M, Huang CL, Yang AC, Tu PC, Yeh HL, Hong C, et al. Effect of bcl-2 rs956572 polymorphisms on age related-gray matter volume changes. PLoS One. 2013; 8(2):e56663.

[87] Bramham CR, Messaoudi E. BDNF function in adult synaptic plasticity: the synaptic consolidation hypothesis. Prog Neurobiol. 2005 Jun; 76(2):99-125.

[88] Post RM. Role of BDNF in bipolar and unipolar disorder: clinical and theoretical implications. J Psychiatr Res. 2007 Dec; 41(12):979-990.

[89] Cunha AB, Frey BN, Andreazza AC et al. Serum brain derived neurotrophic factor is decreased in bipolar disorder during depressive and manic episodes. Neuroscience Lett. 2006 May; 398(3):215-219.

[90] Machado-Vieira R, Dietrich MO, Leke R et al. Decreased plasma brain derived neurotrophic factor levels in unmedicated bipolar patients during manic episode. Biol Psychiatry. 2007 Jan; 61(2):142-144.

[91] Chen G, Manji HK. The extracellular signal-regulated kinase pathway: an emerging promising target of mood stabilizers. Curr Opin Psychiatry. 2006 May; 19(3):313-323.

[92] Engel SR, Creson TK, Hao Y, et al. The extracellular signal-regulated kinase pathway contributes to the control of behavioral excitement. Mol Psychiatry. 2009 Apr; 14(4):448-461.

[93] Dorph-Petersen KA, Lewis DA. Stereological approaches to identifying neuropathology in psychosis. Biol Psychiatr. 2011 Jan; 69(2):113-126.

[94] Gigante AD, Young LT, Yatham LN, Andreazza AC, Nery FG, Grinberg LT, et al. Morphometric post-mortem studies in bipolar disorder: possible association with oxidative stress and apoptosis. Int J Neuropsychopharmacol. 2011 Sep; 14(8):1075-1089.

[95] Otten M, Meeter M. Hippocampal structure and function in individuals with bipolar disorder: a systematic review. J Affect Disord. 2015 Mar 15; 174:113-125.

[96] Soeiro-de-Souza MG, Dias VV, Figueira ML, Forlenza OV, Gattaz WF, Zarate CA Jr, et al. Translating neurotrophic and cellular plasticity: from pathophysiology to improved therapeutics for bipolar disorder. Acta Psychiatr Scand. 2012 Nov; 126(5):332-341.

[97] Brady RO Jr, Masters GA, Mathewa IT, Margolus A, Cohen BM, Öngur D, Keshavan M. State dependent cortico-amygdala circuit dysfunction in bipolar. J Affect Disord. 2016 Sep 1; 201:79-87.

[98] Selek S, Nicoletti M, Zunta-Soares GB, Hatch JP, Nery FG, Matsuo K, et al. A longitudinal study of fronto-limbic brain structures in patients with bipolar I disorder during lithium treatment. J Affect Disord. 2013 Sep 5; 150(2):629-633.

7

Plasticity of Dendritic Spines: Not Only for Cognitive Processes

Ignacio González-Burgos,

Dulce A. Velázquez-Zamora, David González-Tapia,

Nallely Vázquez-Hernández and

Néstor I. Martínez-Torres

Abstract

Excitatory synaptic transmission is associated with the input of "new" information at synaptic junctions established by dendritic spines. The role that each type of spine plays in the transmission of the synaptic impulses is different. Indeed, there is a close relationship between the shape of spines and the differential processing of the excitatory synaptic information that is relayed to them, influencing in turn the transmission of synaptic information related to several psychoneural processes.

The vast majority of the experimental evidence shows that specific plastic interchanges of dendritic spines' shapes are related to specific functional effects in the postsynapse, i.e., the acquisition or learning of new information (thin spines), or to the storage of information in memory (mushroom spines).

Several brain regions are involved in other functions different than those of a cognitive nature, and all projection neurons in these areas possess dendritic spines. However, the functional significance of the changes that the spines of these neurons express has not been studied. Thus, in this Chapter we will discuss experimental evidence supporting the claim that dendritic spines express plastic changes in some brain regions that are not directly related to cognition, and we will also preliminarily approach their possible functional meaning.

Keywords: plasticity, dendritic spines, synapse, cognition

1. Cognition and noncognition: basic concepts

Person A walks down the sidewalk alongside a fence when suddenly, a dog leaps out behind the fence and barks at Person A. Person A, caught off guard, jerks back and then kicks the fence. Coming to his sense, he realizes that the dog is a harmless little Chihuahua, still stuck behind the fence. Now conscious of the situation, he looks around and sees that various passers-by have been watching him and are laughing at his situation. Feeling exposed, Person A continues walking, now blushing furiously.

Looking at this situation, we might ask, if Person A was going to be embarrassed by his actions, why he reacted the way he did in the first place. Why he did not avoid the scare, and with it, the situation? Why did he kick an object without first working through what it was? This type of event—and Person A's type of reaction—is unrelated to cognition, which is the processing of information that permits the abstraction and manipulation of the environment by way of symbols (language and thought, for example) [1]. In this example, Person A could not place the origin of the stimulus nor relate it to as a previous experience, so his reaction had no cognitive component.

Certain *noncognitive* processes express themselves simultaneously with cognitive processes [2]. These processes arise consciously or unconsciously [3], automatically or implicitly [4]. These noncognitive processes do not require attention, perception, learning, memory, language, or thought for their integration; be that as it may, cognitive processes may be present for the regulation or modulation of those noncognitive ones [5].

Izdar [2] explores the role of noncognitive processes in emotional processing. He mentions that there exists a neural basis for the expression of the emotions that escape cognition and which precede the conscious experience of the stimulus. A series of experiments by LeDoux [6] provide experimental evidence for the two-way configuration for the expression of fear: one of them, the faster, permits the organism to generate a reaction to the stimulus without being fully aware of the situation. Person A's situation illustrates this case clearly.

Noncognitive processing has been the object of conceptual debate, since at one time it was thought that all nerve activity was aimed at the expression of processes related to cognition. Lazarus [7] writes that "cognition is the end of all cortical or subcortical activity." Likewise, Lazarus [8] defends that position by arguing that even simple perceptual phenomena (a type of which can be seen in Person A's case) depend on and create meanings or evaluations with respect to the stimulus. Frijda [9] argues that the nervous system is capable of generating emotions, but only when those emotions had been previously acquired through cognition. Frijda [10] argues that "emotions are the result of meaning, and that meaning is the result of inferences about causes and consequences." However, Zajonc [11] responds to Lazarus with experimental evidence wherein he illustrated the primacy of some noncognitive processes that do not themselves attribute meanings to stimuli. Zajonc mentions that even the integration of information from the retinohypothalamic tract is sufficient for the organism to produce a response, "leaving the attribution of the meaning of the stimulus a synapse away" [11].

Izdar [2] talks about the existing predisposition to argue that cognition is anything that goes hand in hand with learning, memory, and, in general, with "mental" life, leaving aside all those instinctive behaviors or those which present without cognitive acquisition or previous experience. An example of this type of behavior is the sucking reflex, the response to aversive stimuli that presents in infants even without prior cognitive processing to give it meaning. Likewise, the expression of circadian rhythms like the sleep-wake cycle. Some of these behaviors come from ancestral information accumulated in the course of a species' evolution, which shapes the brain architecture in the absence of experience with the environment [12] and that establishes itself in the absence of cognitive processing, serving the latter as a potentiator and moderator in later stages of life. It is worth mentioning that the processing of information can take place even in infants without previous experience or learning, that is, without cognitive processing [13]. The above leads to the argument that the processing of information has as much a noncognitive component as a cognitive one.

One can make a distinction between cognitive and noncognitive processes: a cognitive process depends on experience, learning, and memory, whose neural basis is the function of the areas of association of the cerebral cortex, changing stimuli into abstractions, meanings, and manageable symbols [14]. On the other hand, noncognitive processes have as their neural basis the function of subcortical structures such as the hypothalamus [15], the amygdala [6], and the functioning of primary areas of the cerebral cortex [14] that do not depend on learning, on memory, or on previous experience for the expression of certain behaviors, like sexual ones, those based on the emotional fast track [6], and the execution of voluntary movement; among others.

Noncognitive processing generates controversy within psychological epistemology. It creates a heuristic conflict that requires a solution not only from psychology but also from those sciences that provide evidence about the determinants of behavior.

This chapter presents experimental evidence about: the expression of behaviors that do not depend on cognition, as is the case in sexual behavior, which is expressed by virtue of neurophysiological changes in hypothalamic nuclei as well as in the ventromedial nucleus; about the formation of biological rhythms, like the sleep-wake cycle, which depend predominantly on the function of the preoptical area and the suprachiasmatic nucleus of the hypothalamus; about the execution of voluntary motor activity that depends on the function of the primary motor area; and about the expression of emotions through a fast track that is integrated in the nuclei of the amygdala even in the absence of the participation of the cerebral cortex and, therefore, of conscious experience.

2. Neuronal plasticity

The plastic capacity of the structures related to the expression of some of the previously mentioned behaviors that are usually related to cognition. However, as the experimental evidence presented in this chapter will show, the neural structures involved in those cognitive processes also form a part of the repertoire involved in the variable expression "noncognitive" processes through their plastic capacity.

Transmission of excitatory information between neurons is mediated by the activation of receptors located on dendritic spines. These neural substructures exist in all projection neurons, and by virtue of participating in the functional integration of the afferent information by those neurons, they "add" a psychoneural attribute to the conformation of functions integrated into the corresponding neural circuits.

The dendritic spines are cytoplasmic protrusions that cover varying portions of the tubular surface of the dendrites. Depending on the excitatory afferents, the spines show varying densities and distributions along the length of the dendrites. Although the spines generally translate the excitatory information, the way in which they process it depends on their geometric structure. According to their shape, six types of spines have been described: (1) thin; (2) mushroom; (3) stubby; (4) wide; (5) branched; and (6) double [16, 17].

The primary characteristic of these structural distinctions lies in the presence or absence of a neck and a head. The thin spines have a long, narrow neck that results in a bulbous structure, or "head," whose length is shorter than the neck. The mushroom spines have a short, narrow neck that leads to a head whose diameter and length are greater than those of its neck. Stubby spines are protoplasmic protrusions that show no difference between head and neck and whose length is less than their diameter. Similarly, wide spines show neither neck nor head, but their length is greater than their diameter. Branched spines, for their part, display a narrow neck that emerges from the dendrite and which divides into two similar necks before terminating in two similar heads. Double spines have a neck that emerges from the dendrite and forms a head, which then forms another neck, and which finally terminates in a second head.

Typically, the different types of spines show variable amounts between the neurons that host them, but their proportional density remains relatively similar in all neurons: thin > mushroom > fat > wide > branched > double.

Bioelectrically, thin spines have been linked to the rapid transmission of afferent information and are functionally related to the acquisition of new information (learning). Meanwhile, mushroom spines have been related to the slow transmission of afferent synaptic information and with the storage of the same (memory). The other types of spines have not been much studied. There is, however, evidence that suggests that stubby and wide spines could be related to the regulation of the excitability of postsynaptic neurons, while branched spines could be a transformation of other, larger spines (presumably mushroom spines) into two new (branched) spines—hypothetically thin ones. Finally, no functional evidence of the activity of the double spines has been uncovered, although their geometric structure suggests that they represent two independent sites of synaptic contact.

From this chapter's perspective, thin and mushroom spines are particularly relevant. According to the evidence, both are related to the processing of cognitive information: learning from thin spines and memory from mushrooms. However, it is clear that certain lines of projection neurons—like those located in the primary motor cortex, some nuclei of the amygdala, and certain hypothalamic nuclei, like the ventromedial, the preoptic, and the suprachiasmatic—possess dendritic spines that have shown plastic changes, which have been induced experimentally.

3. Neuronal plasticity in cognitive and noncognitive processes

The hypothalamus is a structure that predominantly participates in the regulation of emotion/affective behavior, in the control of visceral functions, and in the maintenance of the body's homeostasis [18]. The hypothalamus is a structure associated with noncognitive functions. It is neuroanatomically divided into several nuclei, among which is the ventromedial nucleus, which participates in the regulation of sexual behavior in females [18–21]. This portion of the hypothalamus receives information primarily from the medial amygdala and passes the information along to other structures, like the periaqueductal gray and the medulla oblongata, provoking the display of female sexual behavior [21].

Research conducted on the ventromedial nucleus of the hypothalamus has shown the presence of adaptive plastic changes in the neurons of this structure. There is evidence that estrogenic activity reduces the density of dendritic spines on the projection neurons of the ventromedial hypothalamus, thereby facilitating lordosis behavior in female rats [22]. Studies in our laboratory [15] have shown plastic changes in projection neurons in the ventrolateral area of the ventromedial nucleus during different stages of the estrous cycle. Among other plastic changes in the neurons, we observed changes in the densities of spines and in the proportional densities of thin and mushroom spines. The density of spines was greater in diestrus, proestrus, and estrus with respect to metestrus, which was reflected in the greater proportional density of thin and mushroom spines in those stages in which the circulating levels of estradiol are higher. We suggest that these changes are associated with neuroendocrine mechanisms, and that they do not respond to any kind of activity related to cognition. Furthermore, these findings evidence that the functional role of the types of spines that have been classically linked to learning (thin spines) and memory (mushroom spines) would also be linked to other neuropsychophysiological events, beyond those related to the expression of cognitive functions.

The largest number of thin spines in stages like those above could be related to the rapid transmission of synaptic information that is, in fact, mediated by spines with the same geometric characteristics as the thin spines [23–25]. Thus, thin spines would then mediate those changes that in the short term influence female behavior in the shorter phases of the reproductive cycle. Meanwhile, the largest proportion of mushroom spines could be related to the changes that may occur slowly in the formation of patterns of sexual behavior by virtue of the fact that the transmission mediated by this type of spine triggers responses mediated by secondary messengers that, when transmitted to the nucleus, generate the synthesis of proteins [16, 17, 26] capable of modifying the psychophysiology of sexual behavior. Thus, the plasticity of dendritic spines in this region unrelated to cognitive activity might be more related to patterns of synaptic activity. Yes, like those related to cognition, but whose functional significance should be associated with the bioelectric activity that is most fundamental to synaptic activity. Consequently, the interpretation of the plastic changes mediated by dendritic spines should be attributed to the very psychophysiological activity of the noncognitive region in question.

Sensory input is of great importance in the deployment of sexual behavior. Olfactory information that has passed through regions such as the olfactory lobe, the amygdala, the stria terminalis, and the medial preoptic area or the hypothalamus has not yet been involved in nervous centers that give that olfactory information a cognitive character. In all of these structures, it has been seen that exposing rodents to the smell of the opposite sex results in an increase in *fos*-protein, which is related to the corresponding increase in metabolic and cellular activity [27]. Thus, the brain generates a plastic response at the molecular level in the presence of relevant sexual stimuli. Studies of brain lesions have shown that massive damage to the medial preoptic area eliminates sexual behavior of male rates throughout the entire life of the individual [28]. In the case of females, the same occurs when the ventromedial hypothalamus is injured [29], a site that, as has already been mentioned, relates to the organization of female sexual behavior.

Despite those findings, there exists in the literature a vast quantity of work, which mentions the role of the prefrontal cortex—an area clearly associated with cognition—in relation to sexual behavior [30–32]. A study by Agmo et al. [33] reported that injuries to the prefrontal cortex and particularly to regions that receive information from the amygdala considerably delay the onset of sexual behavior. However, that same study reported that once male sexual behavior does begin, it then develops normally despite the injury. These data suggest that the prefrontal cortex could be playing an important role in the integration of the information necessary to initiate the approach during sexual arousal. Moreover, other structures participate in the emergence of sexual behavior as sensory receptors, as well as in the expression of copulatory behavior. It is important to highlight that there exists significant gender dimorphism in humans and rodents related to the structures involved in the expression of sexual behavior [27]. This might mark some tendencies about the way processes not directly associated with cognition could differ with the gender of the individuals.

There is experimental evidence that shows a direct relationship between good and bad performance in cognitive tasks and varying levels of hormones such as estradiol and progesterone during the menstrual cycle. It has been observed that in the execution of cognitive tests involving verbal fluency, perceptual speed, fine motor skills, verbal memory, and working memory, performance is higher during the follicular phase, when the greatest amount of estradiol is present in blood plasma. Likewise, when plasma progesterone levels reach their peak in the cycle—halfway through the luteal phase—performance improves on tests of visual memory, in comparison with the menstrual phase [34, 35]. This suggests that there is a differential modulation of cognitive processes by some ovarian hormones, depending on the variation of their concentrations throughout the menstrual cycle. Fernández et al. [36] conducted a longitudinal study that used fMRI to observe the brain activity of young women as they completed cognitive tests focused on language use during different phases of their menstrual cycle. They obtained data that suggested that the neural recruitment necessary to carry out such tasks is very sensitive to the hormonal fluctuations—progesterone and estradiol—of the menstrual cycle. The results likewise showed that the activity of the cortical areas associated with language varies through the different stages of the cycle, and that both progesterone and estradiol were capable of modulating neuronal plasticity of certain areas during the tests. The influence that hormones—which do not imply any cognitive process—have on tasks that are entirely associated with cognition is remarkable.

As in the case of the female reproductive cycle, other hypothalamic structures play a key role in the establishment of some biological rhythms. The suprachiasmatic nucleus and preoptic area of the hypothalamus are associated with the expression of the sleep-wake cycle. This cycle is regulated by the activity of a number of genes, such as the *per*, *clock*, and *tim* genes, which are transcribed cyclically [37, 38]. From the viewpoint of synaptic plasticity, a study from Girardet et al. [39] on rats showed an increase of afferent glutamatergic synapses toward the suprachiasmatic nucleus of the retina, a phenomenon regulated by the input of photic information [40]. That working group also associated with the synaptic arrangements and the configuration of the glia in the suprachiasmatic nucleus with the entrance of photic information that regulates the sleep-wake cycle.

The suprachiasmatic nucleus is comprised of general bipolar small neurons whose dendrites may branch or not. Those dendrites display the presence of dendritic spines whose distribution is irregular [41] and which establish synaptic contact with 33% of all of the synapses in the said nucleus [42]. Despite the relevance of the eventual synaptic plasticity that could implicate the circadian regulation of the sleep-wake cycle, there are no studies that show variations in the synaptology of the suprachiasmatic nucleus, which strongly suggests that investigations ought to be performed.

Some studies discussed the relevance of the use of diverse techniques to establish which circuits are involved in insomnia in human adults [43, 44]. However, it seems clear that the participation of structures associated with cognition (like the prefrontal cortex) is also linked with the adequate establishment of those circuits that govern the sleep-wake cycle. Among these structures, it has been reported that the medial prefrontal cortex reduces its functional connectivity with the medial temporal cortex [45].

It has also been reported that the medial and inferior prefrontal cortex showed a decrease in activity when performing fMRI [46], and, particularly, it has been shown that pyramidal neurons from the infralimbic cortex layer III experience alternating plastic changes during both phases of the cycle: in the nocturnal phase, neurons show a pattern of dendritic arborization that is more profuse, and a greater density of spines in comparison with the diurnal phase, which could relate to the cyclical activity of the liberation of different neurotransmitters, growth factors, and corticosterone, in association with the afferent activities of the fibers of the suprachiasmatic nucleus [47]. Another study showed a decrease in the gray matter of the orbitofrontal cortex and in the parietal cortex [48]. In these studies, the results were associated with the presence of insomnia. Together, these investigations suggest that the sleep-wake cycle, although it is a biological rhythm, could also be regulated by structures associated with cognition.

Voluntary motor activity is the result of a series of mostly cognitive processes in which certain areas of the neocortex such as the prefrontal cortex, the premotor cortex, the parietal posterior cortex, and the primary motor cortex, as well as subcortical areas such as the basal ganglia, the thalamus, and the cerebellum participate [49, 50]. All these structures form different circuits for programming and establishing the commands necessary for the execution of movement. The information that is processed in them is sent through the spinal cord by the pyramidal tract from the Betz pyramidal neurons in the primary motor cortex. These last neurons perform the final step in circuits, integrating all the information that has been processed previously.

The pyramidal neurons in layer V of the primary motor cortex do not perform cognitive processing of the information they receive, but rather represent the final necessary filter for that information before motor function [49–51]. Little has been studied about the plastic capacity of these neurons. However, there is research that shows that after behaviors with a cognitive component, such as motor learning [52] and self-stimulation [53, 54], changes occur in the dendritic arborization of pyramidal neurons in layer V of the primary motor cortex. At the same time, preliminary studies conducted in our laboratory (submitted to publication) showed a greater density of dendritic spines (thin, mushroom, and branched spines) on neurons in the layer V of the motor cortex of mice subjected to forced motor activity over a week under differing levels of intensity using a treadmill device. The increase in branched spines corresponded directly to the increase in thin spines, a phenomenon that could be interpreted as a circumstantial demand for the integration of information coming to those neurons due to the increased demand for motor performance. For its part, the greater proportion of mushroom spines could be interpreted as the establishment of patterns of motor activity, which adjusted throughout the study to meet the increasing demand for physical effort on the part of the rats.

Another necessary component for the performance of voluntary movement is the adjustment of patterns of motor execution at the cerebellar level, a characteristic that, it has been suggested, is not associated with the processing of cognitive information. In this sense, it has been shown that Purkinje cells of the simple lobe of the cerebellum present plastic changes at the level of their dendritic spines during the performance of moderate motor activity. Such modifications consist of an increase in the stubby dendritic spines, which could be due to the input of excessive afferent synaptic information—inherent in the requirements of motor activity—which stimulates the postsynaptic components (the dendritic spines), thus causing the formation of the type of spines that would regulate the hypothetical hyperexcitability of the Purkinje neurons involved [55].

The role of the cerebellum during motor learning, a cognitive process, has also been approached. Those studies have investigated metabolic activity in the cerebellar cortex [56] and the plastic changes of the dendritic spines on the Purkinje neurons, particularly in the region that corresponds with the paramedian lobe [57]. In keeping with the role attributed to the spines in paradigms involving cognitive activity, the study found that there was a particular increase in thin spines (acquisition of new information, or learning) and in mushroom spines (consolidation of acquired information, or memory).

Overall, the results of research related to the functional activity of the cerebellum suggest that differential regions of this brain structure work in concert as much in cognitive processing—motor learning—as in noncognitive processing—motor adjustments. In both cases, there is evidence of plastic events at dendritic spines level underlying these processes.

As mentioned in a previous section, there exists a debate over the role of cognition in the emotions. There are certain brain structures involved in the neural circuits that lead to the expression of emotions, including the amygdala and the prefrontal cortex. In the noncognitive processing of emotion, the amygdala plays a key role. This structure participates in two distinct ways. In the more direct way, the amygdala receives thalamic sensory afferents that provide the information necessary to generate emotional responses and, given their connections with the hypothalamus, that induce autonomic activation. Moreover, the connections of the amygdala with the periaqueductal gray matter and the medulla give way to the responses of "freezing" or fight/flight, respectively. The slower way for the amygdala to participate is an indirect route in which the prefrontal cortex processes information associated with the emotional significance of experiences, providing the amygdaloid complex with the information necessary to trigger the appropriate response [6].

From the above, it can be concluded that the expression of emotions depends on structures that are related both to the organization of cognitive functions—the prefrontal cortex, in the indirect route—and with noncognitive functions—the amygdala, in the direct route. It has been reported that chronic stress induces an increase in dendrite length, in dendritic arborization, and in the density and length of the spines of the neurons in the nuclei of the basolateral amygdala. In turn, acute stress provokes an increase in the density of spines, which could be associated with an increase in elevated circulating levels of glucocorticoids [58], and it is clear that the neuronal cytoarchitecture of the amygdala related to noncognitive processes is also subject to plastic changes.

It is common to think of us processing emotions either "consciously" or "unconsciously" [2]. From a neuroscientific point of view, these two terms are what we have in this chapter referred to as "cognitive" and "noncognitive." A recent review of Lee et al. [59] discusses the importance of the noncognitive processing of information necessary for the expression of emotions, particularly in individuals diagnosed with anxiety disorders, schizophrenia, bipolar disorder, and stress. This paper makes a clear distinction between the perception of the emotions without the involvement of a cognitive process and the analysis of emotion that involves the assignation of meaning and emotional valence. It establishes that the perception of emotion that would involve structures such as the amygdala, the insular cortex, the anterior cingulate, and the primary visual cortex [60, 61] is a phenomenon in which information is processed about the stimulus that provoked an emotion without cognitive attribution [62] almost like an automatic processing of emotions without being aware of their meaning.

Although conflicting data regarding the structures that participate in this first step of the recognition of emotions [63] exists, it seems clear that the set of brain processes that involve emotional processing are not only limited to cognition, but that there exist other structures and previous, noncognitive processes that lead to emotional experience [2, 11, 13].

4. Conclusions

It should be clear that the processing of synaptic information in distinct regions of the brain is independent of the conceptual aspects of the neuropsychological process in question. Thus, the plastic events that underlie the functional organization of "cognitive" and "noncognitive" processes appear to present common neurophysiological and neuromorphological bases. That is, they consist of adaptive changes in different levels of behavioral organization that, more than depending on the plastic events at a cellular level, depend on the structures involved and on the circuits that they establish among themselves in order to result in the expression of behavior.

Based on that, we would propose the following:

1. The intensification of experimental studies of neuronal plasticity related with "noncognitive" processes.

2. The broadening of the criteria of interpretation with regard to the functional significance of such plastic events.

Author details

Ignacio González-Burgos[1*] Dulce A. Velázquez-Zamora[1,2] David González-Tapia[1,2] Nallely Vázquez-Hernández[1] and Néstor I. Martínez-Torres[1]

*Address all correspondence to: igonbur@hotmail.com

1 Laboratorio de Psicobiología, División de Neurociencias, Centro de Investigación Biomédica de Occidente, Instituto Mexicano del Seguro Social, Jalisco, México

2 Universidad Politécnica de la Zona Metropolitana de Guadalajara, Tlajomulco de Zúñiga, Jalisco, México

References

[1] Gardner, H., (1987). The Mind's New Science: A History of the Cognitive Revolution. Basic Books. New York.

[2] Izdar, C., (1993). Four systems for emotion activation: cognitive and noncognitive processes. Pychol. Rev. 100, (1) 68-90.

[3] Kihlstrom, J.F., (1987). The cognitive unconscious. Science. 237, 1445-1452.

[4] Shiffrin, R.M. & Schneider, W., (1977). Controlled and automatic human theory. Psychol. Rev. 84, 127-190.

[5] Izdar, C.E. & Kobak, R.R., (1991). Emotions system functioning an emotion regulation. In: Garber, J. & Dodge, K.A., (Eds). The Development of Emotion Regulation and Dysregulation. Cambridge University Press. England. pp. 303-321.

[6] LeDoux, J., (2000). Emotion circuits in the brain. Annu. Rev. Neurosci. 23, 155-184.

[7] Lazarus, R.S., (1984). On the primacy of cognition. Am. Psychol. 39, 124-129.

[8] Lazarus, R.S., (1991). Cognition and motivation in emotion. Am. Psychol. 46, 352-367.

[9] Frijda, N.H., (1986). The Emotions. Cambridge University Press. England.

[10] Frijda, N.H., (1988). The laws of emotion. Am. Psychol. 43, 349-358.

[11] Zajonc, R.B., (1984). On the primacy of affect. Am. Psychol. 39, 117-123.

[12] Gonzalez-Burgos, I., (2015). Functional neuroanatomy of the memory systems. In: González-Burgos, I. (Ed). Psychobiology of memory: an interdisciplinary view. Bios Médica. México. pp. 15-49.

[13] Izdar, C.E. & Malatesta, C.Z., (1987). Perspectives on emotional development: I. Differential emotions theory of early emotional development. In: Osofsky, J.D., (Ed). Handbook of Infant Development. Second ed. Wiley-Interscience. New York, U.S.A. pp. 494-554.

[14] Olson, C. & Colby, C., (2013). The organization of cognition. In: Kandel, E., et al. (Eds). Principles of Neural Sciences. Fifth ed.. McGraw and Hill. U.S.A. pp. 318-411.

[15] González-Burgos, I., Velázquez-Zamora, D.A., González-Tapia, D., & Cervantes, M., (2015). A golgi study of the plasticity of dendritic spines in the hypothalamic ventromedial nucleus during the estrous cycle of female rats. Neuroscience. 9, (298) 74-80.

[16] González-Burgos, I., (2009). Dendritic spines plasticity and learning/memory processes: theory, evidence and perspectives. In: Baylog, L.R. (Ed). Dendritic Spines. Biochemistry, Modelling and Properties. Neuroscience research progress series. Nova Science Publishers, Inc. New York. pp. 163-186.

[17] González-Burgos, I., (2012). From synaptic transmission to cognition: an intermediary role for dendritic spines. Brain Cogn. 80, (1) 177-183.

[18] Horn, J.P. & Swanson, L.W., (2013). The autonomic motor system and the hypothalamus. In: Kandel, E., Schwartz, J., Jessell, T., Siegelbaum, S., Hudspeth, A.J. (Eds). Principles of Neural Science. Fifth ed. McGraw Hill Professional. U.S.A. pp. 1055-1078.

[19] Rubin, B.S. & Barfield, R.J., (1980). Priming of estrous responsiveness by implants of 17 beta-estradiol in the ventromedial hypothalamic nucleus of female rats. Endocrinology. 106, (2) 504-509.

[20] Rubin, B.S. & Barfield, R.J., (1983). Induction of estrous behavior in ovariectomized rats by sequential replacement of estrogen and progesterone to the ventromedial hypothalamus. Neuroendocrinology. 37, (3) 218-224.

[21] Guillazo, G., Redolar, D.A., Torras, M., Vale, M., (2007). Fundamentals of neuroscience. Soriano, C. (coord.); UOC, Barcelona.

[22] Calizo, L.H. & Flanagan-Cato, L.M., (2002). Estrogen-induced dendritic spine elimination on female rat ventromedial hypothalamic neurons that project to the periaqueductal gray. J. Comp. Neurol. 447, (3) 234-248.

[23] Harris, K.M., Jensen, F.E., Tsao, B., (1992). Three-dimensional structure of dendritic spines and synapses in rat hippocampus (CA1) at postnatal day 15 and adult ages: implications for the maturation of synaptic physiology and long-term potentiation. J. Neurosci. 12, (7) 2685-2705.

[24] Koch, C., Zador, A., Brown, T.H., (1992). Dendritic spines: convergence of theory and experiment. Science. 256, (5059) 973-974.

[25] Koch, C., Zador, A., (1993). The function of dendritic spines: devices subserving biochemical rather than electrical compartmentalization. J. Neurosci. 13, (2) 413-422.

[26] González-Burgos, I., González-Tapia, D., Feria-Velasco, A., (2015). Neuronal plasticity associated to learning and memory. In: González-Burgos, I. (Ed). Psychobiology of memory: an interdisciplinary view. México. Bios Médica. pp. 159-190.

[27] Agmo, A., (2015). Brain circuits relevant to sexual behavior. In: Hernández-González, M., Sanz-Martin, A., & Guevara-Pérez, M.A. (Eds). Brain circuits involved in cognition and behavior. University of Guadalajara. México. pp. 17-46.

[28] Heimer, M. & Larsson, K., (1966). Impairment of mating behavior in male rats following lesions in the preoptic-anterior hypothalamic continuum. Brain Res. 3, 248-263.

[29] Agmo, A., (2007). Functional and Dysfunctional Sexual Behavior. A Synthesis of Neuroscience and Comparative Psychology. Academic Press: San Diego. E.U.A.

[30] Agmo, A., (2015). The role of the prefrontal cortex in male sexual behavior. In: Hernández-González, M., Chacón-Gutiérrez, L., Barradas-Bribiesca, J.A., Guevara-Pérez, M.A. (Eds). Prefrontal cortex. Cognition and behavior. University of Guanajuato. México. pp. 295-328.

[31] Davis, J.F., Loos, M., Di Sebastiano, A.R., Brown, J.L., Lehman, M.N., & Coolen, L.M., (2010). Lesions of the medial prefrontal cortex cause maladaptive sexual behavior in male rats. Biol. Psychiatry. 67, (12) 1199-1204.

[32] Balfour, M.E., Brown, J.L., Yu, L., & Coolen, L.M., (2006). Potential contributions of afferents from medial prefrontal cortex to neural activation following sexual behavior in the male rat. Neuroscience. 137, (4) 1259-1276.

[33] Agmo, A., Villalpando, A., Picker, Z., & Fernández, H., (1995). Lesions of the medial prefrontal cortex and sexual behavior in the male rat. Brain Res. 696, 177-186.

[34] Hausmann, M., (2010). Hormonal effects on the plasticity of cognitive brain functions. Wiley Interdiscip. Rev. Cogn. Sci. 1, (4) 607-612.

[35] Cervantes, J.M., Velázquez-Zamora, D., González-Burgos, I., (2015). Estrogenic modulation of cognitive functions during the menstrual cycle and menopause. In: González-Burgos, I. (Ed). Psychobiology of memory: an interdisciplinary view. México. Bios Médica. pp. 263-290.

[36] Fernández, G., Weis, S., Stoffel-Wagner, B., Tendolkar, I., Reuber, M., Beyenburg, S., Klaver, P., Fell, J., de Greiff, A., Ruhlmann, J., Reul, J., & Elger, C.E., (2003). Menstrual cycle-dependent neural plasticity in the adult human brain is hormone, task, and region specific. J. Neurosci. 23, (9) 3790-3795.

[37] Fort, P., Bassetti, L., & Luppi, T.H., (2009). Alternating vigilance state: new insights regarding neuronal networks and mechanisms. Eur. J. Neurosci. 29, 1741-1753.

[38] King, P. & Takahashi, S., (2000). Molecular genetics of circadian rhythms in mammals. Annu. Rev. Neurosci. 23, 713-742.

[39] Girardet, C., Blanchard, M.P., Ferracci, G., Lévêque, C., Moreno, M., François-Bellan, A.M., Becquet, D., Bosler, O., (2010). Daily changes in synaptic innervation of PVI neurons in the rat suprachiasmatic nucleus: contribution of glutamatergic afferents. Eur. J. Neurosci. 31, (2) 359-370.

[40] Girardet, C., Becquet, D., Blanchard, M.P., François-Bellan, A.M., & Bosler, O., (2010). Neuroglial and synaptic rearrangements associated with photic entrainment of the circadian clock in the suprachiasmatic nucleus. Eur. J. Neurosci. 32, (12) 2133-2142.

[41] Millhouse, O.E., (1979). A Golgi anatomy of the rodent hypothalamus. In: Morgane, P.J., Panksepp, J. (Eds). Handbook of the Hypothalamus. Marcel Dekker. USA. pp. 221-265.

[42] Güldner, F.H., (1976). Synaptology of the rat suprachiasmatic nucleus. Cell Tissue Res. 165, (4) 509-544.

[43] O'Bryne, J.N., Berman-Rosa, M., Gouin, J.P., & Dang-Vu, T.T., (2014). Neuroimaging findings in primary insomnia. Pathol. Biol. Paris. 62, (5) 262-269.

[44] Desseilles, M., Dang-Vu, T., Schabus, B., Sterpenich, V., Maquet, P., & Schwartz, S., (2008). Neuroimaging insights into the patophysiology of sleep disorders. Sleep. 31, (6) 777-794.

[45] Nie, X., Shao, Y., Liu, S.Y., Li, H.J., Wan, A.L., Nie, S., Peng, D.C., & Dai, X.J., (2015). Functional connectivity of paired default mode network subregions in primary insomnia. Neuropsychiatr. Dis. Treat. 11, 3085-3093.

[46] Altena, E., Van Der Werf, Y.D., Sanz-Ariquita, E.J., Voorn, T.A., Rombouts, S.A., Kuijer, J.P., & Van Someren, E.J., (2008). Prefrontal hypoactivation and recovery in insomnia. Sleep. 31, (9) 1271-1276.

[47] Perez-Cruz, C., Simon, M., Flügge, G., Fuchs, E., Czéh, B., (2009). Diurnal rhythm and stress regulate dendritic architecture and spine density of pyramidal neurons in the rat infralimbic cortex. Behav. Brain Res. 205, (2) 406-413.

[48] Altena, E., Vrenken, H., Van Der Werf, Y.D., van den Heuvel, O.A., & Van Someren, E.J., (2010). Reduced orbitofrontal and parietal gray matter in chronic insomnia: a voxel-based morphometric study. Biol. Pshychiatry. 67, (2) 182-185.

[49] Amaral, D, (2013). The functional organization of perception and movement. In: Kandel, E., Schwartz, J., Jessell, T., Siegelbaum, S., Hudspeth, A.J. (Eds). Principles of Neural Science. Fifth ed. McGraw Hill Professional. U.S.A. pp. 356-369.

[50] Kalaska, J.F. & Rizzolatti, G., (2013). Voluntary movement: the primary motor cortex. In: Kandel, E., et al. (Eds). Principles of Neural Sciences. Fifth ed. McGraw and Hill. U.S.A. pp. 835-864.

[51] Noback, R. & Demarest, R., (1975). The Human Nervous System. Basic Principles of Neurobiology. McGraw-Hill. EUA.

[52] Gloor, C., Luft, A.R., & Hosp, J.A., (2015). Biphasic plasticity of dendritic fields in layer V motor neurons in response to motor learning. Neurobiol. Learn. Mem. 125, 189-194.

[53] Rao, B.S., Desiraju, T., Meti, B.L., & Raju, T.R., (1994). Plasticity of hippocampal and motor cortical pyramidal neurons induced by self-stimulation experience. Indian J. Physiol. Pharmacol. 38, (1) 23-28.

[54] Shankaranarayana Rao, B.S., Raju, T.R., & Meti, B.L., (1999). Self-stimulation rewarding experience induced alterations in dendritic spine density in CA3 hippocampal and layer V motor cortical pyramidal neurons. Neuroscience. 89, (4) 1067-1077.

[55] González-Burgos, I., González-Tapia, D., Zamora, D.A., Feria-Velasco, A., & Beas-Zárate, C., (2011). Guided motor training induces dendritic spine plastic changes in adult rat cerebellar purkinje cells. Neurosci. Lett. 491, (3) 216-220.

[56] Ramnani, N., Tini, I., Passingham, R.E., & Haggard, P., (2001). The cerebellum and the parietal cortex play a specific role in coordination: a PET study. Neuro Image, (14) 899-911.

[57] González-Tapia, D., González-Ramírez, M.M., Vázquez-Hernández, N., & González-Burgos, I., The fast period of motor learning is associated with an increase in thin spines on rat cerebellar Purkinje cells. Behav. Brain Res. Submitted to publication.

[58] Leuner, B., Shors, T.J., (2013). Stress, anxiety, and dendritic spines: what are the connections? Neuroscience. 251, 108-119.

[59] Lee, S.A., Kim, C.Y., & Lee, S.H., (2016). Non-conscious perception of emotion in psychiatric disorders: the unsolved puzzle of psychopathology. Psych. Inv. 13, (2) 165-173.

[60] Suslow, T., Kugel, H., Ohrmann, P., Stuhrmann, A., Grotegerd, D., Redlich, R., Bauer, J., Dannlowski, U., (2013). Neural correlates of affective priming effects based on masked facial emotion: an fMRI study. Psychiatry Res. 211, (3) 239-245.

[61] Brooks, S.J., Savov, V., Allzén, E., Benedict, C., Fredriksson, R., Schiöth, H.B., (2012). Exposure to subliminal arousing stimuli induces robust activation in the amygdala, hippocampus, anterior cingulate, insular cortex and primary visual cortex: a systematic meta-analysis of fMRI studies. Neuroimage. 59, (3) 2962-2973.

[62] Tamietto, M., de Gelder, B., (2010). Neural bases of the non-conscious perception of emotional signals. Nat. Rev. Neurosci. 11, (10) 697-709.

[63] Pessoa, L., Japee, S., Sturman, D., Ungerleider, L.G., (2006). Target visibility and visual awareness modulate amygdala responses to fearful faces. Cereb. Cortex. 16, (3) 366-375.

8

Synaptic Behavior in Metal Oxide-Based Memristors

Ping Hu, Shuxiang Wu and Shuwei Li

Abstract

With the end of Moore's law in sight, new computing paradigms are needed to fulfill the increasing demands on data and processing potentials. Inspired by the operation of the human brain, from the dimensionality, energy and underlying functionalities, neuromorphic computing systems that are building upon circuit elements to mimic the neurobiological activities are good concepts to meet the challenge. As an important factor in a neuromorphic computer, electronic synapse has been intensively studied. The utilization of transistors, atomic switches and memristors has been proposed to perform synaptic functions. Memristors, with several unique properties, are exceptional candidates for emulating artificial synapses and thus for building artificial neural networks. In this paper, metal oxide-based memristor synapses are reviewed, from materials, properties, mechanisms, to architecture. The synaptic plasticity and learning rules are described. The electrical switching characteristics of a variety of metal oxide-based memristors are discussed, with a focus on their application as biological synapses.

Keywords: memristor, metal oxide, synapse, neuromorphic computing, synaptic plasticity

1. Introduction

With the aid of modern technology, human society has entered into a new big data era. Meanwhile, it brings a new challenge to humans for data processing. Despite the great success in the past decades, the traditional computer based on Von Neumann architecture and complementary metal oxide semi-conductor (CMOS) technology is still suffering limitations of dealing with big data while it can only deal with well-defined data. These machines cannot compete with the biological system in solving the imprecisely specified problems of the real world which are very simple for biological beings [1, 2]. Even though the digital computers can emulate some functionality of certain animals with comparable speed and complexity, the energy consumptions increase exponentially as the animal hierarchy becomes higher with a very huge volume. Conversely, the biological brain is a compact dense system which can offer parallel processing, self-learning, and adaptivity with a combination of storage and computation in very low power consumption [3]. In these decades, the implementation of Von Neumann architecture computers to mimic biological systems has been in the form of software but such simulations are not comparable to biological systems in terms of efficiency and speed due to the physical limitation of those digital computers. Even the artificial neural networks based on CMOS-integrated circuits are far inadequate for constructing bionic systems. The truly reason for this drawback is the need to transfer data between a memory(storing data) and a processor(computing based on the data). This requirement of data transfer generates an intrinsic delay and inefficiency, which is a bottleneck for all CMOS-based neural networks [4]. In the past decades, the semi-conductive technology has led to great progress under the aid of the rapid development of the electronic industry, which has promoted the steps forward to develop artificial neural networks. In 2011, the supercomputer Watson, with 2880 computing cores [5], won the human-machine contest which proved that supercomputers have their advantages in some aspects [6]. But the important point that has been ignored in this comparison is the energy consumption and the physical volume of the computers. Watson has thousands of cores and requires about 80 kW of power and 20 tons of air-conditioned cooling capacity [7], while the human brain occupies space like a soda bottle and consumes power of 10 W.

Therefore, an alternative approach to building a brain-like or neuromorphic computational system with distributed computing and localized storage in networks becomes an attractive option [1, 8–11]. The brain-like computational system can outperform conventional computers with good performance in handing the real-time processing of unstructured sensory data, such as image, video or voice recognition, navigation, etc. [12–17]. Also, the brain-like computational system has the advantages of architecture and function compared to conventional computers, offering massive parallelism, small area, scalability, power efficiency, the combination of memory and computation, self-learning and adaptivity [3]. Many researches have helped us understand how neurons and synapses function and revealed how essential synapses are to biological computations, especially in memorizing and learning [18–21]. However, building compact neuromorphic computing systems remains as a challenge, especially for the lack of electronic elements which could mimic the biological synapses. In recent decades, the research of neuromorphic systems is renewed by the understanding of biological neural networks and the emergence of new nanodevices. Particularly, the emergence of the fourth electronic element, memristor [22–28], makes it feasible to construct bionic hardware which will lead to effective, high-performance neuromorphic computing hardware.

In this chapter, we will discuss synaptic devices and summarize the recent progress in neuromorphic hardware, which is based on memristors. In particular, we will focus on a few typical devices based on metal oxides and their key properties served as synapses. We will start with a brief description of memory and the learning of synapses in Section 2. In Section 3, we will elaborate more on these oxide-based memristors (TiO_x, WO_x, HfOx, TaOx, NiOx, etc.) with an emphasis on resistive switching (RS) characteristics, which is followed by neuromorphic computing applications and the underlying physical mechanism. We limit this review to metal oxide-based memristive devices for the emulation of synaptic functionalities and will not cover the literature on neuromorphic circuits.

2. Plasticity and learning of the synapse

In the nervous system, neurons and synapses are the basic units for transit information to the whole biological body. In the human brain, it consists of ~10^{11} neurons and an extremely large number of synapses, ~10^{15}, which act as a highly complex interconnection network among the neurons [29]. Neurons consist of three main parts: a soma, dendrites, and an axon. Neurons generate action potentials (spikes), with amplitudes of approximately 100 mV and durations in the range of 0.1–1 ms in their soma. The spikes propagate through the axon and are transmitted to the next neuron through the synapses. A synapse [30] is a 20–40 nm junction between the axon and the dendrites (shown in **Figure 1**) that permits a neuron (or nerve cell) to pass an electrical or chemical signal to another neuron or to the target efferent cell. Each neuron connects with other neurons through 10^3–10^4 synapses to form a complex network. The information transmission between neurons with the synapses is very complicated which

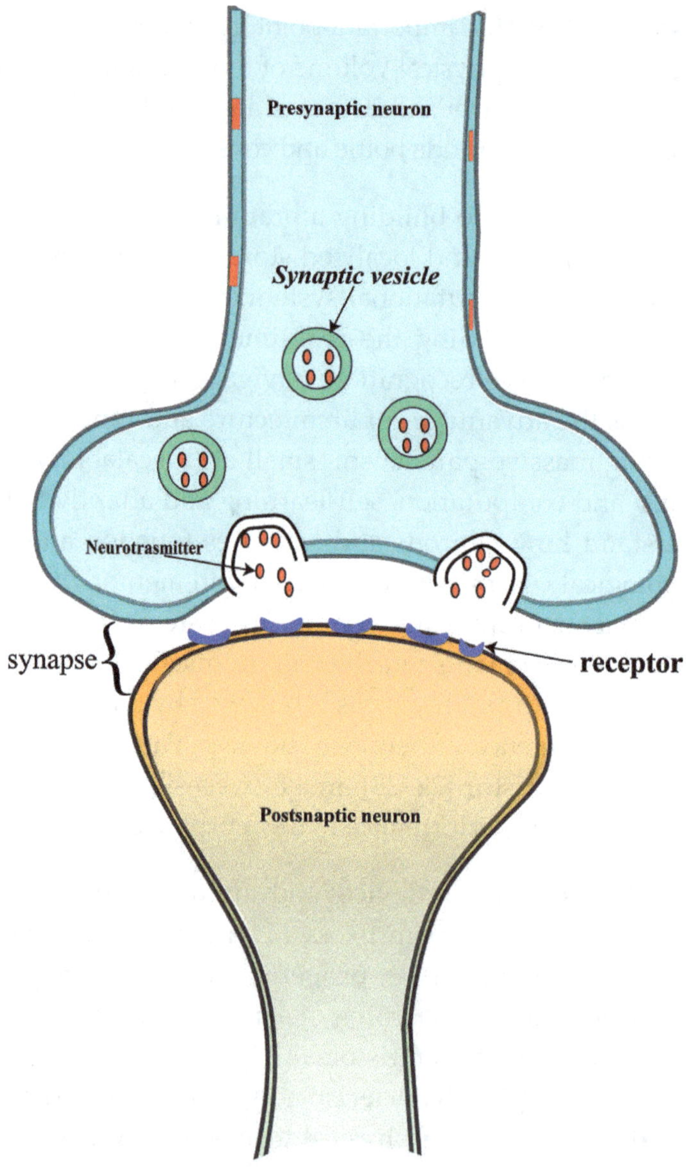

Figure 1. A schematic illustration of synapse.

is excited by the surroundings. At the synapse, the plasma membrane of the signal-passing neuron (the presynaptic neuron) comes into close apposition with the membrane of the target (postsynaptic) cell. Both the presynaptic and postsynaptic sites contain extensive arrays of molecular machinery that links the two membranes together and carries out the signaling process. The presynaptic neuron will open the voltage-gated calcium channels as the action potentials arrive, and then the diffusion of Ca^{2+} ions will make the synaptic vesicle release neurotransmitters to the synaptic junction. Released neurotransmitters bind with their receptor sites of the Na^{+} gated ion channels at postsynaptic neurons, which lead them to open and allow Na^{+} ions to diffuse inside the cell. When the aggregated membrane potential reaches a certain threshold, the neuron generates a spiking. The activation either potentiates or inhibits the postsynaptic neuron. The action potentials propagation, the neurotransmitters release and diffusion, and the neurons spiking activity constitute the ways whereby neurons communicate and transmit information to one another and to nonneuronal tissues [31].

In the biological brain, neurons and synapses are the two basic computational elements connected to each other. To perform different functions including visual, auditory, olfactory, gustatory and tactile means, as well as modulating and regulating a multitude of other physiological processes, the neuron system operates computation by integrating the inputs coming from other neurons and generating spikes across the synapses. In neuron computation, the synapses change their connection strength as a result of neuronal activity, which is known as synaptic plasticity. It is widely accepted that synaptic plasticity is the key mechanism of learning and memorizing for the biological brain [32]. In Hebbian's theory, both pre- and postsynaptic cells are activated coincidently, which results in modifications of synaptic strength between the two cells, thereby creating associative links between them [33]. In other words, the synapse plasticity is triggered by release of neurotransmitters of the presynaptic neurons and by diffusion of calcium ions into postsynaptic neurons, through excitatory amino-acid receptors and possibly voltage-gated calcium channels (VGCCs).

How the brain can achieve learning and memory is a critical question in neuroscience. In 1949 [34], Hebbian postulated a concept of spike-timing-dependent plasticity (STDP), firstly, as a synaptic learning rule which has been demonstrated in various neural circuits over a wide spectrum including insects, animals, and humans, even plants [35–37]. It has attracted considerable interest in neuroscience from experiment to computation [38–41]. According to the asymmetric window of STDP, the synaptic plasticity depends on the order of pre- and postsynaptic spiking within a window of tens of milliseconds. Over the past decades, much progress has been made in understanding the mechanism of STDP. In general, the synapse will be excited (increases in synaptic strength or weight) if repeated presynaptic spikes arrive a few milliseconds before postsynaptic spikes, whereas the synapse will be inhibited (decreases in synaptic strength or weight) if repeated spikes arrive after postsynaptic spikes. In [35], Bi and Poo have plotted a figure of the synaptic weight change as a function of relative timing of pre- and postsynaptic spikes which is called the STDP function or learning window and varies in synapse types. The change of synaptic weight Δw_i depends on the relative timing between presynaptic spike and postsynaptic spikes. A smaller spike timing difference results in a larger increase in synaptic weight. The total weight change Δw_i induced by an impulse with pairs of pre- and postsynaptic spikes is considered as a function [42, 43]:

$$\Delta w_i = \sum_{f=1}^{N}\sum_{n=1}^{N} W\left(t_j^n - t_i^f\right) \tag{1}$$

where $W(x)$ denotes the STDP function, i,j are the notes of the pre- and postsynapses, and t_i^f (t_j^n) labels the firing times of the pre(post)synaptic neuron. An acceptable form of STDP function $W(x)$ is given as

$$\mathrm{W(x)} = \begin{cases} A_+ \exp(-x/\tau_+), & \mathrm{x} > 0 \\ -A_- \exp(x/\tau_-), & \mathrm{x} < 0 \end{cases} \tag{2}$$

The parameters A_+ and A_- depend on the current value of the synaptic weight w_i where τ_+ and τ_- are the time constants in the order of 10 *ms for* biological synapses [36]. Several recent reports have shown the STDP dependencies on rate, higher-order spiking motifs, and dendritic location [39]. This timing-centric view of plasticity is not meant to imply that spike rate is irrelevant. However, this timing-centric view of plasticity is not the only form responsible for synaptic learning in the biological brain. The learning rules may vary with different factors, such as the type, location of a synapse, firing rate, and spiking orders. Several other fundamental learning rules including rate-dependent synaptic plasticity, frequency-dependent synaptic plasticity, and cooperativity have also been studied extensively and believed to be very critical for biological neuron computation.

3. Synaptic devices based on metal oxide memristors

To imitate the learning and memorization of the biological system, new materials as well as architectures exhibiting memristive behavior fit the need well. Memristor, an abbreviation of memory and resistor, is the fourth fundamental passive circuit elements, the others being the resistor, the capacitor, and the inductor, which were proposed theoretically by Professor Leon Chua [22]. It is a kind of a nonlinear, two-terminal element that cannot be replicated with any combination of other fundamental electrical elements. Memristors behaves like a resistor with resistance depending on the history of the current passing through. In fact, it maintains a relationship between the time integrals of current and voltage across a two-terminal element, and the resistance remains in the value as it had earlier when the current stopped. In other words, the memristor has a memory of the current that was last turned on. In 2008, HP Labs realized memristors physically in nanoscale titanium dioxide cross-point resistive switches [24]. In this operation, the device exhibits pinched current-voltage(I-V) hysteresis indicating a resistive memory effect, and the conductive area is adjusted by the concentration of oxygen vacancies, which determine the whole conductive states (resistive switching state), that is, high resistance state (HRS) and low resistance state (LRS). This work invoked a renewable research of new materials and devices that have memristive effects, such as NiO, WO_3 ZrO_2, ZnO, HfO_2, TaO_2, and TiO_2 [44–50] binary oxides, $BiFeO_3$, $SrTiO_3$, $ZnSO_3$, and $LiNbO_3$ [51–54] ternary oxides, and CuO/ZnO, HfO_2/TiO_2 and TaO_x/NiO_x [55–57] heterostructures. **Table 1** gives a summary of the recent work of oxide-based memristors including memristive properties.

Material (architecture)	Endurance (cycles)	Retention	On/off ratio	Reference
$Pt/TiO_2/Pt$	83	10^4s	2	[69]
$Pt/TiO_x/Pt$	8000	—	1.2	[50]
$Pt/Ta_2O_5/Pt$	1000	10 years	10^6	[49]
$Ti/TaO_x/Pt$	120	10^4s	65	[50]
$ITO/WO_3/ITO$	320	2×10^4 s	10	[45]
$Al/WO_3/Pt$	200	3×10^4 s	~50	[79]
$Cu/WO_3/Pt$	150	3×10^4 s	~10	[79]
$Pt/WO_3/Pt$	50	3×10^4 s	~100	[79]
$Cu/WO_{3-x}/ITO$	1000	5×10^4 s	10^5	[80]
Al/ZnO/Al	5	—	54.8	[47]
$Al/ZnO_{1-x}/Al$	5	—	4.8	[47]
Ag/ZnO/Pt	100	10^7s	10^7	[106]
Ti/ZnO/Pt	1000	—	100	[107]
Al/ZnO/Pt	300	10^5s	10^4	[108]
$Pt/ZrO_2/Pt$	200	10^4s	162	[44]
$Cu/ZrO_2/Pt$	50	10^4s	30	[44]
$Ti/ZrO_2/Pt$	100	—	10^4	[109]
$ITO/ZrO_2/ITO$	150	10^3s	~7	[110]
$TiN/ZrO_2/ZrO_{2-x}/TiN$	50	10^4s	40	[110]
$Ta/HfO_2/Pt$	10^{11}	10 years	~100	[111]
$TiN/HfO_2/Pt$	1000	10^4s	~15	[112]
$Ti/HfO_2/Pt$	50	3×10^3 s	100	[100]
$Pt/HfO_2/HfO_{2-x}/TiN$	100	—	1000	[103]
$Pt/BiFeO_3/Pt$	50	2×10^3 s	~100	[51]
$Pt/Ti/Nb:SrTiO_3/Pt$	100	10^5s	~10^3	[105]
$Cu/HfO_2/TiO_2/Pt$	1000	10^3s	10	[56]
$Pt/NiO_x/TiO_2/FTO$	100	10^4s	100	[104]
$Pt/Ti/Ta_2O_5/HfO_2/Pt$	50	2×10^3 s	650	[102]

Table 1. Recent work on metal oxide-based memristors.

Nowadays, the memory is usually referred to as resistive random-access memory (RRAM) devices which can be traced as early as the 1960s [58]. In general, these devices are nanoscale in dimensions and offer excellent performance for data storage in terms of operation speed, nonvolatility, and read/write cycling [59]. Amounts of work have been performed to elucidate types of switching mechanisms that underlie resistive switching phenomena in a broad spectrum of material systems [25–28, 60–62]. According to the switching mechanism, the memristors can be categorized into phase change, valence change, conductive bridge, electrochemical metallization, and ferroelectric devices. Due to the simple structure, biological plausibility, and excellent properties for memory, the scientific researchers explored the application of memristors from data storage to analogy neuromorphic computing for spatial-temporal pattern recognition, sequence learning, navigation, and direction selectivity. As for the human brain-like characteristics, memristor technology could one day lead computer systems to a new state that can remember and associate patterns in a way similar to how people do. Next, we will focus on several kinds metal oxide-based memristors with analog synaptic behavior which are intensively studied for neuromorphic computing.

3.1. TiO_2- and WO_3-based memristors

The first physical instantiation of the memristor was generally acknowledged that was made from TiO_2 by Strukov et al. [24], but as early as in 1968, it was found that the TiO_2 thin-film device shows memristive properties [63]. In literature [63], the work demonstrated that thin films exhibited resistive switching (RS) effects with pinched hysteretic current-voltage (I–V) curves during repeated tests. And also, there are several experimental researches on the RS effect of TiO_2-based devices before 2008, such as Pt/TiO_2/Ru [64] and sputter-deposited Pt/TiO_2/Pt [65] devices. For memristors, the distinctive property is the pinched hysteretic loop indicating no energy dissipation. In [62], the prototype of memristor showed bipolar RS I–V curves with pinched points, which are a result of local stoichiometric change caused by the migration of oxygen vacancies. As oxygen vacancies act as donors in the TiO_2 layer in the depletion zone, the conductance of the device could be modulated by the depletion or accumulation of Vos. Specifically, when the device undergoes a set process from a high resistance state to a low resistance state by the external electric field, the Vos will accumulate resulting in an increase of the conductive layer width. When applying electric pulse with reverse polarity, the Vos will be driven back thereby the conductive layer will become thin. Later it was demonstrated in some studies that the accumulation of Vos in TiO_2 may cause the formation of a new Magneli phase (Ti_4O_7) that is metallic and directly studied by TEM [66, 67]. In 2009 [68], a flexible Al/TiO_2/Al memristor fabricated by solution processing was reported. In this work, it showed that oxygen vacancies were introduced by the aluminum electrodes, and if a noble metal (Au) electrode was used, the form and reversibility of switching will change. The mechanism of the memristive effect strongly depends on the synthesis method, the choice of metal electrodes, and their interfacial properties. Many suggested that an understanding has been put forward through a series of experimental analyses from the view of film composition, microcrystalline structure, and switching zones. It also should be noted that the RS effect of the devices will be affected by device architecture, electrode materials, and layer stacks.

As a prototype of the memristor, TiO_2-based devices show their potential in neuromorphic computing. Seo et al. [69] used titanium oxide as the active material to perform synaptic behavior in the context of analog memory, synaptic plasticity and STDP function. A bilayer of TiO_x and TiO_y structure was fabricated by atomic layer deposition and the sol-gel method, respectively. In the device, the titanium oxide bilayer works as a progressive resistance-changing medium with Al and W as the top and bottom electrodes. The multilevel conductance states were achieved by the movement of oxygen between the TiO_y and the TiO_x layer. In the report, the thickness of the less conductive layer TiO_y was controlled by the applied bias which finally resulted in multi-level conductance and analog memory characteristics. As a positive bias was applied to the top electrode, the oxygen ions were driven from TiO_y to TiO_x and the effective thickness of the TiO_y layer is reduced, which resulted in an increased conductance. Conversely, by applying negative bias to the device, the oxygen ions are moved from TiO_x to TiO_y, which caused a reduction of conductance. Due to the easy controlling of conductance, the analog characteristics of this device have been intensively studied. By applying sets of identical positive (negative) pulses, conductance can be progressively increased (decreased) as well as the potentiation (depression) in biological synapse. **Figure 2** illustrated the continuous potentiating and depressing characteristics of the device which were extremely useful for precisely modulating the device's synaptic weight. Also, the prior conductance state dependence of the subsequent conductance change is shown in **Figure 2b**. The results confirmed that the device showed the behavior as in the biological synaptic STDP model [70]: prior synaptic weight states affect the subsequent weight change. Furthermore, the time dependence of the device conductance change was studied which resembled that of the biological synapse. This indicated the titanium oxide bilayer's resistive switching device had great potential for mimicking biological synapses.

In 2012 [71], Yu fabricated $TiO_x/HfO_x/TiO_x/HfO_x$ multi-layer RRAM stacks and showed that the resistance states of the stacks could be gradually modulated by using identical pulses. The gradual resistance modulation behavior is useful for learning with high fault tolerance. Berdan in 2016 [72] demonstrated that TiO_2 memristors can exhibit non-associative plasticity. The transition between long-term plasticity (LTP) and short-term plasticity (STP) of this device was presented. The rate-limiting volatility in TiO_2 RRAM devices was very essential to capture short-term synaptic dynamics. In addition to Seo's works on the bilayer TiO_x/TiO_y device [69], Bousoulas studied the role of interfaces in TiO_x/TiO_y RRAM structures for high multilevel switching and synaptic properties [73]. A CMOS-memristor architecture composed of the 8*8 array of the neuron was demonstrated by Mostafa [74]. The proposed system comprises CMOS neurons interconnected through TiO_{2-x} memristors and spike-based learning circuits which modulate the conductance of

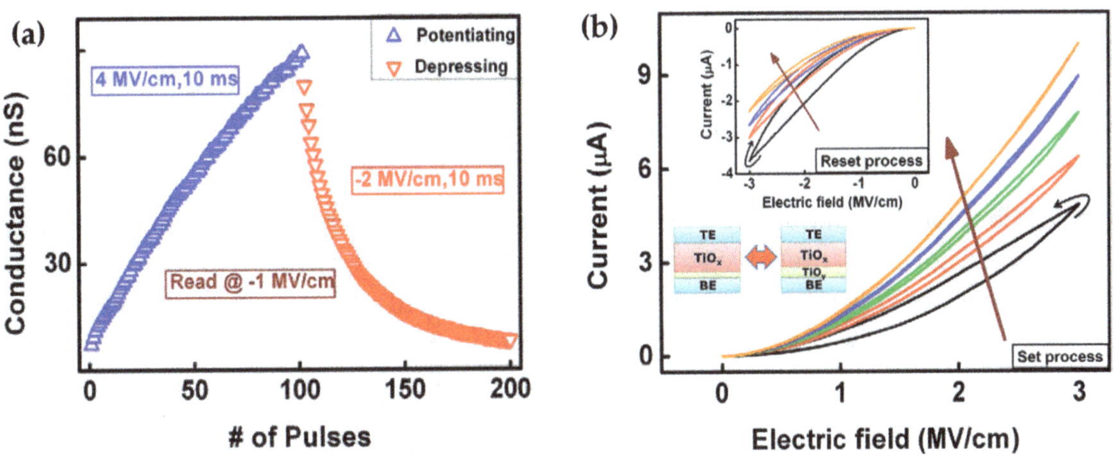

Figure 2. (a) The potentiation and depression for the device and (b) conductance dependence on history. Reprinted with permission from [69].

the memristive synapse elements according to a spike-based perceptron plasticity rule. In 2016, Park developed a Mo-/TiOx-based interface RRAM with 64-level conductance states and proposed a hybrid pulse mode for the synaptic application [75]. Under the stimuli of the hybrid pulse mode, the TiO_{2-x}-based devices show good performance and enhanced pattern recognition accuracy, which was confirmed through synaptic simulation.

Although many investigations have been carried out on the resistive switching mechanism of the TiO_2-based memristor, the demonstration of TiO_2-based memristor for the artificial synapse is still limited when compared to PCMO, HfO_x, and TaO_x materials. In most situations, TiO_x is used in bilayer or multi-layer stacks' synaptic device to optimize the performance. Another great candidate for memristors as artificial synapses is tungsten oxides (WO_x) because of their high endurance, CMOS compatibility, and memorization and learning functions.

Similar to TiO_2, WO_3 is also extensively studied as a memristor due to its CMOS compatibility into standard manufacturing processes [76]. Additionally, WO_3 is a kind of transition metal oxide and can be served as n-type semiconductors depending on its stoichiometry and morphology. Due to its attractive properties, it has been studied for both digital and analog memory. Liu et al. [77] have fabricated Cu/WO_3/Pt structure devices and demonstrated multilevel storage properties by the application of suitable compliance current values. In that study, the device exhibited pronounced RS effects with an endurance of over 100 cycles and a retention of over 10^4 s. During the set process, the conductive filament is modulated by the compliance current between the Cu and WO_3 interface. In addition to the work of Celano [78], the applied positive bias will aid the creation of oxygen vacancies resulting in conductive filaments. The applied negative bias will drive back the oxygen ions to recombine with the vacancies, making the device turn OFF. Meanwhile, the role of electrodes on RS effect has also been studied, such as Ag/WO_3/ITO, W/WO_3/Pd, and Pt/WO_3/ITO [79, 80]. In these studies, no matter the material of the electrodes, the RS effects originate from the formation or annihilation of oxygen vacancies. Under positive bias, the non-inert electrode is oxidized and the ions diffuse toward another electrode to expand a conductive filament and *vice versa*. That is to say, a continuous concentration gradient of oxygen vacancies will be introduced during the oxidation process for the inert electrodes, which can result in low or high resistance states of the devices. In addition, the temperature and humidity impact on the performance of WO_x memristors were studied [81, 82]. The conductance will decrease as the temperature increases due to higher oxygen vacancies' diffusion. In addition to the temperature, the memristive effects of tungsten oxide are also highly humidity dependent. The adsorbed moisture on the surface of WO_3 has resulted in decreasing conductances as the H cation induces an increase in barrier heights.

Synaptic behaviors and modeling of WO_x memristors were reported by Chang [83]. The Pd/WO_x/W memristor shows reliable synaptic operations with robust endurance behavior. The devices can endure at least 10^5 potentiation/depression pulses without degradation which is a necessary characteristic for practical applications in neuromorphic systems. Furthermore, the conductance change is governed by the history of the applied voltage signals, leading to synaptic behaviors including long-term potentiation and depression. The memristor behavior was explained by a novel model that takes both drift and diffusion effects into consideration. **Figure 3** presents the retention loss curve and memory loss in a human memory curve of the Pd/WO_x/W memristor [84]. It was found that the memristor device retention can be improved with the application of repeated stimulations and bears remarkable similarities to the STM-to-LTM transition in biological systems. Among other transition metal oxides, WO_x is a great candidate material for synaptic device application. For further exploring its applications in neuromorphic computing, the enhancement of synaptic operation time (endurance) is of importance.

3.2. Other metal oxide memristor-based synaptic devices

Besides titanium oxide- and tungsten oxide-based memristors discussed above, a variety of other materials has been studied to implement the neural network as a synaptic device. Similar to TiO_x, NiO_x is one of the earliest materials found to exhibit restive switching behavior. Although NiO_x-based RRAM devices have been reported with high endurance (10^6) and retention, its application for neuromorphic computing is restricted due to poor uniformity. Akoh fabricated synaptic devices with bipolar NiO_x memristors [85]. This device also has the ability to update the synaptic conductance according to the difference of pre- and post-neuron spike timing. Hu *et al.* studied the paired-pulse-induced response of an NiOx-based memristor, which is similar to the paired-pulse facilitation(PPF) of biological synapse [86]. In addition to PPF, the synaptic LTP of NiOx-based memristors was also studied by Hu et al. [87]. The LTP effect of the memristor has a dependence on pulse height, width, interval, and number of pulses. An artificial neural network is constructed to realize the associative learning and LTP behavior in the extinction of association in Pavlov's dog experiment.

AlO_x is of interest in memristor materials due to its large band gap (~9 eV) and low RESET current (~ μA). For neuromorphic application, AlO_x can also be used alone or stacked with other RRAM materials to improve the uniformity of the synaptic device characteristics. A GdO_x and Cu-doped MoO_x stack with platinum top and bottom electrodes was reported by Choi [88]. The weighted sum operation was carried out on an electrically modifiable synapse array circuit based on the proposed stacks [89]. The biological synaptic behavior was demonstrated by Chang through integrating SiO_x-based RRAM with Si diodes. The proposed one-diode-one-resistor (1D-1R) architecture not only avoids sneak-path issues and lowers standby power consumption but also helps to realize STDP behaviors [90]. VO_x is a well-known Mott material,

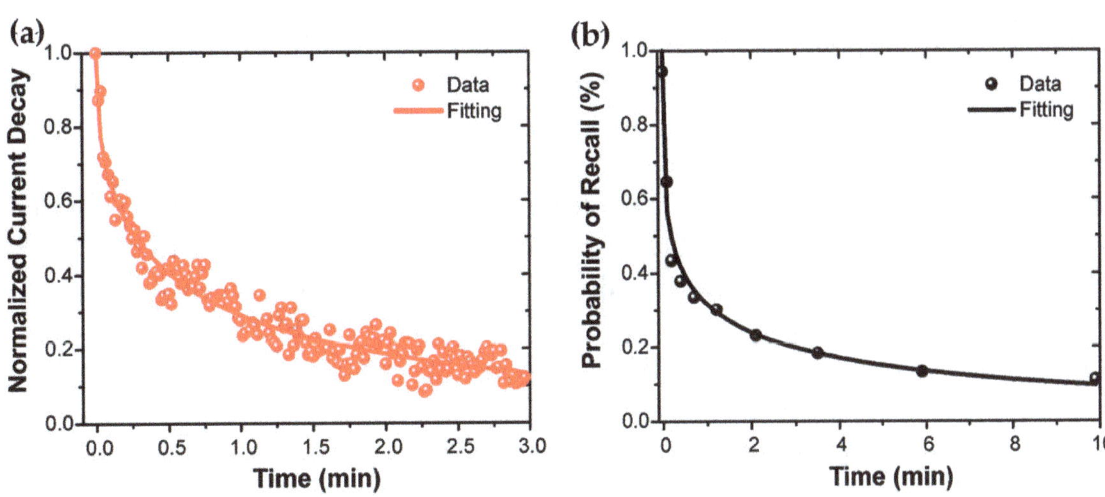

Figure 3. (a) Retention loss curve of Pd/WOx/W-based memristor and (b) forgetting memory of the human memory curve. Reprinted with permission from [44].

which experiences sharp and first-order metal-to-insulator transition (MIT) at the around 68°C [91]. The application of VO_x as RRAM materials had been explored by Drisoll et al. [92] through the sol-gel technique. Nevertheless, most researches on VO_x so far focus on its use for select devices, which can be integrated with the RRAM device to mitigate sneak-path current. The Pt/VO_2/Pt selector has been integrated with NiO unipolar RRAM by Lee et al. [93] in 2007 and ZrO_x/HfO_x bipolar RRAM by Son et al. [94] in 2011. In 2016, 1S-1R configuration of W/VO_2/Pt selection device and Ti/HfO_2/Pt RRAM was demonstrated by zhang et al. [95]. However, thermal instability is a major challenge with VO_2 for practical applications [13].

3.3. Mechanisms

The modulation of the device resistance with memory effects is essential to mimic biological synapse. And the understanding of switching mechanism is also important to incorporate memristors as a bionic synapse into the neuromorphic computing system. Many suggestions have been put forward to elucidate the causes of resistive memory effects of those oxide-based memristors. The most popular views on RS mechanism are taken as ionic diffusion and thermal effect.

For the mechanism of ionic drift and diffusion, under the stimulation of applied bias, the ions will migrate, and the conductance of memristors will be enhanced or depressed [96–98]. Actually, there are two types of ionic drift: cation and or anion drift, which depends on the materials used for active layers and electrodes. For example, for Strukov's [24] TiO_2 memristor, both electrodes have inert Pt; the movement of oxygen vacancies causes the whole active TiO_2 layer to separate into two parts, with one part rich in oxygen vacancies and being more conductive. Hence, the difference in the concentration of oxygen vacancies leads to oxygen ion (anions) diffusion. Oxygen ions move to the anode and more oxygen vacancies are created. The increase of oxygen vacancies then makes the device more conductive to a low resistance state. Meanwhile, there is some evidence that the noninert electrode can hinder the combination of oxygen ions and serve as an oxygen vacancy reservoir. In the set process, the metal is oxidized and the metal ions diffuse into the insulating layer to develop a conducting filament. Under negative bias, the filaments are ruptured by the increase of the electric field.

The second mechanism is about the heating effect [99, 100]. In the set or reset process, the active layer material is changed by the application of an electric field and flowing current heat. As the current is applied, the heat is released and the ions drift, forming an electron path to develop the conductive filament. At the same time, due to the collision of electrons, a new boundary may be created that inhibits the formation of the filament with excess heat [100]. Joule heating effects have been credited both in unipolar and in bipolar switching memories. In unipolar switching, under the high current passing through the memory devices, the heating fuses the conductive filaments in the reset process which is similar to that in bipolar switching. In bipolar switching, Joule heating dissolves the filament when sufficiently high current flows through the device. If this rupture happens in the SET process, it becomes a valid operation since the resistance did not stay in LRS and result in threshold switching [101]. However, large current should be avoided in the device which will introduce bad effects to performance or lead to a permanent failure because large current flowing through the filament will generate severe Joule heating, and a steep increase of the temperature in the filament will finally melt the filament.

Generally, the physical origin of the switching effect in memristors depends on architectures, materials, and interfaces. The comprehensive study of the mechanism is very helpful to the manipulation of memory and to extend the application of memristors. In terms of conductance modulation in memristors, many metal oxide-based memristors can perform not only on digital memory but also on analog memory which is similar to biological functions.

4. Conclusion

In this review, we have outlined an overview of memristor-based synaptic devices, especially for the metal oxide memristors. The neuromorphic approach with oxide-based RRAM devices is promising. Focusing on TiO_x, WO_x-based memristor, the electrical switching characteristics are reviewed. Exploiting the physical mechanisms, the synaptic behaviors of those devices are also discussed. Owing to the magnificent increased computational efficiency, and also increasing compatibility in computer technology and CMOS technology, metal oxide-based synaptic devices are gaining prominent interest. The progress of neuromorphic engineering on devices confirms that the memristive synapses can meet the demand of low energy consumption, high connectivity, and density in neuromorphic devices for efficiently encoding, storing, and processing information. However, challenges still remain for overall oxide-based RRAM materials. Although the inherent fault tolerance of neural network models is able to mitigate the impact of device variation to some extent, the improvement of spatial variation and temporal variation turns out to be one of the greatest challenges on a long-term basis. In addition, the improvement of reliability characteristics of the memristor synaptic devices is another key challenge which is not well studied.

Acknowledgements

This work was supported by National Natural Science Foundation of China (Grant Nos. 61,273,310 and 11,304,399), Natural Science Foundation of Guangdong Province (Grant Nos. 2015A030313121 and 2016A030310234), Scientific Research Fund of Hunan Provincial Education Department (Grant No. 15B203), and the Fundamental Research Funds of Central Universities (Grant No. 17lgpy02).

Author details

Ping Hu[1,2]*, Shuxiang Wu[1] and Shuwei Li[1]*

*Address all correspondence to: huping8@mail.sysu.edu.cn and stslsw@mail.sysu.edu.cn

1 State Key Laboratory of Optoelectronic Materials and Technologies, School of Materials Science and Engineering, Sun Yat-Sen University, Guangzhou, People's Republic of China

2 School of Mathematics and Physics, University of South China, Hengyang, People's Republic of China

References

[1] Mead C. Neuromorphic electronic systems. Proceedings of the IEEE. 1990;**78**:1629-1636

[2] Indiveri G, Liu SC. Memory and information processing in neuromorphic systems. Proceedings of the IEEE. 2015;**103**:1379-1397

[3] Kuzum D, Yu S, Wong H-SP. Synaptic electronics: Materials, devices and applications. Nanotechnology. 2013;**24**:382001. DOI: 10.1088/0957-4484/24/38/382001

[4] Matveyev Y, Egorov K, Markeev A, Zenkevich A. Resistive switching and synaptic properties of fully atomic layer deposition grown TiN/HfO_2/TiN devices. Journal of Applied Physics. 2015;**117**:044901. DOI: 10.1063/1.4905792

[5] Ferrucci D, Brown E, Chu-Carroll J, Fan J, Gondek D, Kalyanpur AA, Lally A, Murdock JW, Nyberg E, Prager J. Building Watson: An overview of the DeepQA project. AI Magazine. 2010;**31**:59-79

[6] Guizzo E. IBM's Watson jeopardy computer shuts down humans in final game. Available from: https://spectrum.ieee.org/automaton/robotics/artificial-intelligence/ibm-watson-jeopardy-computer-shuts-down-humans

[7] Human Watson—IBM. Available from:www-03.ibm.com/systems/hk/resources/systems_zh_hk_IBM_Watson_Human Vs Machine.pdf/

[8] Poon C-S, Zhou K. Neuromorphic silicon neurons and largescale neural networks: Challenges and opportunities. Frontiers in Neuroscience. 2011;**5**:108-108

[9] Modha DS, Ananthanarayanan R, Esser SK, Ndirango A, Sherbondy AJ, Singh R. Cognitive computing. Communications of the ACM. 2011;**54**:62-71

[10] Indiveri G, Linares-Barranco B, Hamilton TJ, van Schaik A, Etienne-Cummings R, Delbruck T, Liu SC, Dudek P, Hafliger P, Renaud S, Wang Y, Boahen K. Neuromorphic silicon neuron circuits. Frontiers in Neuroscience. 2011;**5**:73-73

[11] Pershin YV, Di VM. Neuromorphic, digital, and quantum computation with memory circuit elements. Proceedings of the IEEE. 2011;**100**:2071-2080

[12] Hopfield JJ. Neural networks and physical systems with emergent collective computational abilities. Proceedings of the National Academy of Sciences. 1982;**79**:2554-2558

[13] Rumelhart DE, McClelland JL. Parallel Distributed Processing: Explorations in the Microstructure of Cognition. Volume 1. Foundations. Cambridge, MA: MIT Press; 1986

[14] Kohonen T. Self-Organization and Associative Memory. Springer Series in Information Sciences. 2nd ed. Berlin: Springer; 1988

[15] Hertz J, Krogh A, Palmer RG. Introduction to the Theory of Neural Computation. MA: Addison-Wesley; 1991

[16] Bishop CM. Pattern Recognition and Machine Learning. New York: Springer; 2006

[17] Indiveri G, Horiuchi TK. Frontiers in neuromorphic engineering. Frontiers in Neuroscience. 2011;**5**:118

[18] Rachmuth G, Shouval HZ, Bear MF, Poon C-S. A biophysically-based neuromorphic model of spike rate- and timing-dependent plasticity. Proceedings of the National Academy of Sciences. 2011;**108**:E1266-E1274

[19] Guardiola X, Diaz-Guilera A, Llas M, Perez CJ. Synchronization,diversity, and topology of networks of integrate and fire oscillators. Physical Review E. 2000;**62**:5565-5570

[20] Moreno Y, Pacheco AF. Synchronization of Kuramoto oscillators in scale-free networks. Europhysics Letters. 2004;**68**:603-609

[21] Shouval HZ, Bear MF, Cooper LN. A unified model of NMDA receptor-dependent bidirectional synaptic plasticity. Proceedings of the National Academy of Sciences; **202**(99):10831-10836

[22] Chua LO. Memristor: The missing circuit element. IEEE Transacions on Circuit Theory. 1971;**18**:507-519

[23] Chua LO, Kang SM. Memristive devices and systems. Proceedings of the IEEE. 1976; **64**:209-223

[24] Strukov DB, Snider GS, Stewart DR, Williams RS. The missing memristor found. Nature. 2008;**453**:80-83

[25] Waser R, Aono M. Nanoionics-based resistive switching memories. Nature Materials. 2007;**6**:833-840

[26] Waser R, Dittmann R, Staikov G, Szot K. Redox-based resistive switching memories: Nanoionic mechanisms, prospects, and challenges. Advanced Materials. 2009; **21**:2632-2663

[27] Yang JJ, Strukov DB, Stewart DR. Memristive devices for computing. Nature Nanotechnology. 2013;**8**:13-24

[28] Sawa A. Resistive switching in transition metal oxides. Materials Today. 2008;**11**:28-36

[29] Drachman DA. Do we have brain to spare? Neurology. 2005;**64**:2004-2005

[30] Foster M, Sherrington CS. Textbook of Physiology, Vol. 3. 7th ed. London: Macmillan; 1897. 929 p

[31] Cynthia J. Forehand, The action potential, synaptic transmission, and maintenance of nerve function. Cellular Physiology, Chapter 3, Philadelphia, USA: Wolters Kluwer business; 2009; pp. 38-64

[32] Kandel ER, Schwartz J, Jessell T. Principles of Neural Science. 4th ed. New York; 2000

[33] Raphael L, LeDoux J. Structual plasticity and memory. Neuroscience. 2004;**5**:45-54. DOI: 10.1038/nrn1301

[34] Hebb DO. The Organization of Behavior: A Neuropsychological Theory. New York: Wiley; 1949

[35] Bi G, Poo MM. Synaptic modifications in cultured hippocampal neurons: Dependence on spike timing, synaptic strength, and postsynaptic cell type. The Journal of Neuroscience. 1998;**18**:10464-10472

[36] Zhang LI, Tao HW, Holt CE, Harris WA, Poo M. A critical window for cooperation and competition among developing retinotectal synapses. Nature. 1998;**395**:37-44

[37] Markram H, Lübke J, Frotscher M, Sakmann B. Regulation of synaptic efficacy by coincidence of postsynaptic APs and EPSPs. Science. 1997;**275**:213-215

[38] Song S, Abbott LF. Cortical development and remapping through spike timing-dependent plasticity. Neuron. 2001;**32**:339-350

[39] Song S, Miller KD, Abbott LF. Competitive, Hebbian learning through spike-timing-dependent synaptic plasticity. Nature Neuroscience. 2000;**3**:919-926

[40] Van Rossum MCW, Bi G, Turrigiano G. Stable Hebbian learning from spike timing-dependent plasticity. The Journal of Neuroscience. 2000;**20**:8812-8821

[41] Brader JM, Senn W, Fusi S. Learning real-world stimuli in a neural network with spike-driven synaptic dynamics. Neural Computation. 2007;**19**:2881-2912

[42] Gerstner W, Kempter R, van Hemmen JL. Wagner, H. A neuronal learning rule for sub-millisecond temporal coding. Nature. 1996;**383**:76-78

[43] Kempter R, Gerstner W, van Hemmen JL. Hebbian learning and spiking neurons. Physical Review E. 1999;**59**:4498-4514

[44] Sarkar P, Bhattacharjee S, Barman A, Kanjilal A, Roy A. Nanotechnology. 2016;**27**: 435701

[45] Qian K, Cai G, Nguyen VC, Chen T, Lee PS. Direct observation of conducting filaments in tungsten oxide based transparent resistive switching memory. ACS Applied Materials & Interfaces. 2016;**8**:27885

[46] Zhai H, Kong J, Yang J, Xu J, Xu Q, Sun H, Li A, Wu D. Resistive Switching Properties and Failure Behaviors of (Pt, Cu)/Amorphous ZrO_2/Pt Sandwich Structures. Journal of Materials Science and Technology. 2016;**32**:676

[47] Gul F, Efeoglu H. Bipolar resistive switching and conduction mechanism of an Al/ZnO/Al-based memristor. Superlattices and Microstructures. 2017;**101**:172

[48] Jiang R, Han Z, Du X. Reliability/Uniformity improvement induced by an ultrathin TiO_2 insertion in Ti/HfO_2/Pt resistive switching memories. Microelectronics and Reliability. 2016;**63**:37

[49] Ho P, Hatem F, Almurib HAF, Kumar T. Comparison between Pt/TiO_2/Pt and Pt/TaO_x/TaO_Y/Pt based bipolar resistive switching devices. Journal of Semiconductors. 2016;**37**:064001

[50] Khiat A, Cortese S, Serb A, Prodromakis T. Resistive switching of Pt/TiO_x /Pt devices fabricated on flexible Parylene-C substrates. Nanotechnology. 2017;**28**:025303

[51] Shi T, Yang R, Guo X. Coexistence of analog and digital resistive switching in $BiFeO_3$ -based memristive devices. Solid State Ionics. 2016;**296**:114

[52] Nili H, Ahmed T, Walia S, Ramanathan R, Kandjani AE, Rubanov S, Bhaskaran M. Microstructure and dynamics of vacancy-induced nanofilamentary switching network in donor doped $SrTiO_{3-x}$ memristors. Nanotechnology. 2016;**27**:505210

[53] Siddiqui GU, Rehman MM, Choi KH. Enhanced resistive switching in all-printed, hybrid and flexible memory device based on perovskite $ZnSnO_3$ via PVOH. sPolymer. 2016;**100**:102

[54] Wang S, Wang W, Yakopcic C, Shin E, Subramanyam G, Taha TM. Experimental study of $LiNbO_3$ memristors for use in neuromorphic computing. Microelectronic Engineering. 2017;**168**:37

[55] Huang Y, Shen Z, Wu Y, Xie M, Hu Y, Zhang S, Shi X, Zeng H. CuO/ZnO memristors via oxygen or metal migration controlled by electrodes. AIP Advances. 2016;**6**:025018

[56] Zhou LW, Shao XL, Li XY, Jiang H, Chen R, Yoon KJ, Hwang CS. Interface engineering for improving reliability of resistance switching in Cu/HfO_2/TiO_2/Pt structure. Applied Physics Letters. 2015;**106**:072901

[57] Zhu YB, Zheng K, Wu X, Ang LK. Enhanced stability of filament-type resistive switching by interface engineering. Scientific Reports. 2017;**7**:43664

[58] Simmons JG, Verderbe RR. New conduction and reversible memory phenomena in thin insulating films. Proceedings of the Royal Society of London. Series A, Mathematical and Physical Sciences. 1967;**301**:77-102

[59] Lee M-J, Lee CB, Lee D, Lee SR, Chang M, Kim K. A fast, high-endurance and scalable non-volatile memory device made from asymmetric Ta_2O_{5-x}/TaO_{2-x} bilayer structures. Nature Materials. 2011;**10**:625-630

[60] Jo SH, Kim KH, Lu W. High-density crossbar arrays based on a Si memristive system. Nano Letters. 2009;**9**:870-874

[61] Jo SH, Kim KH, Lu W. Programmable resistance switching in nanoscale two-terminal devices, Nano Letters, 2009;**9**:496-500

[62] Yang JJ, Pickett MD, Li XM, Ohlberg DAA, Stewart DR, Williams RS. Memristive switching mechanism for metal/oxide/metal nanodevices. Nature Nanotechnology. 2008;**3**:429-433

[63] Argall F. Switching phenomena in titanium oxide thin films. Solid State Electronics. 1968;**11**:535-541

[64] Choi BJ. Resistive switching mechanism of TiO_2 thin films grown by atomic-layer deposition. Journal of Applied Physics. 2005;**98**:033715

[65] Jeong DS, Schroeder H, Waser R. Coexistence of bipolar and unipolar resistive switching behaviors in a Pt/ TiO_2/Pt stack. Electrochemical and Solid-State Letters. 2007; **10**:51-53

[66] Kwon DH, Kim KM, Jang JH, Jeon JM, Hwang CS. Atomic structure of conducting nanofilaments in TiO_2 resistive switching memory. Nature Nanotechnology. 2010;**5**:148-153

[67] Strachan JP, Pickett MD, Yang JJ, Aloni S, Kilcoyne ALD, Medeiros-Ribeiro G, Williams RS. Direct identification of the conducting channels in a functioning memristive device. Advanced Materials. 2010;**22**:3573-3577

[68] Gergel-Hackett N, Hamadani B, Dunlap B, Suehle J, Richer C, Hacker C, Gundlach D. A flexible solution-processed memrister. IEEE Electron Device Letters. 2009;**30**:706-708

[69] Seo K, Kim I, Jung S, Jo M, Park S, Hwang H. Analog memory and spike-timing-dependent plasticity characteristics of a nanoscale titanium oxide bilayer resistive switching device. Nanotechnology. 2011;**22**:254023-254025

[70] Gütig R, Aharonov R, Rotter S, Sompolinsky H. The Journal of Neuroscience. 2003;**23**:3697

[71] Yu SM, Gao B, Fang Z, Yu HY, Kang JF, Wong HSP. A neuromorphic visual system using RRAM synaptic devices with sub-pJ energy and tolerance to variability: Experimental characterization and large-scale modeling. In: 2012 IEEE International Electron Devices Meeting (IEDM); 2012

[72] Berdan R, Vasilaki E, Khiat A, Indiveri G, Serb A, Prodromakis T. Emulating short-term synaptic dynamics with memristive devices. Scientific Reports. 2016;**6**:18639. DOI: 10.1038/srep18639

[73] Bousoulas P, Asenov P, Karageorgiou I, Sakellaropoulos D, Stathopoulos S, Tsoukalas D. Engineering amorphous-crystalline interfaces in TiO_{2-x}/TiO_{2-y}-based bilayer structures for enhanced resistive switching and synaptic properties. Journal of Applied Physics. 2016;**120**:154501. DOI: 10.1063/1.4964872

[74] Mostafa H, Khiat A, Serb A, Mayr CG, Indiveri G, Prodromakis T. Implementation of a spike-based perceptron learning rule using TiO_{2-x} memristors. Frontiers in Neuroscience. 2015;**9**:357. DOI: 10.3389/fnins.2015.00357

[75] Park J, Kwak M, Moon K, Woo J, Lee D, Hwang H. TiO_x-based RRAM synapse with 64-levels of conductance and symmetric conductance change by adopting a hybrid pulse scheme for neuromorphic computing. IEEE Electron Device Letters. 2016;**37**:1559-1562. DOI: 10.1109/Led.2016.2622716

[76] Chien WC, Chen YC, Lai EK, Lee FM, Lin YY, Chuang ATH, Chang KP, Yao YD, Chou TH, Lin HM, Lee MH, Shih YH, Hsieh KY, Lu C-Y. A study of the switching mechanism and electrode material of fully CMOS compatible tungsten oxide ReRAM. Applied Physics A: Materials Science & Processing. 2011;**102**:901-907

[77] Li Y, Long S, Liu Q, Wang Q, Zhang M, Lv H, Shao L, Wang Y, Zhang S, Zuo Q, Liu S, Liu M. Nonvolatile multilevel memory effect in Cu/WO_3/Pt device structures. Physica Status Solidi RRL: Rapid Research Letters. 2010;**4**:124-126. DOI: 10.1002/pssr.201004086

[78] Celano U, Yin Chen Y, Wouters DJ, Groeseneken G, Jurczak M, Vandervorst W. Filament observation in metal-oxide resistive switching devices. Applied Physics Letters. 2013;**102**: 121602

[79] Kim J, Inamdar AI, Jo Y, Woo H, Cho S, Pawar SM, Kim H, Im H. Effect of Electronegativity on Bipolar Resistive Switching in a WO_3 Based Asymmetric Capacitor Structure. ACS Applied Materials & Interfaces. 2016;**8**:9499

[80] Ji Y, Yang Y, Lee S-K, Ruan G, Kim T-W, Fei H, Lee S-H, Kim D-Y, Yoon J, Tour JM. Flexible Nanoporous WO_{3-x} Nonvolatile Memory Device. ACS Nano. 2016;**10**:7598

[81] Fan-Yi M, Shu-Kai D, Li-Dan W, Xiao-Fang H, Zhe-Kang D. An improved WOx memristor model with synapse characteristic analysis. Acta Physica Sinica. 2015;**64**(14):148501

[82] Yong Z, Yanling Y, Yuehua P, Weichang Z, Huajun Y, Zhu'ai Q, Binquan L, Yong Z, Dongsheng T. Enhanced memristive performance of individual hexagonal tungsten trioxide nanowires by water adsorption based on Grotthuss mechanism. Materials Research Express. 2014;**1**:025025

[83] Chang T, Jo SH, Kim KH, Sheridan P, Gaba S, Lu W. Synaptic behaviors and modeling of a metal oxide memristive device. Applied Physics A: Materials Science and Engineering. 2011;**102**:857-863. DOI: 10.1007/s00339-011-6296-1

[84] Chang T, Jo SH, Lu W. Short-term memory to longterm memory transition in a nanoscale memristor. ACS Nano. 2011;**5**:7669-7676. DOI: 10.1021/nn202983n

[85] Akoh N, Asai T, Yanagida T, Kawai T, Amemiya Y. A ReRAM-based analog synaptic device having spiketiming-dependent plasticity. IEICE Technical Report. 2010;**110**:23-28

[86] Hu SG, Liu Y, Chen TP, Liu Z, Yu Q, Deng LJ, Yin Y, Hosaka S. Emulating the paired-pulse facilitation of a biological synapse with a NiOx-based memristor. Applied Physics Letters. 2013;**102**:183510. DOI: 10.1063/1.4804374

[87] Hu SG, Liu Y, Liu Z, Chen TP, Yu Q, Deng LJ, Yin Y, Hosaka S. Synaptic long-term potentiation realized in Pavlov's dog model based on a NiO_x-based memristor. Journal of Applied Physics. 2014;**116**:214502. DOI: 10.1063/1.4902515

[88] Choi H, Jung H, Lee J, Yoon J, Park J, Seong DJ, Lee W, Hasan M, Jung GY, Hwang H. An electrically modifiable synapse array of resistive switching memory. Nanotechnology. 2009;**20**:345201. DOI: 10.1088/0957-4484

[89] Guo LQ, Wan Q, Wan CJ, Zhu LQ, Shi Y. Short-term memory to long-term memory transition mimicked in IZO homojunction synaptic transistors. IEEE Electron Device Letters. 2013;**34**:1581-1583. DOI: 10.1109/Led.2013.2286074

[90] Chang YF, Fowler B, Chen YC, Zhou F, Pan CH, Chang TC, Lee JC. Demonstration of synaptic behaviors and resistive switching characterizations by proton exchange reactions in silicon oxide. Scientific Reports. 2016;**6**:21268. DOI: 10.1038/srep21268

[91] Driscoll T, Palit S, Qazilbash MM, Brehm M, Keilmann F, Chae B-G, Yun S-J, Kim H-T, Cho SY, Jokerst NM, Smith DR, Basov DN. Dynamic tuning of an infrared hybrid-metamaterial resonance using vanadium dioxide. Applied Physics Letters. 2008;**93**:024101. DOI: 10.1063/1.2956675

[92] Driscoll T, Kim H-T, Chae B-G, Kim B-J, Lee Y-W, Jokerst NM, Palit S, Smith DR, Di Ventra M, Basov DN. Memory metamaterials. Science. 2009;**325**:1518-1521. DOI: 10.1126/science.1176580

[93] Lee MJ, Park Y, Suh DS, Lee EH, Seo S, Kim DC, Jung R, Kang BS, Ahn SE, Lee CB, Seo DH, Cha YK, Yoo IK, Kim JS, Park BH. Two series oxide resistors applicable to high speed and high density nonvolatile memory. Advanced Materials. 2007;**19**:3919-3923. DOI: 10.1002/adma.200700251

[94] Son M, Lee J, Park J, Shin J, Choi G, Jung S, Lee W, Kim S, Park S, Hwang H. Excellent selector characteristics of nanoscale VO_2 for high-density bipolar ReRAM applications. IEEE Electron Device Letters. 2011;**32**:1579-1581. DOI: 10.1109/LED.2011.2163697

[95] Zhang K, Wang B, Wang F, Han Y, Jian X, Zhang H, Wong HSP. VO_2-based selection device for passive resistive random access memory application. IEEE Electron Device Letters. 2016;**37**:978-981. DOI: 10.1109/LED.2016.2582259

[96] Wong HSP, Lee HY, Yu SM, Chen YS, Wu Y, Chen PS, Lee B, Chen FT, Tsai MJ. Metal-oxide RRAM. Proceedings of the IEEE. 2012;**100**:1951-1970. DOI: 10.1109/Jproc.2012.2190369

[97] Jeong HY, Lee JY, Choi S-Y, Kim JW. Microscopic origin of bipolar resistive switching of nanocale titanium oxide thin films. Applied Physics Letters. 2009;**95**:162108

[98] Kwon D, Jeon J-M, Jang J, Kim K, Hwang C, Kim M. Direct observation of conducting paths in TiO_2 thin film by transmission electron microscopy. Microscopy and Microanalysis. 2009;**7**:996-997

[99] Russo U, Ielmini D, Cagli C, Lacaita AL. Self-Accelerated Thermal Dissolution Model for Reset Programming in Unipolar Resistive-Switching Memory (RRAM) Devices. IEEE Transactions on Electron Devices. 2009;**56**:193

[100] Liu WJ, Tran XA, Yu HY, Sun XW. A Self-Rectifying Unipolar HfOx Based RRAM Using Doped Germanium Bottom Electrode Electronic and Photonic Devices, and Systems. ECS Solid State Letters. 2013;**2**:Q35

[101] Szot K, Speier W, Bihlmayer G, Waser R. Switching the electrical resistance of individual dislocations in singlecrystalline $SrTiO_3$. Nature Materials. 2006;**5**:312-320

[102] Park MR, Abbas Y, Abbas H, Hu Q, Lee TS, Choi YJ, Yoon T-S, Lee H-H, Kang CJ. Resistive switching characteristics in hafnium oxide, tantalum oxide and bilayer devices. Microelectronic Engineering. 2016;**159**:190

[103] Niu G, Schubert M, Sharath S, Zaumseil P, Vogel S, Wenger C, Hildebrandt E, Bhupathi S, Perez E, Alff L. Electron holography on HfO_2/HfO_{2-x} bilayer structures with multilevel resistive switching properties. Nanotechnology. 2017;**28**:215702

[104] Zhou G, Xiao L, Zhang S, Wu B, Liu X, Zhou A. Mechanism for an enhanced resistive switching effect of bilayer NiO_x/TiO_2 for resistive random access memory. Journal of Alloys and Compounds. 2017;**722**:753-759

[105] Nili H, Walia S, Balendhran S, Strukov DB, Bhaskaran M, Sriram S. Nanoscale resistive switching in amorphous perovskite oxide (a-$SrTiO_3$) memristors. Advanced Functional Materials. 2014;**24**:6741

[106] Huang Y, Shen Z, Wu Y, Wang X, Zhang S, Shi X, Zeng H. Amorphous ZnO based resistive random access memory. RSC Advances. 2016;**6**:17867

[107] Jain PK, Salim M, Periasamy C. Switching characteristics in TiO_2/ZnO double layer resistive switching memory device. Materials Research Express. 2017;**4**:065901

[108] Li H, Chen Y, Wu X, Xi J, Huang Y, Ji Z. Studies on structural and resistive switching properties of Al/ZnO/Al structured resistive random access memory. Surface Review and Letters. 2017;**24**:1750048

[109] Parreira P, Paterson G, McVitie S, MacLaren D. Stability, bistability and instability of amorphous ZrO_2 resistive memory devices. Journal of Physics D. 2016;**49**:095111

[110] Huang R, Yan X, Morgan KA, Charlton MD, de Groot CK. Selection by current compliance of negative and positive bipolar resistive switching behavior in ZrO_{2-x}/ZrO_2 bilayer memory. Journal of Physics D. 2017;**50**:175101

[111] Jiang H, Han L, Lin P, Wang Z, Jang MH, Wu Q, Barnell M, Yang JJ, Xin HL, Xia Q. Sub-10 nm Ta channel responsible for superior performance of a HfO_2 memristor. Scientific Reports. 2016;**6**:28525

[112] Chen X, Hu W, Li Y, Wu S, Bao D. Complementary resistive switching behaviors evolved from bipolar TiN/HfO_2/Pt device. Applied Physics Letters. 2016;**108**:053504

9

Plasticity in Damaged Multisensory Networks

Karolina A Bearss and Joseph FX DeSouza

Abstract

This chapter opens by discussing functional and anatomical locations as well as neural networks of unimodal senses: vision, somatosensation, audition, gustation and olfaction. How and where these unimodal sensory systems intersect and interact with multimodal sensory processes to provide a holistic view of how experiencing complex external objects and events lead to a single multimodal percept. Reviews of current neuropsychological research on damage occurring within both unimodal and multimodal sensory networks further explain the association between these networks and how they operate together in perception. Current research reviews on cross-modal plasticity reveal the neural changes that occur in multisensory areas following brain damage and the potential benefits of this plastic reorganization of the cortex.

Keywords: plasticity, multisensory networks, neural damage, unimodal, multimodal integration

1. Introduction

When we actively engage and interact with objects in our surroundings, our brains inherit an enormous amount of information pertaining to the complexity of these objects and features of the external environment itself. Information from the environment is initially collected by our multiple senses, and then processed and interpreted before motor interaction are planned and executed, all occurring within an instance. Perception has been traditionally viewed as a unimodal sensory process with the different sensory modalities operating as independent processes. However, it is obvious that multisensory interactions must occur in various perceptual tasks and events in order to allow one to have proper interactions with the environment. There are numerous brain areas and pathways for multisensory interaction that will be briefly overviewed within this chapter.

External environmental information is received through sensory modalities such as vision, somatosensation, audition, olfaction and gustation. Each of these sensory modalities is comprised of an organ that contains specialized receptive cells, with corresponding receptive fields that respond to external stimuli. The stimulation of a neuron's receptive field initiates a response related to the size and shape of the stimulus; this information travels via sensory pathways sent to the corresponding primary receiving areas of the cerebral cortex. In general, sensory pathways are neurons that link the sensory receptors at the periphery with the spinal cord, brainstem, thalamus and cerebral cortex.

It is essential to clarify how individual pathways work in unison in order to understand the neuronal changes that arise from damage within these systems as a whole. Plasticity of the spared senses can shed light on how the brain changes as a result of damage, providing important insight related to time management and rehabilitation for a variety of neuropsychological disorders.

Next, we will discuss how the senses combine in multisensory networks that enhance our sensory experiences and reactions to external stimuli. Various neuroanatomical techniques are documented in the existing literature, which have been used on nonhuman primates to pinpoint key multimodal cortical sites such as the superior temporal sulcus (STS), intraparietal sulcus, posterior insula, parietopreoccipital cortex, frontal brain regions including the prefrontal, premotor and anterior cingulate (AC) cortex [1–4], and subcortical sites including superior colliculus (SC), claustrum, medial pulvinar nucleus of the thalamus, suprageniculate, hippocampus and the amygdaloid complex [5–7]. The exact functions of these areas and their connections with other multisensory networks will be further examined.

Extensive studies on both animals and humans have shown that during the early stages of development, any environmental alteration or disruption of processing in a single sense results in an enormous fluctuation in favor of neuronal plasticity between multiple senses [8–11]. However, less is known about the potential neuronal changes that arise after damage has occurred to multisensory areas later on in life. Thus, this section will discuss research in cases where damage has occurred within multisensory networks and areas involved in polysensory integration. First, we will describe a study on a patient with Balint's syndrome [12], followed by a report on a case study examining the multisensory effects of damage via infarct in the right primary visual cortex [13]; we will then describe a study which looks at patients with hemianopia and/or neglect in a visual detection task [14]. Lastly, we will describe research on plasticity in multisensory dorsal stream networks involved in nonvisual processing of action [15].

Damage to heteromodal or unimodal sensory areas reduces the effects of multisensory integration that give rise to holistic perception. However, spared multisensory networks have shown to be associated with behavioral benefits through cross-modal plasticity, where the spared heteromodal areas attempt to reconnect the multisensory system and bypass injured areas [9, 11, 14–17].

The final sections of the chapter will discuss some of the research on neuroplastic reorganization that we are currently conducting in our laboratory. In one study, we investigated the effects of long-term professional ballet training on tract fractional anisotropy (FA) lateralization and extent of tract FA. Research indicates that experience and training modulate brain structural parameters including volume and FA [18]; FA is a diffusion tensor imaging (DTI) derived index of water molecule diffusion sensitive to the collective effect of microstructure properties. The effect of long-term ballet training characterized in terms of tract FA lateralization, extent of tract FA and global volume has not been previously reported. We localized these FA parameters in expert dancers relative to controls using DTI, and results indicate that dancers had greater leftward lateralization in the anterior thalamic radiation (ATR), whereas the non-dancers had greater rightward lateralization and that dancers also had higher FA localized to the left cortical spinal tract (CST). Higher dancer FA implies heightened axonal ability to communicate. The large percentages of variability shared by dancer years of training and the structural metrics FA and global volume implicate a substantive impact of dance training on brain structure.

In another study, we investigated the structural and functional plasticity associated with dance expertise in a cross-sectional pilot study, comparing ballet dancers to controls. Using functional magnetic resonance imaging (fMRI), whole-brain functional activation maps of dancers and controls were compared, while they engaged in motor imagery of dance movements. Anatomically the results reveal that dancers exhibited greater cortical thickness in areas such as the inferior occipital gyrus, inferior frontal gyrus and superior temporal gyrus. We also found years of dance training to be positively correlated with cortical thickness in various regions, including the fusiform gyrus and parahippocampal gyrus. These preliminary results suggested that dance expertise is associated with a functional reorganization that corresponds to reduced activity reported in other motor expertise groups.

Lastly, our lab has investigated the impacts that dance intervention has on people with Parkinson's disease (PwPD) and healthy controls. Dance has been shown to have a positive effect on motor functioning in PwPD, but less well understood are the effects of dance on mood and associated brain activity observed within PwPD. Our aim was to examine the effects of dance on both motor and nonmotor functioning and correlate these potential effects to onsite recordings of resting state electroencephalogram (rsEEG) within the alpha rhythm (6–12 Hz), collected immediately before and after a single dance class. Precisely, we aim to examine and potentially construct brain-related plasticity mechanism(s) as a function of dance. As expected, the preliminary results show an overall improvement in motor impairment after a single dance class in PwPD. We also found differential effects of dance on negative and positive mood for both PwPD and HC. Finally, we show an increase in global alpha power after a single dance intervention. These findings imply that dance promotes changes in affect through its overwhelming positivity, use of imagery, use of imagination, the presence of music and a sense of bonding through partner work. These results are of importance as their implications may allow researchers to better correlate and understand the positive behavioral and physiological benefits of dance for PD, and perhaps can aid in the implementation of dance as a form of rehabilitation for PwPD. We are currently leading a follow-up study examining the results of participation in multiple dance classes overtime in conjunction with our ongoing rsEEG research, which will provide an account for the observed neural changes in global alpha power.

Taken together, these investigations on neural plasticity following dance will supplement the earlier studies discussed in the section on damaged multisensory networks. They provide compelling evidence that plasticity occurs in both healthy and clinical populations following learning, exposure to training and greater experience with a particular task.

2. Unimodal and multimodal sensory systems

2.1. Visual perception

The eye is considered the primary sensory organ for the modality of vision. All external information from both eyes has to travel to the very back of the brain, the primary visual receiving area known as the occipital lobes, before it begins to the process toward conscious vision. Libet's famous study, deriving from direct stimulation of the somatosensory cortex (postcentral gyrus), suggests that at threshold intensity for a sensation, visual information can guide actions within one-fifth of a second (200 ms) and that takes about half a second (500 ms) for us to see an object consciously [19, 20].

Most neurons from the retina and lateral geniculate nucleus (LGN) of the thalamus terminate onto the striate cortex (area V1) where initial cortical processing of all visual information first occurs in the perceptual process. Two retinal ganglion cells exist and create two separate pathways, magnocellular (M) and parvocellular (P). M and P pathways become segregated within the LGN, where the bottom two layers consist of M cells, and the upper four layers are made up of P cells. Neural signaling is converted faster by the M cells for the functions of visual motion perception and eye movements, whereas P cells contribute more toward object recognition and face recognition and thus represent more constant stimulus presence. The M and P pathways remain segregated beyond the striate cortex where the M pathway continues along the dorsal stream of the cortex and the P pathway along the ventral stream of the extrastriate cortex (V2) [21]. The dorsal stream passes through area V2, then area V4, and leads to the posterior parietal cortex (PPC), Brodmann's areas 5 and 7, and the middle temporal area (MT). Research on monkeys has shown that MT is responsible for motion processing, representation of object location, control of the eyes and arms for action and is thus referred to as the "where pathway" [21, 22]. Ventral stream begins at V1 then travels through V2–V4 and finally terminates in the inferior temporal area (IT). The ventral stream is devoted to fine analysis of the visual scene and to the perception of color, features and form on an object and is thus referred to as the "what pathway" [21, 22].

Finally, there is still unsatisfactory evidence as to whether these two separate systems converge onto a mutual pathway that explains the neurological basis of visual perception. One way to explore this further is to examine multimodal processing areas and their association with each of the senses.

2.2. Somatosensory systems

Somatic sensibility has four major modalities that provide us with information of objects in the external world: touch (via physical contact with the skin), proprioception (through the position and movement of our body), nociception (such as pain and itch) and temperature (such as feeling warmth and cold) [23]. Each of these modalities begins at a somatosensory organ with distinct receptors and pathways that lead to the brain; however, all share common sensory neurons known as the dorsal root ganglia neurons (DRG). Tactile and limb proprioception are transmitted to the ventral posterolateral (VPL) nucleus of the thalamus via the dorsal column of the spinal cord known as the medial lemniscus pathway. These neurons project to the primary somatosensory cortex (SI) in the postcentral gyrus located on the parietal lobe where information is processed regarding the perception of your body and the external environment [24], whereas pain and temperature information terminate in the intralaminar nuclei of the thalamus through the anterolateral pathway [25]. These afferents also project to SI, specifically the dorsal anterior insular cortex and to the anterior cingulate gyrus where both deep pain and dull pain are processed [23].

SI performs the initial stage of cortical processing, and an overlap of information from any of the four somatosensory modalities may intermingle in higher cortical areas leading to complexity in neural responses. SI is subdivided into 4 Brodmann's area: 3a, 3b, 1 and 2. Most of the thalamic afferents project to areas 3a and 3b and these areas in turn extensively innervate their axons to areas 2 and 1 [23]. These four regions are differentiated according to their functionality; areas 3b and 1 receive somatosensory information from areas on the skin, whereas areas 3a and 2 receive proprioceptive information from receptors that belong to muscles and joints [23]. Research on monkeys has shown that much of SI projections innervate a secondary brain region, the secondary somatic sensory cortex (SII), which projects to areas responsible for tactile memory within the temporal lobe [26]. Lastly, Brodmann's area 5 receives input from SI and pulvinar and is known to be responsible for the integration of tactile and proprioceptive information [23]. Projections from the PPC innervate motor areas in the frontal lobe which play a role in the sensory initiation and guidance of movement [23].

2.3. Audition

Auditory perception gives rise to the ability to perceive sound in our environments by detecting vibrations and changes in pressure in the air. The ear is considered the organ for auditory perception; however, it also assists us in determining balance of our bodies [23]. The eighth cranial nerve travels and branches onto the cochlear nuclear complex located within the brainstem. From here, axons project to the inferior colliculus within the midbrain and to the nucleus of the lateral lemniscus located within the pons where further processing of sound occurs [23]. All of these afferents then move to the medial geniculate nucleus of the thalamus and end up in the superior temporal gyrus a part of the primary auditory cortex (Brodmann's areas 41 and 42). Once action potentials reach here, the conscious perception and processing of sound occur.

2.4. Olfaction and gustation

The olfactory system, also known as the sense of smell, aids humans in distinguishing an enormous amount of odors that are categorized into various groups; spicy, floral, burnt, resin, fruit and putrid [27]. Mitral and tufted cells act as relay cells from the olfactory bulb to the olfactory cortex which is subdivided into five areas: (1) anterior olfactory nucleus (AON), an area responsible for the processing of odors [28]; (2) amygdala for memory associated with specific odors; (3) olfactory tubercle mediating multisensory integration of olfactory information; (4) piriform cortex, responsible for olfactory processing; and finally (5) entorhinal cortex (EC) for preprocessing familiar odors [23]. The latter four parts relay information to the orbitofrontal cortex (OFC) via the thalamus and are an area responsible for decision making for expected rewards or punishments given a certain situation. In addition, the olfactory cortex makes direct connection to the frontal cortex itself for value judgments of odors [23].

Gustatory perception, otherwise known as taste, begins with its essential organ, the tongue. There are a total of five basic tastes that the gustatory system distinguishes, and a combination of these basic tastes gives rise to more complex, established tastes: sour, salty, sweet, bitter and umami [23]. Chorda tympani (cranial nerve VII) innervate the anterior two-third of the tongue and soft palate, the glossopharyngeal (cranial nerve IX) innervates the posterior one-third of the tongue, and lastly, both the vagus (cranial nerve X) and glossopharyngeal nerves innervate the epiglottis and the pharynx [23]. These afferent nerves enter the solitary tract and synapse with secondary neurons in the gustatory area of the medulla [23]. These second order afferent neurons project to the ventral posterior medial nucleus of the thalamus [23]. Finally, they project to the gustatory cortex, between the anterior insula and frontal operculum in the ipsilateral cerebral cortex, to provide conscious perception and discrimination of taste [23].

2.5. Multisensory interaction: anatomical and synaptic levels

Objects and situations that we experience in our everyday lives are embedded within rich and complex environment that contain an enormous amount of information. Perceiving, planning and responding to these complex scenarios involve more than a single, isolated sense. Instead a holistic gathering of information across multiple sensory modalities must occur in order to have successful interactions with the external world. This ability to combine sensory information across different modalities enhances both detection and discrimination of external objects [29]. For example, visual sensitivity can be enhanced with the presence of an auditory or tactile stimulus in healthy participants [30]. In this part of the chapter, we will discuss the neural pathways from primary unimodal sensory areas to multimodal association areas involved in sensory integration. After each multimodal description, we will present cases where damage occurred within these areas to provide explanations of their particular functions.

Unimodal association areas discussed above project to multimodal sensory association areas including the parietotemporal and prefrontal cortices, cingulate gyrus, hippocampus and amygdala [23, 31]. In order to plan and compute a movement toward an external object, the multimodal sensory association areas project to multimodal motor association areas where these converging sensory inputs are transformed into planned motor commands or movements [23, 31]. Execution of movement is initiated when the multimodal motor association areas project to premotor (motor preparation) and primary motor (movement execution) cortices [23].

Our knowledge of the nature and localization of neural mechanisms underlying multimodal sensory processing has stemmed from studies involving different animal species while using a variety of neuroscience techniques. Studies on nonhuman primates using direct cortical recordings have shown convergence of unimodal afferents onto heteromodal cortical sites within the superior temporal sulcus (STS), intraparietal sulcus, posterior insula, parietopreoccipital cortex, and frontal regions including the prefrontal, premotor and anterior cingulate (AC) cortices [1–4]. Heteromodal sites have also been found in subcortical structures such as the SC, claustrum, medial pulvinar nucleus of the thalamus, suprageniculate, hippocampus and the amygdaloid complex [5–7].

Each multisensory neuron located within the SC contains a map of sensory space corresponding to the senses of audition, vision and tactile sensation. These multimodal sensory maps overlap each other, eliciting activation in the same region of the SC where different sensory modalities innervate the same spatial location on the SC [32]. Research has also shown that multisensory neurons within the SC not only respond to multiple sources of sensory information but are also capable of combining them into an integrated form, when two or more afferent sensory neurons appear in close temporal and spatial proximity. The firing rate of these multisensory neurons sums the impulses for each individual modality and thus increases the firing rate of these cells, in turn resulting in a multimodal neuronal response [33]. In contrast, studies have shown that responses to a stimulus from another sensory modality can substantially lessen a vigorous unimodal sensory response in a different sensory modality [34]. Thus, the SC, both at the population and synaptic level, has shown cross-modal integration mediating attentive and orientation behaviors to external stimuli [33].

Neuroimaging studies in humans have been a bit more convoluted with respect to their findings as the description of the different networks involved in multisensory perception has shown to depend on the type of stimuli being integrated and the demands of the task [35]. Multisensory cortical areas in humans include superior temporal sulcus (STS), intraparietal sulcus (IPS) including the ventral (VIP) and lateral (LIP) intraparietal sulcus, parieto-occipital cortex, posterior insula and frontal regions which include the premotor and prefrontal cortices, parietal cortex and the lateral occipital tactile-visual area [36]. With regard to the subcortical level, multisensory activity has been shown in thalamus [37], ventral and dorsal regions of the cochlear nucleus [38], SC [39] and basal ganglia (BG) [40].

Studies in monkey parietal cortex have shown that area VIP receives multimodal sensory inputs from visual, somatosensory, auditory and polysensory areas [41]; in addition, area LIP connects with areas dealing with spatial vision (visual area MT and the auditory caudiomedial) along with the frontal eye field (FEF) [42] and with inferotemporal cortex (ventral visual pathway) [43]. Also, studies on STS show its connection with the visual occipital cortex and with the auditory association area [44]. In addition, the prefrontal cortex receives projections from auditory and visual cortices, essentially playing the role in temporal integration [45]. Lastly, studies on monkeys have shown interconnected multisensory networks in the putamen, VIP, premotor cortex, and parietal area 7b in the perception of visual, tactile and auditory stimuli presented in peripersonal space (a part of external space that is close to the body or a particular body part) [39, 46].

3. Damage in multisensory networks and plasticity

In this part of the chapter, we will introduce patient cases where damage has occurred in particular areas within multisensory networks at both the local brain regions and synaptic levels that will shed light on the mechanisms behind neural plasticity and cortical reorganization.

One study conducted on a patient with a rare affliction known as Balint's syndrome, observed the effects of spatial visuotactile interactions [12]. Balint's syndrome is a very rare neuropsychological impairment resulting from two or more strokes in the parietal lobes in each hemisphere. The symptoms present themselves as a severe disturbance of external space representation with clinical signs of simultanagnosia (inability to perceive the visual field as a whole), oculomotor apraxia (difficulty in fixating the eyes) and optic ataxia (inability to move hand extremities to a specific external object guided by vision) [47]. Within this study, visuotactile interactions were examined during a tactile discrimination task where spatially congruent or incongruent visual cues were simultaneously presented in either the same or the opposite side as the tactile object near the patient's hand. The results for healthy comparison subjects showed that irrelevant visual events elicited a strong and involuntary orientation of spatial attention during concurrent discrimination of tactile stimuli at the same location that was not observed in the Balint's syndrome patient [47]. This finding explains how the posterior parietal cortex (PPC) contributes to spatial processing of exogenous shifts in attention. In the patient with Balint's syndrome, severe spatial deficits were observed affecting the left hemispace in the visual tasks. More precisely, when stimulating the patient's left hand in the left side of visual space, visuotactile interactions were not modulated by spatially congruent conditions. However, when the right hand was stimulated on the right side of space, performance was affected where improvement in responses occurred when the visual cue was presented on the right side, whereas a visual stimulus near the opposite hand caused an interference [47]. In addition, to dissociate the effects on somatotopic and spatiotopic coordinates, the patient crossed their hands during unimodal tactile discriminations. The results indicated that tactile performance of the left hand was improved when it was crossed over into the right hemispace, whereas no significant changes were found with the crossed over left hand into the right hemispace. The results of the study suggested that from the bilateral PPC damage what was lost was the spatial selectivity of the visuotactile effects, the effects produced from the crossing over of the hands suggest a deficit in egocentric spatial coding with respect to the left tactile stimulus. These results indicate the critical role that the PPC has in the integration of both visual and tactile sensory information.

A case study was conducted on a patient with damage to their right primary visual cortex sustaining loss in their left visual hemifield, left hemianopia [13]. In this study, the researchers performed a visual detection task to compare abilities while varying the position of the patients left arm in space. Variation in the presentation of visual stimuli in space included a baseline condition where the patient's left hand was on their lap, while other conditions presented visual stimuli in various reaching space locations, in locations well out of reach, and lastly a condition where the patient held a tennis racket in their hand in order to extend their reach. The results indicated that the patient's ability to detect visual stimuli in their left blind field was significantly improved with the extension of their contralesional arm into the blind field [13]. This arm-mediated visual enhancement was restricted to visual stimuli being presented in reaching distance of the hand. Similar results have been reported in cortical activity of VIP and LIP regions in the monkey, regions related to bimodal visuotactile integration of the hand [1]. In humans, these bimodal neurons contain receptive fields that are located directly on the surface of the skin and extend outward into peripersonal space. Thus, any external stimuli approaching the body, for example the hand, will elicit responses in cells that are responsible for that particular receptive field. This recruitment of activity is present even without the person observing the object coming in closer proximity to the hand [15]. Together these findings indicate that the extension of the arm in space enhances visual processing in the presence of degraded visual information.

As mentioned earlier in the chapter, primary visual cortex projects onto several other areas of the brain. Thus, any loss of neurons in the primary visual cortex could be compensated for by the activity of other higher-order visual association areas that remain stimulated by visual input in the presence of damage to V1, such as in hemianopia. In fact, researchers proposed the existence of compensatory synaptic changes for the neuronal loss seen in primary visual cortex where some patients tend to exhibit blindsight. The hypothesis of blindsight is that subcortical pathways bypass the primary visual cortex and directly project onto secondary visual areas such as V5 (for motion detection), thalamus, brain stem, hypothalamus and/or the amygdala (for emotional response). In fact, this hypothesis was confirmed based on anatomical data acquired from fMRI studies where extrastriate activations in the damaged hemisphere of a hemianopic patient were observed during a forced-choice task known to elicit blindsight [48]. The results of this study support the notion of possible changes occurring at the synaptic level between spared and damaged visual networks based on clinical patients.

Another study investigated whether bimodal audiovisual interactions affect visual processing in patients with hemianopia, visuospatial attention deficit (i.e., neglect) and with both conditions presented visual stimuli in the impaired field in two conditions [14]. The patients underwent a visual detection task with unimodal (i.e., vision only) and cross-modal conditions, with the latter presenting a simultaneous auditory stimulus with the visual target that was either spatially congruent or incongruent. The results of the study showed that in patients with hemianopia or neglect, temporally congruent audiovisual stimuli improved the ability to consciously detect the contralesional visual stimuli in comparison with unimodal visual stimuli only. However, these results were not seen in patients that exhibited both hemianopia and neglect [14]. These findings can be explained by considering the functional characteristics of the multisensory neurons found within SC. As described previously, stimuli from multiple sensory modalities interact at close spatial proximity within the SC, which in turn, produces an enhancement of multisensory integration and responses relative to when stimuli are spatially disparate in the environment and SC receptive fields, and there is no integration. The lack of enhancement in patients with both hemianopia and neglect could be explained by the idea that an auditory cue alone can produce improvement in visual detection, but if both hemianopia and neglect are simultaneously present, the effect of the auditory cue may be inhibited. Also, when the lesion was within fronto-temporo-parietal areas (seen in patients with neglect) or to the occipital cortex (seen in patients with hemianopia), both visual and auditory stimuli were integrated. However, in patients with hemianopia and neglect that have damage to both anatomical areas, the visual and auditory stimuli were not integrated [14].

Using functional magnetic resonance imaging (fMRI) and psychophysical methods, researchers have investigated action control and space perception in congenitally blind and sighted adults while performing active and passive hand movements without any visual feedback information. Congenital blindness is defined as an absence of vision from the time of birth and can be caused by a number of factors including environment, genetic or improper development [17]. In this study, participants were blindfolded in the fMRI scanner, while they performed kinesthetic guided hand movements in a delayed recognition task. Participants were asked to draw three different line patterns one after the other with a stylus, in their right hand, and maintain a mental representation of their hand movements across a variable delay, while their right hand rested. After the delay, a movement recognition trial was initiated where participants were asked to trace a single probe line pattern and press one of the two buttons with their left hand to indicate whether the last line pattern matched one of the stimulus items [16]. The results indicated that both groups did not differ in their task performance. Interestingly, however, kinesthetically guided hand movements activated the bilateral primary somatosensory cortex, left anterior intraparietal sulcus and the left superior parietal lobe [16]. As explained in the previous section on multisensory integration within the brain, this area is part of the dorsal stream pathway which is responsible for visually guided movements. The fact that this pathway was activated in congenitally blind patients indicates that the functions pertaining to this stream arise even in the absence of visual experience [16]. Sighted participants showed greater activation in areas that are responsible for tactile object localization and processing of spatial coordinates (i.e., precuneus) and pre-supplementary motor area associated with higher-order motor control in comparison with congenitally blind participants. This finding indicates that sighted participants have less experience with in nonvisual movement control creating higher task-related demands on these networks [16]. Unlike the sighted participants, congenitally blind participants rely heavily on their remaining senses to guide their movements, and this is evident in the findings where stronger activation in the extrastriate cortex and auditory cortex was present in congenitally blind participants while performing the kinesthetically guided hand movements. These coactivations imply heteromodal plasticity in the auditory cortex due to visual loss [16]. Taken together, these results suggest that the dorsal stream pathway is not only responsible for visual action directed movements but also for somatosensory guidance of movements and that spared sensory areas may manage the loss of function from the preexisting damaged areas.

In summary, there are a number of studies that indicate the integration of multisensory modalities within particular damaged brain regions. Damage to heteromodal association areas, such as the PPC, and independent unimodal sensory cortices, such as the occipital cortex, indicates how these areas are essential for multisensoroy integration and the clinical signs that occur postdamage to them, among other polysensory areas described above. Damage to either any of the heteromodal sensory areas or unimodal sensory areas reduces the effects of multisensory integration that give rise to holistic perception. However, spared multisensory networks have shown behavioral benefits by cross-modal plasticity, both at the cortical level and synaptic level, where spared heteromodal areas attempt to reconnect the multisensory system via bypassing existing injured brain areas thus creating alternative routes in the system.

4. Plasticity research in the lab

In this section of the chapter, we will discuss some of the research on neuroplastic reorganization that we are currently conducting in our laboratory.

4.1. Leftward heightened lateralized fractional anisotropy measures in professional ballet dancers

In one study, we investigated the effects of long-term professional ballet training on tract fractional anisotropy (FA) lateralization and extent of tract FA [49]. Sensorimotor and cognitive training have been associated with altered tract properties as well as altered brain volume. Research indicates that experience and training modulate brain structural parameters including volume and FA [50]. FA is a diffusion tensor imaging (DTI) derived index of water molecule diffusion highly sensitive to the collective effect of microstructure properties, is a putative index of anatomical connectivity and thus is an indicator of microstructural tissue changes.

A single study involving professional ballet dancers and healthy age-matched controls studied whether brain plasticity in either reflex and/or perceptual vestibular processing had discrete neural basis [51]. The authors emphasized that studying brain plasticity while observing changes in gray matter (GM) and white matter (WM) within the vestibular system is of importance as both reflexive and perceptual processing can be assessed while investigating the potential effects of training. Here, the authors correlated GM density and WM microstructure in both groups while simultaneously measuring vestibular psychophysical parameters [51]. Results showed reduction in GM volume in the posterior bilateral vestibular cerebellum negatively correlated with years of dance experience where dancers demonstrated reduced GM volume relative to controls [51]. These results suggested that brain changes within the vestibular cerebellum as a function of dance training affect processing of vestibular perception [51]. Due to the fact that this study reported changes in global volume, our study aimed to investigate changes in FA specifically while secondarily observing global volume changes within dancers and healthy controls.

The effects of long-term ballet training characterized in terms of tract FA lateralization (calculated by tbss_sym script was used [52]), extent of tract FA and global volume have not been previously reported in existing literature and thus was the primary concern for this study. We localized tract FA lateralization and extent of tract FA in expert ballet dancers ($n_{male} = 9$, $M_{age} = 23.00$, $SD = 10.21$) relative to healthy controls ($n_{male} = 5$, $M_{age} = 24.89$, $SD = 1.70$) using DTI. The results indicated that dancers had greater leftward lateralization in the anterior thalamic radiation (ATR), whereas healthy controls had greater rightward lateralization and that dancers also had higher FA localized to the left cortical spinal tract (CST). Refer to **Table 1** for significantly lateralized FA voxels; p-values; and effect sizes (Cohen's d).

Voxels	Max X	Max Y	Max Z	Structures	*d*	$p < 0.10$
260	−15	−56	28	JHU: 11% left Ci; JH: 10% left CB WM	2.00	0.052
49	−17	22	41	HOC: 8% left SFG WM	1.89	0.079
48	−21	−55	39	JHU: 3% left ATR	1.83	**0.038**
29	−18	33	31	JHU: 3% left IFOF; 3% left ATR	2.25	0.059
25	−7	−67	34	JHU: 3% left Ci	2.34	0.069
5	−19	27	33	JHU: 3% left ATR; HOC: 4% WM of left SFG	1.19	0.099
1	−14	47	27	JHU: 29% left FMi; 3% left ATR	1.65	0.100

ATR = anterior thalamic radiation; CB = callosal body; Ci = cingulum; *d* = Cohen's *d;* FMi = forceps minor; IFOF = inferior fronto-occiptal fasciculus; ILF = inferior longitudinal fasciculus; SFG = superior frontal gyrus; HCs = healthy controls. Percentages represent the probability identity of a structure as estimated by the HOC = Harvard-Oxford Cortical, JHU = JHU-ICBM White-Matter Tractography and JH = Juelich Histological Atlases; WM = white matter.

Table 1. MNI coordinates of dancer leftward FA asymmetry.

In addition to the FA lateralization found in our expert ballet dancers, we also showed that substantive variability in FA was shared with ballet training (32–35%) implicating a relatively large effect of training on tract alteration and enhanced tract conductivity. Overall, the results of our study imply that higher dancer FA reflects heightened axonal ability to communicate. The large percentages of variability shared by dancer years of training, and the structural metrics FA and global volume implicate a substantive impact of dance training on change in brain structure.

4.2. Functional and neural correlates of dance expertise

In a different study, we investigated structural and functional plasticity associated with dance expertise in a cross-sectional pilot study, comparing ballet dancers to healthy controls [53]. Using functional magnetic resonance imaging (fMRI), whole-brain functional activation maps of dancers and controls, while they engaged in motor imagery of dance movements, were compared. Brain plasticity has been studied through a wide variety of experimental paradigms. With respect to humans, one of the most influential models to study experience-related plasticity has been that of probing the structural and functional changes that occur as a result of motor skill learning and expertise [54, 55] through complex motor skills that take extensive time and practice to learn, focused on expert groups whose motor expertise is commonly restricted to finger or single limb movements. Thus, there has been a noted lack of studies, particularly in the context of functional neuroimaging, that have investigated the plasticity associated with motor expertise in skills that require whole-body movements [56, 57]. An expert group that may be used to investigate questions on plasticity associated with expertise in complex whole-body movements is that of professional dancers, which were investigated within our current study.

To investigate the above structural and functional neural changes, we had both ($n = 17$) expert ballet dancers ($n_{male} = 11$, $M_{age} = 19.00$, $SD = 1.17$, dance experience $M = 11.25$, $SD = 3.21$ years) and ($n = 5$) controls ($n_{male} = 3$, $M_{age} = 26.00$, $SD = 10.07$, with no self-reported dance experience) perform motor imagery of dance movements while undergoing 8 min of functional neuroimaging. Due to dance being a highly complex motor and cognitive task, both groups were expected to recruit an extensive functional network that included motor-related cortical and subcortical areas, as well as frontoparietal regions during motor imagery [57]. We also investigated the structural correlates associated with dance expertise by comparing cortical thickness between dancers and controls. Various studies have reported motor learning and expertise to be associated with alterations in gray matter, with the common finding being an increase in gray matter in regions believed to be task relevant [58, 59]. Prior to the fMRI scanning procedure, participants received a 20–45 min tutorial on motor visualization, in which they learned the difference between visualizing movements from an internal (kinesthetic motor imagery) and external (visual motor imagery) perspective; this was done to ensure that the participants engaged in the motor imagery task from an internal perspective. Participants were then placed in the MRI scanner and were instructed to visualize themselves dancing to the music from an internal perspective. Scanning followed a block design, consisting of five 60-s-long dance imagery task blocks, interleaved by Six 30-s long rest blocks [68].

Anatomically the results revealed that dancers exhibited greater cortical thickness in areas such as the inferior occipital gyrus, inferior frontal gyrus and superior temporal gyrus ($p < 0.01$). We also found years of dance training to be correlated with cortical thickness in various regions, including positive correlations being reported in the fusiform gyrus and parahippocampal gyrus ($p < 0.01$).

Functionally, controls were found to exhibit significantly greater activity in areas such as superior frontal and medial gyrus, anterior cingulate cortex, hippocampus, precuneus and left cerebellum during motor imagery of dance movements when compared to the expert dancers.

Dance training involves learning and correction of movements, thus leading to the consistent recruitment of regions that are related to functions such as motor control, timing and synchronization, visuomotor imagery, spatial transformations, and action observation and imitation; our results showed cortical differences between dancers and controls in brain regions whose functions are those listed above. It is possible that dancers, who are skilled imaginers due to their training extensively recruit regions such as the precuneus when they are engaged in visual imagery of dance movements. The precuneus in particular has been shown to be implicated in various types of mental imagery tasks, including in motor imagery, where it is believed to be involved in the processing of spatial relationships for body movement control.

These preliminary results suggest that dance expertise is associated with a functional and structural reorganization that corresponds to the reduced activity reported in other motor expertise groups.

Lastly, final studies in the lab investigate the impacts that dance intervention has on people with Parkinson's disease (PwPD) and healthy controls [60–66]. Dance has been shown to have positive effects on motor functioning in PwPD [65, 67], but less well understood are the neural effects and changes of dance on motor skills and nonmotor skills and associated brain activity observed within PwPD. Our aim was to examine the effects of dance on both motor and non-motor functioning and correlate these potential effects to onsite recordings of resting state electroencephalogram (rsEEG) alpha rhythm recordings, collected immediately before and after participation in a single dance class. Precisely, we aimed to examine and potentially construct brain-related plasticity mechanism(s) as a function of dance. We compared changes in motor (using the standardized MDS-UPDRS Part-III), non-motor (using PANAS-X) and rsEEG in both PwPD ($n = 17$; $N_{Males} = 12$, $M_{age} = 68.82$, $SD = 8.95$) and healthy controls ($n = 19$; $N_{Males} = 6$, $M_{age} = 52.78$, $SD = 17.30$) before (PRE) and after (POST) voluntary participation in a single 1.25-h dance class for the dance with Parkinson's program at Canada's National Ballet School (NBS) [60].

As expected, our preliminary results showed overall motor impairment improved after a single dance class in PwPD ($p < 0.001$). We also found differential effects of dance on negative and positive mood for both PwPD and HC ($p < 0.01$). We are in the continual process of data collection and correlating these behavioral effects with rsEEG recordings.

Thus far, these findings imply that dance promotes changes in motor functioning and affects through its overwhelming positivity, use of imagery, use of imagination, the presence of music and a sense of bonding through partner work. These results are of importance as its implications may allow researchers to better correlate and understand the positive behavioral and physiological benefits of dance for PD, and perhaps will aid in the implementation of dance as a form of rehabilitation for PwPD. Currently, we are leading a follow-up study examining these potential results from participation in multiple dance classes overtime. This is in conjunction with our ongoing rsEEG research and will provide a better understanding behind the observed neural changes seen in global alpha power. Further examination of whether the music being played at multiple frequencies would somehow influence these changes in neural alpha band rhythms observed after class is needed to help explain the increases in alpha power observed in our findings.

5. Conclusion and future directions

Overall, it seems reasonable to conclude that in the context of multisensory or unimodal damage or deprivation, the brain recognizes these losses in function and reorganizes to exploit the remaining intact unimodal or multimodal senses at its disposal. The presented set of reviewed literature on plasticity in multisensory networks may have important implications regarding teaching, learning and rehabilitation strategies in persons with damage to the above described brain areas. These findings indicate that the brain is capable of plastic changes throughout the lifespan, and even in healthy individuals, the brain seems to be always changing as a function of training and expertise.

However, it is essential to make note that plasticity changes are intrinsic properties of the central nervous system, and thus, neural plastic changes do not always lead to a behavioral gain, but instead could be deleterious. Thus, more research should be focused on modulation of neural plasticity for optimal behavioral gain across all different types of individuals.

Author details

Karolina A Bearss[1] and Joseph FX DeSouza[1,2*]

*Address all correspondence to: desouza@yorku.ca

1 Department of Psychology, Centre for Vision Research, York University, Toronto, ON, Canada

2 Biology and Interdisciplinary Studies, York University, Toronto, ON, Canada

References

[1] Graziano MS. A system of multimodal areas in the primate brain. Neuron. 2001;29:4–6.

[2] Jones EG, Powell TP. An anatomical study of converging sensory pathways within the cerebral cortex of the monkey. Brain. 1970;93:793–820.

[3] Chavis DA, Pandya DN. Further observations on corticofrontal connections in the rhesus monkey. Brain Research. 1976;117:369–386.

[4] Seltzer B, Pandya DN. Converging visual and somatic sensory cortical input to the intraparietal sulcus of the rhesus monkey. Brain Research. 1980;192:339–351.

[5] Mufson EJ, Mesulam MM. Thalamic connections of the insula in the rhesus monkey and comments on the paralimbic connectivity of the medial pulvinar nucleus. Journal of Comparative Neurology. 1984;227:109–120.

[6] Fries W. Cortical projections to the superior colliculus in the macaque monkey: a retrograde study using horseradish peroxidase. Journal of Comparative Neurology. 1984;230:55–76.

[7] Turner BH, Mishkin M, Knapp M. Organization of the amygdalopetal projections from modality-specific cortical association areas in the monkey. Journal of Comparative Neurology. 1980;191:515–543.

[8] Shimojo S, Shams L. Sensory modalities are not separate modalities: plasticity and interactions. Current Opinion in Neurobiology. 2001;11:505–509.

[9] Majewska AK, Sur M. Plasticity and specificity of cortical processing networks. Trends in Neuroscience. 2006;29:323–329.

[10] Sleigh MJ, Lickliter R. Augmented prenatal auditory stimulation alters postnatal perception, arousal, and survival in bobwhite quail chicks. Development Psychobiology. 1997;30:201–212.

[11] Bavelier D, Neville HJ. Cross-modal plasticity: where and how? Nature Reviews Neuroscience. 2002;3:443–452.

[12] Valenza N, Murray MM, Ptak R, Vuilleumier P. The space of senses: impaired cross-modal interactions in a patient with Balint syndrome after bilateral parietal damage. Neuropsychology. 2004;42:1737–1748.

[13] Schendel K, Robertson LC. Reaching out to see: arm position can attenuate human visual loss. Journal of Cognitive Neuroscience. 2004;16:935–943.

[14] Frassinetti F, Bolognini N, Bottari D, Bonora A, Ladavas E. Audiovisual integration in patients with visual deficit. Journal of Cognitive Neuroscience. 2005;17:1442–1452.

[15] Graziano MSA, Gandhi S. Location of the polysensory zone in the precentral gyrus of anesthesized monkeys. Experimental Brain Research. 2000:135:259–266.

[16] Fiehler K, Rosler F. Plasticity of multisensory dorsal stream functions: evidence from congenitally blind and sighted adults. Restorative Neurology and Neuroscience. 2010;28:193–205.

[17] Shaper M, Cline D, Hofstetter HW. In Dictionary of Visual Science (2nd ed), vol. 81. Chilton Book Company; Philadelphia 1968.

[18] Halwani GF, Loui P, Ruber T, Schlaug G. Effects of practice and experience on the arcuate fasciculus: comparing singers, instrumentalists, and non-musicians. Frontiers in Psychology. 2011;2:2–9.

[19] Libet B. The neural time factor in conscious and unconscious events. Experimental and theoretical studies of consciousness, Ciba Foundation Symposium 174. Chichester: Wiley; 1993.

[20] Libet B. The timing of mental events: Libet's experimental findings and their implications. Consciousness and Cognition. 2002;11:291–299.

[21] Goodale MA, Milner AD. Separate pathways for perception and action. Trends in Neuroscience. 1992;15:20–25.

[22] Ungerleider LG, Mishkin M. Two cortical visual systems. In D. J. Ingle, M. A. Goodale, & R. J. W. Mansfield (Eds.) Analysis of Visual Behavior. Cambridge: MA; 1982. pp. 549–586

[23] Kandel ER, Schwartz JH, Jessell TM. Principles of Neural Science. 4th ed. McGraw-Hill; New York 1991. pp. 508–510.

[24] Gasser HS. The classification of nerve fibers. Ohio Journal of Science. 1941;41:145.

[25] Dubin AE, Patapoutian A. Nociceptors: the sensors of the pain pathway. Journal of Clinical Investigation. 2010;120:3760–3772.

[26] Murray EA, Miskin M. Relative contributions of SII and area 5 to tactile discrimination in monkeys. Behavioral Brain Research. 1984;11:67–83.

[27] Bartoshuk LM, Beauchamp GK. Chemical senses. Annual Review Psychology. 1994;45:419–449.

[28] Brunjes PC, Illig KR, Meyer EA. A field guide to the anterior olfactory nucleus (cortex). Brain Research Reviews. 2005;50:305–335.

[29] Stein BE, Meredith MA, Huneycutt WS, McDade L. Behavioural indices of multisensory integration: orientation to visual cues is affected by auditory stimuli. Journal of Cognitive Neuroscience. 1989;1:12–24.

[30] Bolognini N, Frassinetti F, Serino A, Ladavas E. Acoustical vision of below threshold stimuli: interaction among spatially converging audiovisual inputs. Experimental Brain Research. 2005a;160:273–282.

[31] Jones EG, Powell TP. An anatomical study of converging sensory pathways within the cerebral cortex of the monkey. Brain. 1970;93:793–820.

[32] King AJ, Palmer AR. Integration of visual and auditory information in bimodal neurones in the guinea-pig superior colliculus. Experimental Brain Research. 1985;60:492–500.

[33] Calvert GA. Crossmodal processing in the human brain: Insights from functional neuroimaging studies. Cerebral Cortex. 2001;11:1110–1123.

[34] Kadunce DC, Vaughan JW, Wallace MT, Benedek G, Stein BE. Mechanisms of within- and cross-modality suppression in the superior colliculus. Journal of Neurophysiology. 1997;78:2834–2847.

[35] Bolognini N, Convento S, Rossetti A, Meraber LB. Multisensory porcessing after a brain damage: clues on post-injury crossmodal plasticity from neuropsychology. Neuroscience and Behavioral Review. 2013;37:269–278.

[36] Driver J, Noesselt T. Multisensory interplay reveals crossmodal influences on 'sensory-specific' brain regions, neural responses, and judgments. Neuron. 2008;57:11–23.

[37] Cappe C, Morel A, Barone P, Rouiller EM. The thalamocortical projection systems in primate: an anatomical support for multisensory and sensorimotor interplay. Cerebral Cortex. 2009;19:2025–2037.

[38] Shore SE, Koehler S, Oldakowski M, Hughes LF, Syed S. Dorsal cochlear nucleus responses to somatosensory stimulation are enhanced after noiseinduced hearing loss. European Journal of Neuroscience. 2008;27:155–168.

[39] Bell AH, Corneil BD, Meredith MA, Munoz DP. The influence of stimulus properties on multisensory processing in the awake primate superior colliculus. Canadian Journal of Experimental Psychology. 2001;55:123–132.

[40] Nagy A, Eordegh G, Paroczy Z, Markus Z, Benedek G. Multisensory integration in the basal ganglia. European Journal of Neuroscience. 2006;24:917–924.

[41] Duhamel JR, Colby CL, Goldberg ME. Ventral intraparietal area of the macaque: congruent visual and somatic response properties. Journal of Neurophysiology. 1998;79:126–136.

[42] Andersen RA, Snyder LH, Bradley DC, Xing J. Multimodal representation of space in the posterior parietal cortex and its use in planning movements. Annual Review of Neuroscience. 1997;20:303–330.

[43] Cappe C, Rouiller EM, Barone P. Multisensory anatomical pathways. Hearing Research. 2009;258:28–36.

[44] Seltzer B, Pandya DN. Parietal, temporal, and occipital projections to cortex of the superior temporal sulcus in the rhesus monkey: a retrograde tracer study. Journal of Comparative Neurology. 1994;343:445–463.

[45] Fuster JM, Bodner M, Kroger JK. Cross-modal and cross-temporal association in neurons of frontal cortex. Nature. 2000;405:347–351.

[46] Graziano MSA, Gross CG. Spatial maps for the control of movement. Current Opinion in Neurobiology. 1998;8:195–201.

[47] Robertson LC. Binding, spatial attention and perceptual awareness. Nature Review Neuroscience. 2003;4:93–102.

[48] Goebel R, Muckli L, Zanella FE, Singer W, Stoerig P. Sustained extrastriate cortical activation without visual awareness revealed by fMRI studies of hemianopic patients. Vision Research. 2001;41:1459–1474.

[49] Leger C, DeSouza JFX. Professional Ballet Training Induces Heightened and Lateralized Fractional Anisotropy Measures [thesis]. Toronto, ON: York University; 2014.

[50] Halwani GF, Loui P, Ruber T, Schlaug G. Effects of practice and experience on the arcuate fasciculus: comparing singers, instrumentalists, and non-musicians. Frontiers in Psychology. 2011;2:2–9.

[51] Nigmatullina Y, Hellyer PJ, Nachev P, Sharp DJ, Seemungal BM. The neuroanatomical correlates of training-related perceptuo-reflex uncoupling in dancers. Cerebral Cortex. 2013;25:667–679.

[52] Smith SM, Jenkinson M, Johansen-Berg H, Rueckert D, Nichols TE, Mackay CE, et al. Tract-based spatial statistics: voxelwise analysis of multi-subject diffusion data. Neuroimage. 2006;31:1487–1505.

[53] Dhami P, DeSouza JFX. Investigating the functional and structural neural correlates associated with dance expertise [thesis]. Toronto, ON: York University; 2016.

[54] Hamaide J, De Groof G, Van der Linden A. Neuroplasticity and MRI: a perfect match. NeuroImage. 2015;131:13–28.

[55] Luft AR, Buitrago MM. Stages of motor skill learning. Molecular Neurobiology. 2005;32:205–216.

[56] Bezzola L, Mérillat S, Jäncke L. The effect of leisure activity golf practice on motor imagery: an fMRI study in middle adulthood. Frontiers in Humam Neuroscience. 2012;6:67.

[57] Hetu S, Grégoire M, Saimpont A, Coll MP, Eugène F, Michon PE, Jackson PL. The neural network of motor imagery: an ALE meta-analysis. Neuroscience and Biobehavioral Reviews. 2013;37:930–949.

[58] Bezzola L, Mérillat S, Gaser C, Jäncke L. Training-induced neural plasticity in golf novices. The Journal of Neuroscience. 2011;31:12444–12448.

[59] Draganski B, Gaser C, Busch V, Schuierer G, Bogdahn U, May A. Neuroplasticity: changes in grey matter induced by training. Nature. 2004;427:311–312.

[60] Bearss K, Simone S, Maguire S, Martin K-L, Nsamba Luabeya G, Owe B, Dhami P Smith K, Bar RJ, DeSouza JFX. Investigating behavioural and EEG effects of dance on people with Parkinson's Disease (PwPD). 4th World Parkinson Congress, Portland, Oregon; 2016.

[61] Barnstaple R, Rabinovich D, DeSouza JFX. Dancing with the Brain—New Evidence for Neurorehabilitation associated with Dance. American Dance Therapy Conference, San Diego; 2015.

[62] Levkov GR, Di Noto PM, Montefusco-Siegmund R, Bar RJ, DeSouza JFX. Global alpha slowing in individuals with Parkinson's disease and dance-induced increases in frontal alpha synchronization. Neuroscience Meeting Planner. Washington, DC: Society for Neuroscience Abstracts; 2014 [Online].

[63] DeSouza JFX, McDonald KC. Dance intervention for people with Parkinson's disease: investigating short-term impact of a 12-week dance with Parkinson's class on motor functions and quality of life. McMaster NeuroMusic Conference, 10; 2014.

[64] DeSouza JFX, Bar RJ, Tehrani H. Brain networks involved in dance: a model mechanism for examining plasticity during dance therapy. World Parkinson Congress. Journal of Parkinson's Disease. Vol. 3, Supplement 1, 2013.

[65] McDonald KC, Bar RJ, DeSouza JFX. A dance intervention for people with Parkinson's Disease: investigating short-term and long-term impacts of dance on physical functioning and quality of life. Collaborative Program In Neuroscience (CPIN) Research, Toronto, ON; 2014.

[66] Levkov GR, DeSouza JFX. The effects of dance on motor and non-motor functions, and resting state electroencephalography in individuals with Parkinson's Disease and age-matched controls [thesis]. Toronto, ON: York University; 2016.

[67] Heiberger L, Maurer C, Amtage F, Mendez-Balbuena I, Schulte-Mönting J, Hepp-Reymond MC, Kristeva R. Impact of a weekly dance class on the functional mobility and on the quality of life of individuals with Parkinson's disease. Frontiers in Aging Neuroscience. 2011;3:1–15.

[68] Bar RJ, DeSouza JFX. Tracking Plasticity: Effects of long-term rehearsal in expert dancers encoding music to movement. PLoS ONE 2016;11,1:e0147731.

10

Mitochondrial Regulators of Synaptic Plasticity in the Ischemic Brain

Han-A Park and Elizabeth A. Jonas

Abstract

Synaptic plasticity is a process by which neurons adapt or alter the strength of information transfer, and it is known to play a role in memory formation, learning, and recovery after injury. In this chapter, we describe how ischemic insults alter neuronal intracellular mechanisms and signaling pathways, and we discuss how, after neuronal injury, synaptic plasticity is regulated prior to and during death or rehabilitation and recovery. In addition, recently described regulators of synaptic plasticity will be introduced.

Keywords: ischemia, mitochondrial metabolism, neuroprotection, Bcl-xL, ATP synthase

1. Cellular mechanisms after cerebral ischemia

Cerebral ischemia occurs as a result of a lack of, or insufficiency of, blood supply to the brain, which results in the failure to meet neuronal metabolic demands. Thrombotic or embolic stroke (focal), and cardiac arrest or cardiac surgery (global) are common causes of cerebral ischemia. The loss of oxygen and glucose flow to the brain eventually leads to neuronal energy deficits. These energy deficits result in the failure of adenosine triphosphate (ATP)-dependent ion pumps expressed on the neuronal plasma membrane, permitting an unregulated surge of ion influx into the neuronal cytoplasm [1–3]. Calcium influx induces the release of neurotransmitters from presynaptic neurons and activation of postsynaptic glutamate receptors such as N-methyl-D-aspartate (NMDA) receptors and α-amino-3-hydroxy-5-methyl-4-isoxazolepropionic acid (AMPA) receptors [4–6]. Uncontrolled opening of postsynaptic receptors provokes failure of intracellular ion homeostasis, resulting in excessive postsynaptic entrance of calcium or sodium through NMDA- or AMPA-regulated channels; this initiates signaling pathways.

Calcium is a trigger for a number of important cell-signaling pathways. Increased levels of intracellular calcium activate phospholipase C, which hydrolyzes phosphatidylinositol 4,5-bisphosphate (PIP_2) and forms diacylglycerol (DAG) and inositol 1,4,5-triphosphate (IP_3) [1]. The hydrophobic DAG molecule is expressed on the cell membrane, and recruits protein kinase C (PKC) from the cytosol. PKC regulates synaptic function by phosphorylating ion channels [7–9] and glutamate receptors [10, 11], and enhancing neuronal outgrowth [12, 13]. On the other hand, hydrophilic IP_3 travels into the cytosol and binds with the IP_3 receptor expressed on the endoplasmic reticulum (ER). The ER membrane-embedded IP_3 receptor releases calcium from the ER to mitochondria, depolarizing mitochondrial inner membranes and further compromising ATP production.

Ischemic conditions also activate death receptors (e.g., Fas, tumor necrosis factor (TNF)αR, DR) that cause caspase activation and ultimately lead to neuronal apoptosis [14, 15]. Death receptor-ligand binding releases caspase 8, which directly cleaves either caspase 3 (which can activate downstream death-inducing enzyme pathways) or BH3 interacting-domain death agonist (Bid) to form truncated tBid [16, 17]. tBid translocates to the mitochondria and initiates activation of the pro-apoptotic proteins Bax and Bak. Oligomerization of Bax on the mitochondrial membrane causes cytochrome c release. Cytochrome c forms an apoptosome complex made up of cytochrome c, apoptotic protease-activating factor 1 (APAF 1), and caspase 9. Caspase 9 cleaves and activates effectors such as caspase 3 and caspase 6 which results in neuronal apoptosis. Numerous proteins are subjected to caspase-mediated cleavage [18] including regulators for synaptic function such as glutamate receptors [19, 20], synaptic adhesion molecules [21], ion channels [2], neuronal growth/pruning regulators [22, 23], and inflammatory cytokines [24, 25].

In addition, ischemic stimulation increases the permeability of the blood-brain barrier, and activates neuroinflammatory responses in the brain. Inflammatory infiltration such as the entrance of leukocytes (e.g. neutrophils, macrophages, and lymphocytes) activates microglia and astrocytes which then release inflammatory regulators, including cytokines (e.g. interleukin-1β (IL-1β), IL-6), tumor necrosis factor α, chemokines (e.g. chemokine C-C motif ligand 2 (CCL2), CXC-chemokine ligand 1 (CXCL1)), nitric oxide, reactive oxygen species (ROS), and growth factors [26–29]. Neuroinflammation is a dual-purpose response that can hasten neuronal death or facilitate repair depending on the circumstances. For example, TNF-α is one of the most well-studied pro-inflammatory cytokines increased by ischemic events; it is clearly responsible in large part for ischemia-induced brain injury [30]. However, TNF-α also enhances synaptic strength by increasing the expression of AMPA receptors [31] and through the regulation of the transcription factor, NFκB [32], increasing the expression of anti-apoptotic proteins (Bcl2, and Bcl-xL) and facilitating the production of neurotrophic factors such as nerve growth factor (NGF) and brain-derived neurotrophic factor (BDNF) [33, 34] which play a role in neuroprotection [35]. Taken together, ischemia triggers a multifunctional and complex process in the brain that can lead to neuronal death or facilitate the defense system to rescue the brain against neurotoxic stimulation.

2. Synaptic plasticity in the ischemic brain

The process of early neuronal growth and neurite elongation is critical for synapse formation and neuronal network development. Projection of filopodia, where actin and microtubules become polymerized and attach to substrates, anchors a growth cone and guides a peripheral domain within the thin outer edge of the growth cone known as the lamellipodium. After the lamellipodium contacts the substrate, the central domain of the growth cone, where actin is reorganized and microtubules predominate, moves toward its target [36–38]. These steps occur repeatedly during neurite sprouting and branching. When the tip of the axon reaches its target (either dendrite, soma, or another axon), it differentiates to become suitable for neurotransmission. Presynaptic terminals contain a high density of mitochondria, presynaptic vesicles, and endosomes to enhance communication within the synapse. The target of presynaptic contact is the postsynapse, which matures by the expression of neurotransmitter receptors. Neurexin-neuroligin, N-cadherin, ephrin, and synaptic cell-adhesion molecules play a role in the interaction between presynaptic and postsynaptic neurons [37, 39–42].

Neuronal development is far from static in the mature brain. Recent studies have found that neurons are capable of plasticity during the entire human lifespan [43–46]. Mature neurons have the ability to repair their synaptic network after neurotoxic insults. Stroke induces changes in numerous genes including the ones involved in axonal sprouting in both young and aged animals [47]. Alteration of neuronal connectivity and degradation of neurites are well described after ischemic stroke [47–49], and strategies to strengthen the synaptic network to regain neuronal function and enhance brain repair after episodes of brain injury have been reported [47, 50]. Our study demonstrates examples of the dynamic and adaptive changes that occur in neurites after glutamate neurotoxic challenge. Neurite branches initially become fragmented and damaged (**Figure 1A** and **D**), but then neurites regain structure (**Figure 1B**and **C**) over time, or undergo degradation if severely damaged; in some case collateral sprouting occurs to compensate for lost neurites and to regain synaptic connectivity with healthy neighboring cells (**Figure 1D–F**).

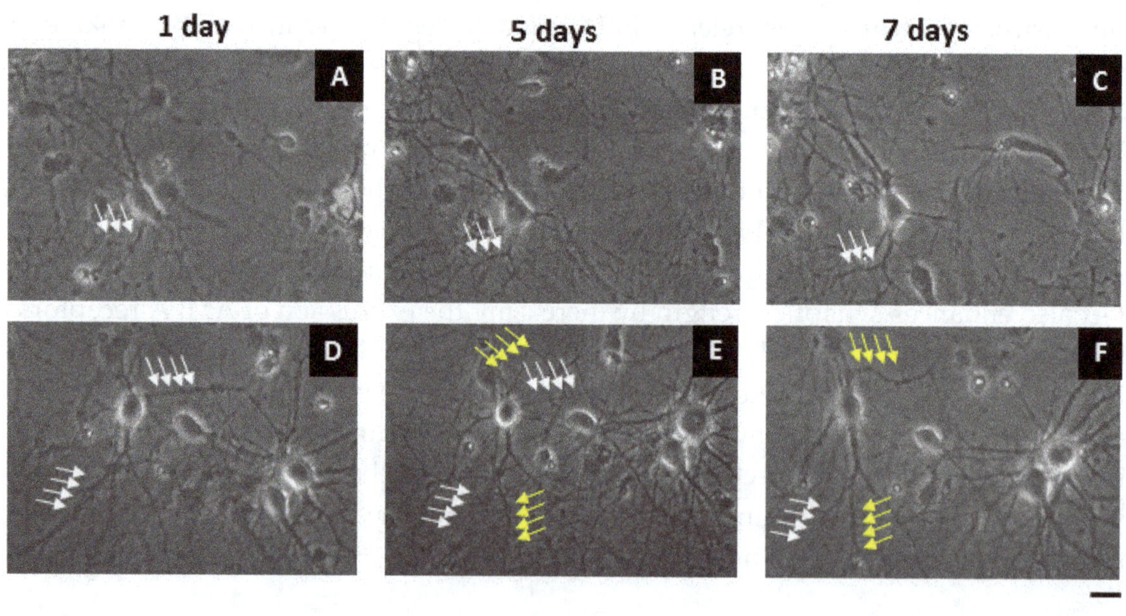

Figure 1. Adaptation of neurite sprouting and pruning after glutamate-induced neurotoxicity. Primary hippocampal neurons were treated with 20 μM glutamate and then imaged at days 1, 5 and 7 after introduction of the insult. Bar, 20 μm. (A) Damaged and fragmented neurite at 1 day after insult (white arrows). (B) Early recovery of injured neurite at day 5 (white arrows). (C) Thickening of recovering neurite at day 7 (white arrows). (D) Fragmented and damaged neurites at day 1 (white arrows) are cleared at day 5 (E, white arrows), but strengthening of collateral branches was found at day 7 (F, yellow arrows) to supplement synaptic networking.

Numerous studies have reported the modification of synaptic plasticity during or after ischemic events. Some studies describe synaptic modification as a part of death signaling; on the other hand, other studies suggest changes in synaptic function as a mechanism of protection or rehabilitation. Synaptic plasticity plays a role in the decision for the neuron to live or die. Synaptic transmission demands high levels of energy production [51]. Failure to control neurotransmitter release [6, 52], and abnormalities of synaptic transmitter release due to lack of energy supply after ischemic insult are well described previously [53]. Regulation of the postsynaptic receptor is critical to control synaptic plasticity [54, 55], and studies have reported that NMDAR or AMPAR are subject to alterations after ischemic events. Earlier studies have shown that brains of animals undergoing four vessel occlusion (4VO)-induced global ischemia show impaired voltage-dependent NMDAR responses, display NMDA-mediated hyperexcitability and loss of long-term potentiation (LTP), and manifest morphological changes of pyramidal neurons prior to the onset of delayed death in the CA1 region of hippocampus [56, 57]. Recent studies expand on these mechanisms and distinguish roles for individual ion channel subunits [58–61]. Studies have reported that ischemia is responsible for the alteration of AMPA receptor expression, especially the GluR2 subunit, transforming a non-calcium permeable into a calcium-permeable AMPA receptor, thereby further mediating calcium entry into CA1 neurons after global ischemia. Although this role contributes to delayed neuronal death in the globally ischemic rodent brain [62–65], these changes may also occur during normal events in synaptic plasticity [54, 66]. Despite the close relationship between ischemia-induced neuronal death and NMDA receptor activation, the application of NMDAR antagonists fails to prevent stroke-related brain injury in clinical trials [67] perhaps indicating involvement of NMDAR in neuronal survival. Indeed, functioning NMDARs are required for synaptogenesis, and the NMDAR plays a neuroprotective role against apoptotic stimulation and oxidative stress [61, 68–70]. In summary, synaptic changes that occur during ischemia may be protective or detrimental depending on the severity and temporal sequence of ischemic events.

2.1. Synaptic failure may lead to ischemic death

Structural damage including degradation of axons or dendrites, and loss of synaptic connectivity associated with synaptic dysfunction are described in various cerebral ischemic models [53, 71]. Animals undergoing ischemic surgery exhibit a reduction of the total neuronal population and an increased appearance of degenerating neurons and apoptotic cells [72–76]. Shy of frank cell demise, axonal morphological changes after brain ischemia have been reported within a variety of brain regions including cortex, striatum, and hippocampus. Degenerating axons exhibit swelling and the appearance of varicosities in both an acute and chronic manner; changes are observed over a period between 6 h and 4 weeks after ischemia reperfusion [49]. Cerebral ischemic insults also lead to cytoskeletal disruption in neurites such as a reduction in the amount of microtubule-associated protein (MAP2), an enhancement in neurofilament proteolysis and an alteration of tau in some neurons [77–79]. Ischemia causes an increase in intracellular calcium levels and ROS production [15] and triggers neuronal death by mechanisms such as enhancing mitochondrial permeability which can facilitate both apoptotic and necrotic death and neuritic degeneration [80]. Therefore, ischemia is one of the major causes of structural and functional failure of both somata and neuronal processes during stroke.

2.2. Synaptic repair after ischemic events

Although ischemic stroke induces neuronal death that leads to functional disability, studies have reported evidence for synaptic plasticity contributing to recovery after stroke [81]. Rats undergoing neocortical ischemia had induction of the growth-associated protein 43 (GAP-43) which is enriched in the growth cone, promoting synaptogenesis and behavioral recovery [82, 83]. Axonal sprouting and plasticity in the intracortical circuitry was observed in post-ischemic brain regions [84, 85]. Plasticity was not limited to neurons but also occurred in other cells including reorganization of vascular structures. Enhancement of the dendritic network such as increased dendritic density has been reported in post-ischemic brain [86, 87]. Moreover, the brain is capable of generating new neurons. The subventricular zone (SVZ) of the lateral ventricles and the subgranular zone (SGZ) of the dentate gyrus are reported to be the site of neurogenesis, exhibiting therapeutic potential for the treatment of brain diseases [88]. In particular, studies have shown that stroke increases neuronal progenitor cell populations in the brain [89, 90], and enhances cell proliferation in the SVZ [91] and in the ischemic penumbra of stroke patients [92]. These studies indicate that ischemia-induced signaling, even denervation itself, may act as a stimulus for the functional and structural recovery of synapses.

2.3. Preconditioning in synaptic potentiation

Despite the possibility of severe ischemia to trigger adaptive responses on its own, studies have also reported that non-noxious, lower levels of injury (preconditioning) may augment ischemic tolerance. Moderate levels of neurotoxic stimuli such as glutamate, ROS, or inflammation initiate survival mechanisms without impairing brain function. Thus, preconditioning builds a latent neuroprotective environment in the brain and provides for a reprogrammed defense response when the truly injurious stimulation occurs [93, 94].

Zukin's group has reported that ischemic preconditioning downregulates AMPA receptors, and blocks mitochondrial release of death molecules such as Smac and DIABLO without altering the pro-survival inhibitor of apoptosis (IAP) family, therefore attenuating ischemia-induced damage in rodent hippocampal neurons [95, 96]. Neuroprotective mechanisms of preconditioning are further evidenced as a change in dynamics of mitochondrial proteins. Preconditioning prevents translocation of the pro-apoptotic protein Bad, enhances the availability of the pro-survival protein Bcl-xL, blocks activation of caspase 3, decreases release of Smac, DIABLO, and cytochrome *c*, and prevents large conductance mitochondrial channel activity, eventually rescuing hippocampal neurons after ischemic insult [72]. In addition, mitochondrial Bcl2 protein family [97–99], redox regulators [100, 101], and transcription factors such as hypoxia-inducible factor (HIF) [102, 103], NFκB [104, 105], c-Fos [106], CREB [97, 105], Nrf2 [101, 107], and AP1 [108] are involved in gene regulation after preconditioning, further modifying neuronal functions such as neurotransmitter release, channel activity, and synaptic networking by regulating the expression of new proteins.

3. Regulators of mitochondrial function and synaptic plasticity

Ischemic insults damage the mitochondrial electron transport chain, decrease mitochondrial ATP production, impair ATP-dependent transporters, and allow intracellular calcium entrance that triggers opening of the mitochondrial permeability transition pore (mPTP) [80, 109, 110]. Ischemia also impairs electron transfer and causes ROS generation from mitochondrial proteins such as complex I and III [111]; ROS greatly contributes to mPT-mediated responses in the mitochondrial membrane [112]. On the other hand, ischemia alters proteins that resides in the mitochondria, and changes levels of transcription factors that target the promoter regions of mitochondrial and nuclear genes. Thus, mitochondria are an essential organelle in ischemia-mediated neuronal responses. There are several regulators that modify mitochondrial function and plasticity to either enhance synaptic recovery after injury or signal for synaptic decline prior to neuronal death. We describe these individually and then show how they work together to support synaptic function during stress.

3.1. Mitochondrial reactive oxygen species

Oxidative phosphorylation is the metabolic process that produces ATP, but it is also the main source of production of superoxide in the mitochondria that can be converted into hydrogen peroxide. Due to the high metabolic rate of neurons, ROS is highly produced in the brain. However, the brain is also more vulnerable than other organs to ROS-induced damage, because it is rich in polyunsaturated fatty acids, and lacking in catalase activity [113, 114]. Indeed, ROS is one of the main causes of mPTP opening, release of mitochondrial death molecules and cell death in ischemic brain [15]. Although numerous studies have reported that an ischemia-induced surge of ROS causes functional and structural injury to neurons, ROS plays multifunctional roles. Physiological levels of ROS regulate synaptic signaling. Approaches that block production or enhance clearance of superoxide using depletion of NADPH oxidase, or overexpression of superoxide dismutase (SOD), respectively, failed to allow for LTP in hippocampal slice [115–117]. Moreover, SOD-overexpressing mice demonstrate defective hippocampal memory formation as measured by water maze learning and fear conditioning [117, 118].

Nitric oxide synthase (NOS) is an enzyme that generates nitric oxide (NO) gas from arginine. NO is considered to be a ROS, due to its ability to generate highly reactive peroxynitrite [119]. Indeed, 4VO-induced global ischemia causes induction of NO in various regions of the brain including hippocampus, cortex, striatum, and cerebellum [120]. Excessive NO production is reported to be neurotoxic as it damages mitochondria, and exacerbates excitotoxicity [121–123]. However, NO is also required for synaptic transmission and synaptic plasticity [124, 125]. NADPH oxidase (NOX) is a cell membrane-bound enzymatic complex that generates superoxide from NADPH, and it also expresses in the mitochondria [126]. NOX contributes to ROS-induced neuroinflammation and apoptosis [127, 128]. Studies reported an upregulation of NOX mRNA and protein level in response to experimental stroke [129, 130]. Inhibition of NOX using the pharmacological inhibitor apocynin improved ischemia-induced brain damage and mortality [131, 132]. However, mice lacking NOX subunits had impaired long-term potentiation and manifested hippocampus-mediated memory deficits, indicating that a physiological level of NOX and ROS may be required for synaptic plasticity and memory formation [114, 115].

3.2. Mitochondrial permeability transition pore (mPTP) and ATP synthase

Ischemia-induced death signaling opens a calcium-sensitive inner mitochondrial membrane pore called mPTP, causing permeabilization of the mitochondrial inner membrane [80, 109, 110]. Loss of mitochondrial inner membrane integrity leads to leakage of intermembrane molecules such as cytochrome *c*, Smac, and DIABLO into the cytoplasmic space, facilitates death-signaling cascades, and results in the impairment of mitochondrial outer membrane structure and cell death. Thus, mPTP is recognized as an important target for neuroprotection; inhibition of mPTP opening may delay or prevent mitochondrial-mediated cell death. Since the discovery of the calcium-induced mitochondrial membrane permeability transition (PT) [133, 134], several molecular participants in mPTP structure or formation have been reported. However, the identification of mPTP is still under investigation.

Cyclophilin D (Cyp D) is a peptidyl-prolyl *cis/trans* isomerase that is localized to the mitochondrial matrix. Cyp D has been considered as a main element of mPTP. However, recent studies have reported that depletion of Cyp D did not eliminate mPTP [135–137] indicating it may not be the critical component of pore opening. One target of Cyp D is a complex of proteins that includes the voltage-dependent anion channel (VDAC), localized to the mitochondrial outer membrane, and the adenine nucleotide translocase (ANT), an ADP/ATP translocator localized to the mitochondrial inner membrane. Therefore, this protein complex was widely studied for its possible role in forming mPTP [138]. Studies showed that mitochondrial swelling after stimulation facilitates the formation of VDAC and ANT complexes along with Cyp D binding, leading to opening of pores in the mitochondrial inner and outer membranes [139–143]. Studies have continuously reported new participants of Cyp D-ANT-VDAC complex: the mitochondrial phosphate carrier binds to Cyp D and ANT [144], spastic paraplegia 7 forms a heterooligomeric complex with VDAC [145], and hexokinase binds to VDAC [146, 147]. However, a recent study revealed that animals lacking VDAC genes did not show improvement of mPTP-mediated mitochondrial stress. They exhibited equivalent levels of cytochrome c release, caspase activation, and cell death compared to control animals [135]. In addition, mitochondria from mice lacking ANT also displayed mPT and cytochrome c release at similar rates compared to wild-type controls [148]. These studies indicate that further investigations are required to clarify the roles of VDAC and ANT in mPTP activation.

In contrast to the studies of VDAC and ANT, knockdown of the membrane-embedded portion (c-subunit) of the F_1F_0 ATP synthase does regulate the ability of mitochondria to undergo PT. Several recent studies have reported that F_1F_0 ATP synthase is an important candidate to form mPTP [149–157]. F_1F_0 ATP synthase is localized in the mitochondrial inner membrane (F_0 unit) and matrix (F_1 unit), and produces ATP by using the potential energy of the hydrogen ion gradient. F_1F_0 ATP synthase gained attention as a putative candidate for mPTP when it was found that it binds CypD [152] and when it was reported to regulate the efficiency of mitochondrial energy metabolism via controlling an inner mitochondrial membrane ion leak

[158]; the c-subunit of the ATP synthase was found to be required for mPTP [149]; the c-subunit of ATP synthase was revealed to form a voltage-sensitive channel, the opening of which is correlated with PT and neuronal death [155]. Bonora and Alavian also showed that shRNA-mediated c-subunit depletion protects neurons from PT-induced cell death, such as excitotoxic and oxidative stress. Together, the findings suggest that the c-subunit forms the pore component of mPTP [155]. Moreover, the depletion of c-subunit of F_1F_0 ATP synthase causes resistance to calcium-induced mPTP opening, while overexpression of c-subunit accelerates calcium-mediated responses, decreases mitochondrial potential, and promotes mitochondrial fragmentation [149, 155]. In addition to the role of the ATP synthase monomer, dimerization of F_1F_0 ATP synthase in mPTP has been correlated with the onset of mPT [151, 159–161].

3.3. B-cell lymphoma-extra large (Bcl-xL) and other Bcl2 family proteins regulate the synapse

Bcl-xL is a member of the Bcl-2 family of proteins. It is traditionally known for anti-apoptotic properties through its role to inhibit the activation/oligomerization of pro-apoptotic Bax and Bak on mitochondrial membranes [162, 163], and its ability to block mitochondria-mediated cytochrome c release and cell death [164]. However, recent studies have reported multifunctional roles of Bcl-xL in the brain. Bcl-xL facilitates reorganization and biogenesis of mitochondria by regulation of fission and fusion [165–167]. Inhibition of Bcl-xL decreases neuronal ATP levels but increases oxygen flux, indicating that Bcl-xL enhances the efficiency of mitochondrial metabolism by preventing the wasteful leak of H^+ ions through the inner membrane [158, 168]. Inefficient leakage of H^+ through a mitochondrial inner membrane pore prevents ATP production. These latter studies provided the first evidence for a functional role for Bcl-xL at the mitochondrial inner membrane and F_1F_0ATP synthase. Bcl-xL interacts with α- and β-subunits [158, 169] of F_1F_0ATP synthase in the mitochondrial matrix. These protein-protein interactions may cause conformational changes of the Bcl-xL-F_1F_0ATP synthase complex, favoring closure of the c-subunit channel (putative mPTP), enhanced mitochondrial energy metabolism, and increased ATP production with minimal oxygen use (decreased inner membrane uncoupling).

It is therefore not surprising that Bcl-xL is an important player in energy-demanding processes such as neuronal outgrowth [74, 170] and synapse formation [167, 171]. Depletion of Bcl-xL in primary hippocampal neurons impairs neuronal branching and elongation [74]. Abnormalities of neurite sprouting caused by Bcl-xL depletion do not induce immediate cytotoxicity, but cause delayed neuronal death, presumably as more synapses fail. Despite their low propensity toward death in the absence of stress, neurons depleted of Bcl-xL are significantly vulnerable to hypoxic insult compared with control neurons, presumably due to failure of synaptic connections and impaired metabolism. In contrast to depletion, Bcl-xL overexpression increases levels of pre- and postsynaptic markers on axons and on the opposing dendrites and enhances the number of mitochondria and synaptic vesicles in the presynaptic bouton [167]. Bcl-xL also enhances synaptic vesicle recycling during presynaptic plasticity, by forming a complex of clathrin, Bcl-Xl, and Drp1 which is necessary for normal or enhanced endocytosis [171]. In addition, Bcl-xL is reported to have multiple binding partners besides those of traditional Bcl2 family proteins that regulate apoptotic pathways (**Table 1**); thus, additional functions of Bcl-xL in synaptic plasticity need to be further investigated.

Protein	Roles	References
Bcl2 family protein		
Bak	Regulates apoptosis	[163, 208]
Bax	Regulates apoptosis	[209–211]
Beclin 1	Prevents autophage	[212]
Bad	Regulates apoptosis and cell cycle	[213–215]
Bim	Regulates apoptosis	[216, 217]
Bid	Regulates apoptosis	[217]
PUMA	Regulates apoptosis	[209, 218]
Non-Bcl2 family proteins		
Apoptotic protease-activating factor 1 (Apaf-1)	Regulates caspase 9-mediated apoptosis	[219, 220]
Apoptosis regulatory protein Siva (Siva-1)	Sequestrates Bcl-xL and induces apoptosis	[221]
F_1F_0 ATP synthase	Regulates mitochondrial energy metabolism	[158, 169]
Aven	Stabilizes Bcl-xL and regulates caspase-dependent apoptosis	[222, 223]
Dynamin-related protein 1 (Drp1)	Regulates synaptic vesicle endocytosis	[165, 167, 171]
IP3 receptor	Regulates calcium signaling and apoptosis	[224, 225]
Phosphoglycerate mutase family 5 (PGAM5)	Enhances Keap1-dependent degradation	[226, 227]
PTEN-induced putative kinase 1 (PINK1)	Regulates phosphorylation of Bcl-xL to prevent its cleavage	[228]
Voltage-dependent anion channel (VDAC)	Regulates mitochondrial calcium, cytochrome c release, ATP release	[164, 229, 230]
Tumor protein p53	Regulates cytochrome c release and apoptosis	[231, 232]

Table 1. List of proteins that bind to Bcl-xL.

In contrast to its neuroprotective properties, Bcl-xL is also capable of decreasing synaptic strength [172, 173] and inducing neurotoxicity [73, 174]. Bcl-xL is subject to caspase-mediated fragmentation [174–176], and forms N-terminus truncated ΔN-Bcl-xL. The N-terminally localized BH4 region has been reported as the functional domain that carries out the anti-apoptotic role of Bcl-xL [177, 178], and cleavage of Bcl-xL to remove this domain gives pro-apoptotic characteristics to this molecule. ΔN-Bcl-xL is reported to induce large channel activity in the synaptic mitochondria [172], to cause decline of the amplitude of post synaptic potentials [173], and to increase cytochrome c release [179]. Studies show that transient global ischemia induces ΔN-Bcl-xL formation prior to delayed neuronal death in the CA1 region of hippocampus [72, 73]. The strategies to block ΔN-Bcl-xL formation such as administration of pharmacological inhibitors, or mutation of the caspase cleavage site protect rodent brains against ischemic injury [73, 172].

Bcl-2-associated x protein (Bax) is a pro-apoptotic member of the Bcl2 family containing BH1, BH2, and BH3 domains but lacking the BH4 domain found in many anti-apoptotic family members. Bax forms channel activity in lipid bilayers [180], induces cytochrome c release [162, 181], and cooperates with mPTP candidates such as ANT and VDAC [138, 164]. Interestingly, although it is mostly known as a pro-apoptotic protein, it also has important functions in healthy synapses undergoing plasticity. Injection of Bax protein into the presynaptic terminal induces enhanced neurotransmitter release, similarly to effects of pro-survival Bcl-xL, indicating that Bax is capable of supporting normal synaptic plasticity in unstressed neurons [182]. In healthy hippocampal neurons, Bax is necessary for the formation of synaptic plasticity known as NMDA receptor-dependent LTD. Despite comparable expression of NMDA receptors in Bax knockout animals, these animals fail to demonstrate hippocampal LTD induction [183].

Bid is a pro-apoptotic BH3 only protein. Bid is normally expressed in the cytoplasm, but during cytotoxic stimulation, caspase cleaves Bid into truncated Bid (tBid) which activates other members of the pro-apoptotic Bcl2 family [184] or antagonizes anti-apoptotic Bcl2 proteins [17]. tBid contributes to the mobilization of cytochrome c by Bax and alters mitochondrial cristae independent of its function to activate Bax, and it opens mitochondrial intermembrane spaces [185]. Bid enhances mitochondrial membrane permeabilization, cooperates with mPT or Bax, and mediates large-channel conductances [186]. Studies show that Bid is an important activator in ischemia-induced brain injury [187, 188]. Cleavage of Bid was also found after middle cerebral artery occlusion (MCAO)-induced stroke in mouse. Bid knockout animals show decreased levels of cytochrome c release and infarct volume [187, 188].

3.4. Hypoxia-inducible factor 1 (HIF1-α)

HIF1-α is a transcriptional factor activated in response to hypoxia. In normoxic conditions, HIF1-α is generally degraded by prolyl hydroxylases (PHD)-mediated ubiquitination, but hypoxia inhibits PHD activity and leads to stabilization of HIF1-α which then is translocated to the nucleus and regulates gene expression. Although HIF1-α is not generally considered as a mitochondrial protein, HIF1-α is reported as an important player in mitochondrial function [189–191]. HIF1-α directly binds with the promoter region of Bcl-xL [192] and targets the expression of BNIP3, a BH3-only protein member of the Bcl2 family that mediates hypoxia-induced mitochondrial autophagy [193–195]. HIF1- α regulates a subunit of cytochrome c oxidase [196] which is an essential member in the mitochondrial electron transport chain. In addition, a recent study showed localization of HIF1-α to both the nucleus and mitochondria after hypoxia [197].

Since ischemia is closely related to hypoxic stimulation, there are studies reporting functions of HIF1-α in models of cerebral ischemia. HIF1-α is enhanced by MCAO-induced stroke in rodent brains, and co-regulated with death-signaling molecules such as caspases, inflammatory cytokines, and apoptotic molecules [198–202]. On the other hand, the neuroprotective role of HIF1-α has been studied by several groups during the past decade [203–205]. Impairment of dopaminergic differentiation and reduction of vascular endothelial growth factor are reported in a HIF-1α knockout model [206]. Tomita et al. reported that neuron-specific-HIF1-α knockout mice have reduced numbers of neurons and impaired spatial memory [207]. Therefore, understanding both physiological and pathological roles of HIF-1α and its targets is important to understand synaptic plasticity in cerebral ischemia.

4. Conclusion

Mitochondria are the center of intracellular energy production, and the executor of cellular fate. Ischemic injury triggers or is caused by mitochondria-mediated signaling pathways. We have discussed in this chapter the intracellular signals activated during and after episodes of ischemia, the alteration in the dynamics of structural components of the synapse, and how these elements play a role in attenuation of synaptic plasticity or recovery of synaptic responses. Since after ischemia, increased energy demands are inherent in the formation of new synapses and repair of the normal operation of existing synapses, we are particularly focused on mitochondrial components that regulate mPTP and neuronal energy metabolism. Although details of the structure of mPTP are still in question, it is clear that prevention of mPT and conservation of energy are critical in management of ischemia-induced damage in the brain. We have also highlighted non-canonical roles of mitochondrial Bcl2 family proteins in the synapse besides their known functions in apoptosis; these roles should be further studied to elucidate the crucial functions of mitochondria in synaptic plasticity.

Author details

Han-A Park and Elizabeth A. Jonas*

*Address all correspondence to: elizabeth.jonas@yale.edu

Department of Internal Medicine, Section of Endocrinology, Yale University, New Haven, CT, USA

References

[1] F. B. Meyer (1989) Calcium, neuronal hyperexcitability and ischemic injury. Brain Res Brain Res Rev 14:227–243.

[2] B. L. Schwab, D. Guerini, C. Didszun, D. Bano, E. Ferrando-May, E. Fava, J. Tam, D. Xu, S. Xanthoudakis, D. W. Nicholson, E. Carafoli and P. Nicotera (2002) Cleavage of plasma membrane calcium pumps by caspases: a link between apoptosis and necrosis. Cell death and differentiation 9:818–831.

[3] D. Bano, K. W. Young, C. J. Guerin, R. Lefeuvre, N. J. Rothwell, L. Naldini, R. Rizzuto, E. Carafoli and P. Nicotera (2005) Cleavage of the plasma membrane Na+/Ca2+ exchanger in excitotoxicity. Cell 120:275–285.

[4] D. W. Choi (1987) Ionic dependence of glutamate neurotoxicity. The Journal of neuroscience: the official journal of the Society for Neuroscience 7:369–379.

[5] K. Szydlowska and M. Tymianski (2010) Calcium, ischemia and excitotoxicity. Cell Calcium 47:122–129.

[6] Y. Nishizawa (2001) Glutamate release and neuronal damage in ischemia. Life Sci 69:369–381.

[7] Y. Zhang, J. S. Helm, A. Senatore, J. D. Spafford, L. K. Kaczmarek and E. A. Jonas (2008) PKC-induced intracellular trafficking of Ca(V)2 precedes its rapid recruitment to the plasma membrane. The Journal of neuroscience: the official journal of the Society for Neuroscience 28:2601–2612.

[8] C. M. Macica, C. A. von Hehn, L. Y. Wang, C. S. Ho, S. Yokoyama, R. H. Joho and L. K. Kaczmarek (2003) Modulation of the kv3.1b potassium channel isoform adjusts the fidelity of the firing pattern of auditory neurons. The Journal of neuroscience: the official journal of the Society for Neuroscience 23:1133–1141.

[9] Y. Chen, A. R. Cantrell, R. O. Messing, T. Scheuer and W. A. Catterall (2005) Specific modulation of Na+ channels in hippocampal neurons by protein kinase C epsilon. The Journal of neuroscience: the official journal of the Society for Neuroscience 25:507–513.

[10] T. A. Macek, H. Schaffhauser and P. J. Conn (1998) Protein kinase C and A3 adenosine receptor activation inhibit presynaptic metabotropic glutamate receptor (mGluR) function and uncouple mGluRs from GTP-binding proteins. The Journal of neuroscience: the official journal of the Society for Neuroscience 18:6138–6146.

[11] S. Kawabata, R. Tsutsumi, A. Kohara, T. Yamaguchi, S. Nakanishi and M. Okada (1996) Control of calcium oscillations by phosphorylation of metabotropic glutamate receptors. Nature 383:89–92.

[12] J. L. Bixby (1989) Protein kinase C is involved in laminin stimulation of neurite outgrowth. Neuron 3:287–297.

[13] R. Zeidman, U. Troller, A. Raghunath, S. Pahlman and C. Larsson (2002) Protein kinase Cepsilon actin-binding site is important for neurite outgrowth during neuronal differentiation. Mol Biol Cell 13:12–24.

[14] K. Matsushita, Y. Wu, J. Qiu, L. Lang-Lazdunski, L. Hirt, C. Waeber, B. T. Hyman, J. Yuan and M. A. Moskowitz (2000) Fas receptor and neuronal cell death after spinal cord ischemia. The Journal of neuroscience: the official journal of the Society for Neuroscience 20:6879–6887.

[15] B. R. Broughton, D. C. Reutens and C. G. Sobey (2009) Apoptotic mechanisms after cerebral ischemia. Stroke; a journal of cerebral circulation 40:e331–339.

[16] H. Li, H. Zhu, C. J. Xu and J. Yuan (1998) Cleavage of BID by caspase 8 mediates the mitochondrial damage in the Fas pathway of apoptosis. Cell 94:491–501.

[17] X. Luo, I. Budihardjo, H. Zou, C. Slaughter and X. Wang (1998) Bid, a Bcl2 interacting protein, mediates cytochrome c release from mitochondria in response to activation of cell surface death receptors. Cell 94:481–490.

[18] U. Fischer, R. U. Janicke and K. Schulze-Osthoff (2003) Many cuts to ruin: a comprehensive update of caspase substrates. Cell death and differentiation 10:76–100.

[19] S. L. Chan, W. S. Griffin and M. P. Mattson (1999) Evidence for caspase-mediated cleavage of AMPA receptor subunits in neuronal apoptosis and Alzheimer's disease. J Neurosci Res 57:315–323.

[20] G. W. Glazner, S. L. Chan, C. Lu and M. P. Mattson (2000) Caspase-mediated degradation of AMPA receptor subunits: a mechanism for preventing excitotoxic necrosis and ensuring apoptosis. The Journal of neuroscience: the official journal of the Society for Neuroscience 20:3641–3649.

[21] I. Hunter, D. McGregor and S. P. Robins (2001) Caspase-dependent cleavage of cadherins and catenins during osteoblast apoptosis. J Bone Miner Res 16:466–477.

[22] F. G. Gervais, D. Xu, G. S. Robertson, J. P. Vaillancourt, Y. Zhu, J. Huang, A. LeBlanc, D. Smith, M. Rigby, M. S. Shearman, E. E. Clarke, H. Zheng, L. H. Van Der Ploeg, S. C. Ruffolo, N. A. Thornberry, S. Xanthoudakis, R. J. Zamboni, S. Roy and D. W. Nicholson (1999) Involvement of caspases in proteolytic cleavage of Alzheimer's amyloid-beta precursor protein and amyloidogenic A beta peptide formation. Cell 97:395–406.

[23] A. Nikolaev, T. McLaughlin, D. D. O'Leary and M. Tessier-Lavigne (2009) APP binds DR6 to trigger axon pruning and neuron death via distinct caspases. Nature 457:981–989.

[24] L. Tong, G. A. Prieto, E. A. Kramar, E. D. Smith, D. H. Cribbs, G. Lynch and C. W. Cotman (2012) Brain-derived neurotrophic factor-dependent synaptic plasticity is suppressed by interleukin-1beta via p38 mitogen-activated protein kinase. The Journal of neuroscience: the official journal of the Society for Neuroscience 32:17714–17724.

[25] N. A. Thornberry, H. G. Bull, J. R. Calaycay, K. T. Chapman, A. D. Howard, M. J. Kostura, D. K. Miller, S. M. Molineaux, J. R. Weidner, J. Aunins and et al. (1992) A novel heterodimeric cysteine protease is required for interleukin-1 beta processing in monocytes. Nature 356:768–774.

[26] A. H. Jacobs, B. Tavitian and I. N. consortium (2012) Noninvasive molecular imaging of neuroinflammation. Journal of cerebral blood flow and metabolism: official journal of the International Society of Cerebral Blood Flow and Metabolism 32:1393–1415.

[27] M. V. Sofroniew (2015) Astrocyte barriers to neurotoxic inflammation. Nat Rev Neurosci 16:249–263.

[28] M. L. Block (2014) Neuroinflammation: modulating mighty microglia. Nat Chem Biol 10:988–989.

[29] D. N. Xanthos and J. Sandkuhler (2014) Neurogenic neuroinflammation: inflammatory CNS reactions in response to neuronal activity. Nat Rev Neurosci 15:43–53.

[30] T. Liu, R. K. Clark, P. C. McDonnell, P. R. Young, R. F. White, F. C. Barone and G. Z. Feuerstein (1994) Tumor necrosis factor-alpha expression in ischemic neurons. Stroke; a journal of cerebral circulation 25:1481–1488.

[31] E. C. Beattie, D. Stellwagen, W. Morishita, J. C. Bresnahan, B. K. Ha, M. Von Zastrow, M. S. Beattie and R. C. Malenka (2002) Control of synaptic strength by glial TNFalpha. Science 295:2282–2285.

[32] M. Tamatani, Y. H. Che, H. Matsuzaki, S. Ogawa, H. Okado, S. Miyake, T. Mizuno and M. Tohyama (1999) Tumor necrosis factor induces Bcl-2 and Bcl-x expression through NFkappaB activation in primary hippocampal neurons. The Journal of biological chemistry 274:8531–8538.

[33] R. N. Saha, X. Liu and K. Pahan (2006) Up-regulation of BDNF in astrocytes by TNF-alpha: a case for the neuroprotective role of cytokine. J Neuroimmune Pharmacol 1:212–222.

[34] Y. Takei and R. Laskey (2008) Tumor necrosis factor alpha regulates responses to nerve growth factor, promoting neural cell survival but suppressing differentiation of neuroblastoma cells. Mol Biol Cell 19:855–864.

[35] I. Figiel (2008) Pro-inflammatory cytokine TNF-alpha as a neuroprotective agent in the brain. Acta Neurobiol Exp (Wars) 68:526–534.

[36] D. M. Suter and P. Forscher (1998) An emerging link between cytoskeletal dynamics and cell adhesion molecules in growth cone guidance. Curr Opin Neurobiol 8:106–116.

[37] L. A. Lowery and D. Van Vactor (2009) The trip of the tip: understanding the growth cone machinery. Nature reviews. Molecular cell biology 10:332–343.

[38] K. Kalil and E. W. Dent (2014) Branch management: mechanisms of axon branching in the developing vertebrate CNS. Nat Rev Neurosci 15:7–18.

[39] A. M. Craig and Y. Kang (2007) Neurexin-neuroligin signaling in synapse development. Curr Opin Neurobiol 17:43–52.

[40] T. C. Sudhof (2008) Neuroligins and neurexins link synaptic function to cognitive disease. Nature 455:903–911.

[41] M. Takeichi (2007) The cadherin superfamily in neuronal connections and interactions. Nat Rev Neurosci 8:11–20.

[42] M. B. Dalva, A. C. McClelland and M. S. Kayser (2007) Cell adhesion molecules: signalling functions at the synapse. Nat Rev Neurosci 8:206–220.

[43] A. Nissant, C. Bardy, H. Katagiri, K. Murray and P. M. Lledo (2009) Adult neurogenesis promotes synaptic plasticity in the olfactory bulb. Nat Neurosci 12:728–730.

[44] P. M. Lledo, M. Alonso and M. S. Grubb (2006) Adult neurogenesis and functional plasticity in neuronal circuits. Nat Rev Neurosci 7:179–193.

[45] C. R. Bramham and E. Messaoudi (2005) BDNF function in adult synaptic plasticity: the synaptic consolidation hypothesis. Prog Neurobiol 76:99–125.

[46] A. Pascual-Leone, A. Amedi, F. Fregni and L. B. Merabet (2005) The plastic human brain cortex. Annu Rev Neurosci 28:377–401.

[47] S. Li, J. J. Overman, D. Katsman, S. V. Kozlov, C. J. Donnelly, J. L. Twiss, R. J. Giger, G. Coppola, D. H. Geschwind and S. T. Carmichael (2010) An age-related sprouting transcriptome provides molecular control of axonal sprouting after stroke. Nat Neurosci 13:1496–1504.

[48] J. D. Hinman, M. N. Rasband and S. T. Carmichael (2013) Remodeling of the axon initial segment after focal cortical and white matter stroke. Stroke; a journal of cerebral circulation 44:182–189.

[49] Q. Zhang, T. Gao, Y. Luo, X. Chen, G. Gao, X. Gao, Y. Zhou and J. Dai (2012) Transient focal cerebral ischemia/reperfusion induces early and chronic axonal changes in rats: its importance for the risk of Alzheimer's disease. In: PloS one 7:e33722.

[50] B. P. Liu, W. B. Cafferty, S. O. Budel and S. M. Strittmatter (2006) Extracellular regulators of axonal growth in the adult central nervous system. In: Philos Trans R Soc Lond B Biol Sci 361:1593–1610.

[51] J. J. Harris, R. Jolivet and D. Attwell (2012) Synaptic energy use and supply. Neuron 75:762–777.

[52] D. J. Rossi, T. Oshima and D. Attwell (2000) Glutamate release in severe brain ischaemia is mainly by reversed uptake. Nature 403:316–321.

[53] J. Hofmeijer and M. J. van Putten (2012) Ischemic cerebral damage: an appraisal of synaptic failure. Stroke; a journal of cerebral circulation 43:607–615.

[54] J. T. Isaac, M. C. Ashby and C. J. McBain (2007) The role of the GluR2 subunit in AMPA receptor function and synaptic plasticity. Neuron 54:859–871.

[55] S. Cull-Candy, L. Kelly and M. Farrant (2006) Regulation of Ca2+-permeable AMPA receptors: synaptic plasticity and beyond. Curr Opin Neurobiol 16:288–297.

[56] N. Hori and D. O. Carpenter (1994) Functional and morphological changes induced by transient in vivo ischemia. Exp Neurol 129:279–289.

[57] N. Hori, N. Doi, S. Miyahara, Y. Shinoda and D. O. Carpenter (1991) Appearance of NMDA receptors triggered by anoxia independent of voltage in vivo and in vitro. Exp Neurol 112:304–311.

[58] H. Y. Wu, E. Y. Yuen, Y. F. Lu, M. Matsushita, H. Matsui, Z. Yan and K. Tomizawa (2005) Regulation of N-methyl-D-aspartate receptors by calpain in cortical neurons. The Journal of biological chemistry 280:21588–21593.

[59] Y. Liu, T. P. Wong, M. Aarts, A. Rooyakkers, L. Liu, T. W. Lai, D. C. Wu, J. Lu, M. Tymianski, A. M. Craig and Y. T. Wang (2007) NMDA receptor subunits have differential roles in mediating excitotoxic neuronal death both in vitro and in vivo. The Journal of neuroscience: the official journal of the Society for Neuroscience 27:2846–2857.

[60] M. Chen, T. J. Lu, X. J. Chen, Y. Zhou, Q. Chen, X. Y. Feng, L. Xu, W. H. Duan and Z. Q. Xiong (2008) Differential roles of NMDA receptor subtypes in ischemic neuronal cell death and ischemic tolerance. Stroke; a journal of cerebral circulation 39:3042–3048.

[61] K. Yashiro and B. D. Philpot (2008) Regulation of NMDA receptor subunit expression and its implications for LTD, LTP, and metaplasticity. Neuropharmacology 55:1081–1094.

[62] J. A. Gorter, J. J. Petrozzino, E. M. Aronica, D. M. Rosenbaum, T. Opitz, M. V. Bennett, J. A. Connor and R. S. Zukin (1997) Global ischemia induces downregulation of Glur2 mRNA

and increases AMPA receptor-mediated Ca2+ influx in hippocampal CA1 neurons of gerbil. The Journal of neuroscience: the official journal of the Society for Neuroscience 17:6179–6188.

[63] P. L. Peng, X. Zhong, W. Tu, M. M. Soundarapandian, P. Molner, D. Zhu, L. Lau, S. Liu, F. Liu and Y. Lu (2006) ADAR2-dependent RNA editing of AMPA receptor subunit GluR2 determines vulnerability of neurons in forebrain ischemia. Neuron 49:719–733.

[64] S. Liu, L. Lau, J. Wei, D. Zhu, S. Zou, H. S. Sun, Y. Fu, F. Liu and Y. Lu (2004) Expression of Ca(2+)-permeable AMPA receptor channels primes cell death in transient forebrain ischemia. Neuron 43:43–55.

[65] T. Opitz, S. Y. Grooms, M. V. Bennett and R. S. Zukin (2000) Remodeling of alpha-amino-3-hydroxy-5-methyl-4-isoxazole-propionic acid receptor subunit composition in hippocampal neurons after global ischemia. Proceedings of the National Academy of Sciences of the United States of America 97:13360–13365.

[66] D. L. Hunt and P. E. Castillo (2012) Synaptic plasticity of NMDA receptors: mechanisms and functional implications. Curr Opin Neurobiol 22:496–508.

[67] C. Ikonomidou and L. Turski (2002) Why did NMDA receptor antagonists fail clinical trials for stroke and traumatic brain injury? Lancet Neurol 1:383–386.

[68] G. E. Hardingham (2009) Coupling of the NMDA receptor to neuroprotective and neurodestructive events. Biochem Soc Trans 37:1147–1160.

[69] S. Papadia, F. X. Soriano, F. Leveille, M. A. Martel, K. A. Dakin, H. H. Hansen, A. Kaindl, M. Sifringer, J. Fowler, V. Stefovska, G. McKenzie, M. Craigon, R. Corriveau, P. Ghazal, K. Horsburgh, B. A. Yankner, D. J. Wyllie, C. Ikonomidou and G. E. Hardingham (2008) Synaptic NMDA receptor activity boosts intrinsic antioxidant defenses. Nat Neurosci 11:476–487.

[70] M. Sheng, J. Cummings, L. A. Roldan, Y. N. Jan and L. Y. Jan (1994) Changing subunit composition of heteromeric NMDA receptors during development of rat cortex. Nature 368:144–147.

[71] J. T. Wang, Z. A. Medress and B. A. Barres (2012) Axon degeneration: molecular mechanisms of a self-destruction pathway. The Journal of cell biology 196:7–18.

[72] T. Miyawaki, T. Mashiko, D. Ofengeim, R. J. Flannery, K. M. Noh, S. Fujisawa, L. Bonanni, M. V. Bennett, R. S. Zukin and E. A. Jonas (2008) Ischemic preconditioning blocks BAD translocation, Bcl-xL cleavage, and large channel activity in mitochondria of postischemic hippocampal neurons. Proceedings of the National Academy of Sciences of the United States of America 105:4892–4897.

[73] D. Ofengeim, Y. B. Chen, T. Miyawaki, H. Li, S. Sacchetti, R. J. Flannery, K. N. Alavian, F. Pontarelli, B. A. Roelofs, J. A. Hickman, J. M. Hardwick, R. S. Zukin and E. A. Jonas (2012) N-terminally cleaved Bcl-xL mediates ischemia-induced neuronal death. In: Nat Neurosci, 2012/03/01 Edition 15:574–580.

[74] H. A. Park, P. Licznerski, K. N. Alavian, M. Shanabrough and E. A. Jonas (2015) Bcl-xL Is Necessary for Neurite Outgrowth in Hippocampal Neurons. Antioxidants & redox signaling 22:93–108.

[75] H. A. Park, N. Kubicki, S. Gnyawali, Y. C. Chan, S. Roy, S. Khanna and C. K. Sen (2011) Natural vitamin E alpha-tocotrienol protects against ischemic stroke by induction of multidrug resistance-associated protein 1. Stroke; a journal of cerebral circulation 42:2308–2314.

[76] W. A. Pulsinelli, J. B. Brierley and F. Plum (1982) Temporal profile of neuronal damage in a model of transient forebrain ischemia. Ann Neurol 11:491–498.

[77] D. F. Matesic and R. C. Lin (1994) Microtubule-associated protein 2 as an early indicator of ischemia-induced neurodegeneration in the gerbil forebrain. Journal of neurochemistry 63:1012–1020.

[78] K. Kitagawa, M. Matsumoto, M. Niinobe, K. Mikoshiba, R. Hata, H. Ueda, N. Handa, R. Fukunaga, Y. Isaka, K. Kimura and et al. (1989) Microtubule-associated protein 2 as a sensitive marker for cerebral ischemic damage–immunohistochemical investigation of dendritic damage. Neuroscience 31:401–411.

[79] J. Aronowski, K. H. Cho, R. Strong and J. C. Grotta (1999) Neurofilament proteolysis after focal ischemia; when do cells die after experimental stroke? Journal of cerebral blood flow and metabolism: official journal of the International Society of Cerebral Blood Flow and Metabolism 19:652–660.

[80] C. P. Baines (2009) The mitochondrial permeability transition pore and ischemia-reperfusion injury. Basic Res Cardiol 104:181–188.

[81] T. H. Murphy and D. Corbett (2009) Plasticity during stroke recovery: from synapse to behaviour. Nat Rev Neurosci 10:861–872.

[82] R. P. Stroemer, T. A. Kent and C. E. Hulsebosch (1995) Neocortical neural sprouting, synaptogenesis, and behavioral recovery after neocortical infarction in rats. Stroke; a journal of cerebral circulation 26:2135–2144.

[83] R. P. Stroemer, T. A. Kent and C. E. Hulsebosch (1998) Enhanced neocortical neural sprouting, synaptogenesis, and behavioral recovery with D-amphetamine therapy after neocortical infarction in rats. Stroke; a journal of cerebral circulation 29:2381–2393; discussion 2393–2385.

[84] S. T. Carmichael (2003) Plasticity of cortical projections after stroke. Neuroscientist 9:64–75.

[85] S. T. Carmichael, L. Wei, C. M. Rovainen and T. A. Woolsey (2001) New patterns of intracortical projections after focal cortical stroke. Neurobiology of disease 8:910–922.

[86] C. E. Brown, P. Li, J. D. Boyd, K. R. Delaney and T. H. Murphy (2007) Extensive turnover of dendritic spines and vascular remodeling in cortical tissues recovering from stroke. The Journal of neuroscience: the official journal of the Society for Neuroscience 27:4101–4109.

[87] R. Mostany, T. G. Chowdhury, D. G. Johnston, S. A. Portonovo, S. T. Carmichael and C. Portera-Cailliau (2010) Local hemodynamics dictate long-term dendritic plasticity in peri-infarct cortex. The Journal of neuroscience: the official journal of the Society for Neuroscience 30:14116–14126.

[88] C. Zhao, W. Deng and F. H. Gage (2008) Mechanisms and functional implications of adult neurogenesis. Cell 132:645–660.

[89] J. Macas, C. Nern, K. H. Plate and S. Momma (2006) Increased generation of neuronal progenitors after ischemic injury in the aged adult human forebrain. The Journal of neuroscience: the official journal of the Society for Neuroscience 26:13114–13119.

[90] O. Lindvall and Z. Kokaia (2015) Neurogenesis following Stroke Affecting the Adult Brain. Cold Spring Harb Perspect Biol 7:1–19.

[91] J. Marti-Fabregas, M. Romaguera-Ros, U. Gomez-Pinedo, S. Martinez-Ramirez, E. Jimenez-Xarrie, R. Marin, J. L. Marti-Vilalta and J. M. Garcia-Verdugo (2010) Proliferation in the human ipsilateral subventricular zone after ischemic stroke. Neurology 74:357–365.

[92] K. Jin, X. Wang, L. Xie, X. O. Mao, W. Zhu, Y. Wang, J. Shen, Y. Mao, S. Banwait and D. A. Greenberg (2006) Evidence for stroke-induced neurogenesis in the human brain. Proceedings of the National Academy of Sciences of the United States of America 103:13198–13202.

[93] J. M. Gidday (2006) Cerebral preconditioning and ischaemic tolerance. Nat Rev Neurosci 7:437–448.

[94] U. Dirnagl, K. Becker and A. Meisel (2009) Preconditioning and tolerance against cerebral ischaemia: from experimental strategies to clinical use. Lancet Neurol 8:398–412.

[95] H. Tanaka, A. Calderone, T. Jover, S. Y. Grooms, H. Yokota, R. S. Zukin and M. V. Bennett (2002) Ischemic preconditioning acts upstream of GluR2 down-regulation to afford neuroprotection in the hippocampal CA1. Proceedings of the National Academy of Sciences of the United States of America 99:2362–2367.

[96] H. Tanaka, H. Yokota, T. Jover, I. Cappuccio, A. Calderone, M. Simionescu, M. V. Bennett and R. S. Zukin (2004) Ischemic preconditioning: neuronal survival in the face of caspase-3 activation. The Journal of neuroscience: the official journal of the Society for Neuroscience 24:2750–2759.

[97] R. Meller, M. Minami, J. A. Cameron, S. Impey, D. Chen, J. Q. Lan, D. C. Henshall and R. P. Simon (2005) CREB-mediated Bcl-2 protein expression after ischemic preconditioning. Journal of cerebral blood flow and metabolism: official journal of the International Society of Cerebral Blood Flow and Metabolism 25:234–246.

[98] C. Wu, H. Fujihara, J. Yao, S. Qi, H. Li, K. Shimoji and H. Baba (2003) Different expression patterns of Bcl-2, Bcl-xl, and Bax proteins after sublethal forebrain ischemia in C57Black/Crj6 mouse striatum. Stroke; a journal of cerebral circulation 34:1803–1808.

[99] L. Y. Wu, A. S. Ding, T. Zhao, Z. M. Ma, F. Z. Wang and M. Fan (2004) Involvement of increased stability of mitochondrial membrane potential and overexpression of Bcl-2 in enhanced anoxic tolerance induced by hypoxic preconditioning in cultured hypothalamic neurons. Brain Res 999:149–154.

[100] S. A. Stroev, T. S. Gluschenko, E. I. Tjulkova, G. Spyrou, E. A. Rybnikova, M. O. Samoilov and M. Pelto-Huikko (2004) Preconditioning enhances the expression of mitochondrial antioxidant thioredoxin-2 in the forebrain of rats exposed to severe hypobaric hypoxia. J Neurosci Res 78:563–569.

[101] K. F. Bell, J. H. Fowler, B. Al-Mubarak, K. Horsburgh and G. E. Hardingham (2011) Activation of Nrf2-regulated glutathione pathway genes by ischemic preconditioning. Oxid Med Cell Longev 2011:689524.

[102] M. Liu and N. J. Alkayed (2005) Hypoxic preconditioning and tolerance via hypoxia inducible factor (HIF) 1alpha-linked induction of P450 2C11 epoxygenase in astrocytes. Journal of cerebral blood flow and metabolism: official journal of the International Society of Cerebral Blood Flow and Metabolism 25:939–948.

[103] N. M. Jones and M. Bergeron (2001) Hypoxic preconditioning induces changes in HIF-1 target genes in neonatal rat brain. Journal of cerebral blood flow and metabolism: official journal of the International Society of Cerebral Blood Flow and Metabolism 21:1105–1114.

[104] A. Ravati, B. Ahlemeyer, A. Becker, S. Klumpp and J. Krieglstein (2001) Preconditioning-induced neuroprotection is mediated by reactive oxygen species and activation of the transcription factor nuclear factor-kappaB. Journal of neurochemistry 78:909–919.

[105] E. Rybnikova, T. Gluschenko, E. Tulkova, A. Churilova, O. Jaroshevich, K. Baranova and M. Samoilov (2008) Preconditioning induces prolonged expression of transcription factors pCREB and NF-kappa B in the neocortex of rats before and following severe hypobaric hypoxia. Journal of neurochemistry 106:1450–1458.

[106] E. Rybnikova, T. Glushchenko, E. Tyulkova, K. Baranova and M. Samoilov (2009) Mild hypobaric hypoxia preconditioning up-regulates expression of transcription factors c-Fos and NGFI-A in rat neocortex and hippocampus. Neurosci Res 65:360–366.

[107] K. F. Bell, B. Al-Mubarak, J. H. Fowler, P. S. Baxter, K. Gupta, T. Tsujita, S. Chowdhry, R. Patani, S. Chandran, K. Horsburgh, J. D. Hayes and G. E. Hardingham (2011) Mild oxidative stress activates Nrf2 in astrocytes, which contributes to neuroprotective ischemic preconditioning. Proceedings of the National Academy of Sciences of the United States of America 108:E1–2; author reply E3–4.

[108] K. Kapinya, R. Penzel, C. Sommer and M. Kiessling (2000) Temporary changes of the AP-1 transcription factor binding activity in the gerbil hippocampus after transient global ischemia, and ischemic tolerance induction. Brain Res 872:282–293.

[109] P. Bernardi and F. Di Lisa (2015) The mitochondrial permeability transition pore: molecular nature and role as a target in cardioprotection. Journal of molecular and cellular cardiology 78:100–106.

[110] E. A. Jonas (2009) Molecular participants in mitochondrial cell death channel formation during neuronal ischemia. Exp Neurol 218:203–212.

[111] K. M. Holmstrom and T. Finkel (2014) Cellular mechanisms and physiological consequences of redox-dependent signalling. Nature reviews. Molecular cell biology 15:411–421.

[112] A. J. Kowaltowski, R. F. Castilho and A. E. Vercesi (2001) Mitochondrial permeability transition and oxidative stress. FEBS Lett 495:12–15.

[113] B. Halliwell (1992) Reactive oxygen species and the central nervous system. Journal of neurochemistry 59:1609–1623.

[114] C. A. Massaad and E. Klann (2011) Reactive oxygen species in the regulation of synaptic plasticity and memory. Antioxidants & redox signaling 14:2013–2054.

[115] K. T. Kishida, C. A. Hoeffer, D. Hu, M. Pao, S. M. Holland and E. Klann (2006) Synaptic plasticity deficits and mild memory impairments in mouse models of chronic granulomatous disease. Mol Cell Biol 26:5908–5920.

[116] E. Klann (1998) Cell-permeable scavengers of superoxide prevent long-term potentiation in hippocampal area CA1. J Neurophysiol 80:452–457.

[117] E. Thiels, N. N. Urban, G. R. Gonzalez-Burgos, B. I. Kanterewicz, G. Barrionuevo, C. T. Chu, T. D. Oury and E. Klann (2000) Impairment of long-term potentiation and associative memory in mice that overexpress extracellular superoxide dismutase. The Journal of neuroscience: the official journal of the Society for Neuroscience 20:7631–7639.

[118] E. Gahtan, J. M. Auerbach, Y. Groner and M. Segal (1998) Reversible impairment of long-term potentiation in transgenic Cu/Zn-SOD mice. Eur J Neurosci 10:538–544.

[119] R. Radi, J. S. Beckman, K. M. Bush and B. A. Freeman (1991) Peroxynitrite oxidation of sulfhydryls. The cytotoxic potential of superoxide and nitric oxide. The Journal of biological chemistry 266:4244–4250.

[120] S. P. Olesen, A. Moller, P. I. Mordvintcev, R. Busse and A. Mulsch (1997) Regional measurements of NO formed in vivo during brain ischemia. Acta Neurol Scand 95:219–224.

[121] V. L. Dawson, T. M. Dawson, E. D. London, D. S. Bredt and S. H. Snyder (1991) Nitric oxide mediates glutamate neurotoxicity in primary cortical cultures. Proceedings of the National Academy of Sciences of the United States of America 88:6368–6371.

[122] J. P. Bolanos, A. Almeida and J. M. Medina (1998) Nitric oxide mediates brain mitochondrial damage during perinatal anoxia. Brain Res 787:117–122.

[123] J. P. Bolanos, S. Peuchen, S. J. Heales, J. M. Land and J. B. Clark (1994) Nitric oxide-mediated inhibition of the mitochondrial respiratory chain in cultured astrocytes. Journal of neurochemistry 63:910–916.

[124] E. M. Schuman and D. V. Madison (1991) A requirement for the intercellular messenger nitric oxide in long-term potentiation. Science 254:1503–1506.

[125] J. P. Bolanos and A. Almeida (1999) Roles of nitric oxide in brain hypoxia-ischemia. Biochimica et biophysica acta 1411:415–436.

[126] K. A. Graham, M. Kulawiec, K. M. Owens, X. Li, M. M. Desouki, D. Chandra and K. K. Singh (2010) NADPH oxidase 4 is an oncoprotein localized to mitochondria. Cancer Biol Ther 10:223–231.

[127] S. P. Tammariello, M. T. Quinn and S. Estus (2000) NADPH oxidase contributes directly to oxidative stress and apoptosis in nerve growth factor-deprived sympathetic neurons. The Journal of neuroscience: the official journal of the Society for Neuroscience 20:RC53.

[128] C. Cheret, A. Gervais, A. Lelli, C. Colin, L. Amar, P. Ravassard, J. Mallet, A. Cumano, K. H. Krause and M. Mallat (2008) Neurotoxic activation of microglia is promoted by a nox1-dependent NADPH oxidase. The Journal of neuroscience: the official journal of the Society for Neuroscience 28:12039–12051.

[129] P. Vallet, Y. Charnay, K. Steger, E. Ogier-Denis, E. Kovari, F. Herrmann, J. P. Michel and I. Szanto (2005) Neuronal expression of the NADPH oxidase NOX4, and its regulation in mouse experimental brain ischemia. Neuroscience 132:233–238.

[130] H. Li, Y. Wang, D. Feng, Y. Liu, M. Xu, A. Gao, F. Tian, L. Zhang, Y. Cui, Z. Wang and G. Chen (2014) Alterations in the time course of expression of the Nox family in the brain in a rat experimental cerebral ischemia and reperfusion model: effects of melatonin. J Pineal Res 57:110–119.

[131] X. N. Tang, B. Cairns, N. Cairns and M. A. Yenari (2008) Apocynin improves outcome in experimental stroke with a narrow dose range. Neuroscience 154:556–562.

[132] H. Chen, Y. S. Song and P. H. Chan (2009) Inhibition of NADPH oxidase is neuroprotective after ischemia-reperfusion. Journal of cerebral blood flow and metabolism: official journal of the International Society of Cerebral Blood Flow and Metabolism 29:1262–1272.

[133] R. A. Haworth and D. R. Hunter (1979) The Ca2+-induced membrane transition in mitochondria. II. Nature of the Ca2+ trigger site. Arch Biochem Biophys 195:460–467.

[134] D. R. Hunter and R. A. Haworth (1979) The Ca2+-induced membrane transition in mitochondria. I. The protective mechanisms. Arch Biochem Biophys 195:453–459.

[135] C. P. Baines, R. A. Kaiser, T. Sheiko, W. J. Craigen and J. D. Molkentin (2007) Voltage-dependent anion channels are dispensable for mitochondrial-dependent cell death. Nat Cell Biol 9:550–555.

[136] T. Nakagawa, S. Shimizu, T. Watanabe, O. Yamaguchi, K. Otsu, H. Yamagata, H. Inohara, T. Kubo and Y. Tsujimoto (2005) Cyclophilin D-dependent mitochondrial permeability transition regulates some necrotic but not apoptotic cell death. Nature 434:652–658.

[137] E. Basso, L. Fante, J. Fowlkes, V. Petronilli, M. A. Forte and P. Bernardi (2005) Properties of the permeability transition pore in mitochondria devoid of Cyclophilin D. The Journal of biological chemistry 280:18558–18561.

[138] C. Brenner, H. Cadiou, H. L. Vieira, N. Zamzami, I. Marzo, Z. Xie, B. Leber, D. Andrews, H. Duclohier, J. C. Reed and G. Kroemer (2000) Bcl-2 and Bax regulate the channel activity of the mitochondrial adenine nucleotide translocator. Oncogene 19:329–336.

[139] I. Szabo, V. De Pinto and M. Zoratti (1993) The mitochondrial permeability transition pore may comprise VDAC molecules. II. The electrophysiological properties of VDAC are compatible with those of the mitochondrial megachannel. FEBS Lett 330:206–210.

[140] I. Szabo and M. Zoratti (1993) The mitochondrial permeability transition pore may comprise VDAC molecules. I. Binary structure and voltage dependence of the pore. FEBS Lett 330:201–205.

[141] M. Crompton (1999) The mitochondrial permeability transition pore and its role in cell death. The Biochemical journal 341 (Pt 2):233–249.

[142] K. M. Debatin, D. Poncet and G. Kroemer (2002) Chemotherapy: targeting the mitochondrial cell death pathway. Oncogene 21:8786–8803.

[143] K. Woodfield, A. Ruck, D. Brdiczka and A. P. Halestrap (1998) Direct demonstration of a specific interaction between cyclophilin-D and the adenine nucleotide translocase confirms their role in the mitochondrial permeability transition. The Biochemical journal 336 (Pt 2):287–290.

[144] A. W. Leung, P. Varanyuwatana and A. P. Halestrap (2008) The mitochondrial phosphate carrier interacts with cyclophilin D and may play a key role in the permeability transition. In: The Journal of biological chemistry 283:26312–26323.

[145] S. Shanmughapriya, S. Rajan, N. E. Hoffman, A. M. Higgins, D. Tomar, N. Nemani, K. J. Hines, D. J. Smith, A. Eguchi, S. Vallem, F. Shaikh, M. Cheung, N. J. Leonard, R. S. Stolakis, M. P. Wolfers, J. Ibetti, J. K. Chuprun, N. R. Jog, S. R. Houser, W. J. Koch, J. W. Elrod and M. Madesh (2015) SPG7 Is an Essential and Conserved Component of the Mitochondrial Permeability Transition Pore. Mol Cell 60:47–62.

[146] H. Azoulay-Zohar, A. Israelson, S. Abu-Hamad and V. Shoshan-Barmatz (2004) In self-defence: hexokinase promotes voltage-dependent anion channel closure and prevents mitochondria-mediated apoptotic cell death. The Biochemical journal 377: 347–355.

[147] J. G. Pastorino and J. B. Hoek (2008) Regulation of hexokinase binding to VDAC. J Bioenerg Biomembr 40:171–182.

[148] J. E. Kokoszka, K. G. Waymire, S. E. Levy, J. E. Sligh, J. Cai, D. P. Jones, G. R. MacGregor and D. C. Wallace (2004) The ADP/ATP translocator is not essential for the mitochondrial permeability transition pore. Nature 427:461–465.

[149] M. Bonora, A. Bononi, E. De Marchi, C. Giorgi, M. Lebiedzinska, S. Marchi, S. Patergnani, A. Rimessi, J. M. Suski, A. Wojtala, M. R. Wieckowski, G. Kroemer, L. Galluzzi and P. Pinton (2013) Role of the c subunit of the FO ATP synthase in mitochondrial permeability transition. Cell Cycle 12:674–683.

[150] M. Bonora, M. R. Wieckowski, C. Chinopoulos, O. Kepp, G. Kroemer, L. Galluzzi and P. Pinton (2015) Molecular mechanisms of cell death: central implication of ATP synthase in mitochondrial permeability transition. Oncogene 34:1475–1486.

[151] V. Giorgio, S. von Stockum, M. Antoniel, A. Fabbro, F. Fogolari, M. Forte, G. D. Glick, V. Petronilli, M. Zoratti, I. Szabo, G. Lippe and P. Bernardi (2013) Dimers of mitochondrial ATP synthase form the permeability transition pore. Proceedings of the National Academy of Sciences of the United States of America 110:5887–5892.

[152] V. Giorgio, E. Bisetto, M. E. Soriano, F. Dabbeni-Sala, E. Basso, V. Petronilli, M. A. Forte, P. Bernardi and G. Lippe (2009) Cyclophilin D modulates mitochondrial F0F1-ATP synthase by interacting with the lateral stalk of the complex. The Journal of biological chemistry 284:33982–33988.

[153] T. S. Azarashvili, J. Tyynela, I. V. Odinokova, P. A. Grigorjev, M. Baumann, Y. V. Evtodienko and N. E. Saris (2002) Phosphorylation of a peptide related to subunit c of the F0F1-ATPase/ATP synthase and relationship to permeability transition pore opening in mitochondria. J Bioenerg Biomembr 34:279–284.

[154] T. Azarashvili, I. Odinokova, A. Bakunts, V. Ternovsky, O. Krestinina, J. Tyynela and N. E. Saris (2014) Potential role of subunit c of F0F1-ATPase and subunit c of storage body in the mitochondrial permeability transition. Effect of the phosphorylation status of subunit c on pore opening. Cell Calcium 55:69–77.

[155] K. N. Alavian, G. Beutner, E. Lazrove, S. Sacchetti, H. A. Park, P. Licznerski, H. Li, P. Nabili, K. Hockensmith, M. Graham, G. A. Porter, Jr. and E. A. Jonas (2014) An uncoupling channel within the c-subunit ring of the F1FO ATP synthase is the mitochondrial permeability transition pore. Proceedings of the National Academy of Sciences of the United States of America 111:10580–10585.

[156] E. A. Jonas, G. A. Porter and K. N. Alavian (2014) Bcl-xL in neuroprotection and plasticity. Front Physiol 5:355.

[157] S. Couoh-Cardel, Y. C. Hsueh, S. Wilkens and L. Movileanu (2016) Yeast V-ATPase Proteolipid Ring Acts as a Large-conductance Transmembrane Protein Pore. Sci Rep 6:24774.

[158] K. N. Alavian, H. Li, L. Collis, L. Bonanni, L. Zeng, S. Sacchetti, E. Lazrove, P. Nabili, B. Flaherty, M. Graham, Y. Chen, S. M. Messerli, M. A. Mariggio, C. Rahner, E. McNay, G. C. Shore, P. J. Smith, J. M. Hardwick and E. A. Jonas (2011) Bcl-xL regulates metabolic efficiency of neurons through interaction with the mitochondrial F1FO ATP synthase. Nat Cell Biol 13:1224–1233.

[159] F. Minauro-Sanmiguel, S. Wilkens and J. J. Garcia (2005) Structure of dimeric mitochondrial ATP synthase: novel F0 bridging features and the structural basis of mitochondrial cristae biogenesis. Proceedings of the National Academy of Sciences of the United States of America 102:12356–12358.

[160] B. Daum, A. Walter, A. Horst, H. D. Osiewacz and W. Kuhlbrandt (2013) Age-dependent dissociation of ATP synthase dimers and loss of inner-membrane cristae in mitochondria. Proceedings of the National Academy of Sciences of the United States of America 110:15301–15306.

[161] P. Bernardi (2013) The mitochondrial permeability transition pore: a mystery solved? Front Physiol 4:95.

[162] J. M. Jurgensmeier, Z. Xie, Q. Deveraux, L. Ellerby, D. Bredesen and J. C. Reed (1998) Bax directly induces release of cytochrome c from isolated mitochondria. In: Proceedings of the National Academy of Sciences of the United States of America 95:4997–5002.

[163] M. Sattler, H. Liang, D. Nettesheim, R. P. Meadows, J. E. Harlan, M. Eberstadt, H. S. Yoon, S. B. Shuker, B. S. Chang, A. J. Minn, C. B. Thompson and S. W. Fesik (1997) Structure of Bcl-xL-Bak peptide complex: recognition between regulators of apoptosis. Science 275:983–986.

[164] S. Shimizu, M. Narita and Y. Tsujimoto (1999) Bcl-2 family proteins regulate the release of apoptogenic cytochrome c by the mitochondrial channel VDAC. Nature 399:483–487.

[165] S. B. Berman, Y. B. Chen, B. Qi, J. M. McCaffery, E. B. Rucker, 3rd, S. Goebbels, K. A. Nave, B. A. Arnold, E. A. Jonas, F. J. Pineda and J. M. Hardwick (2009) Bcl-x L increases mitochondrial fission, fusion, and biomass in neurons. The Journal of cell biology 184:707–719.

[166] P. Delivani, C. Adrain, R. C. Taylor, P. J. Duriez and S. J. Martin (2006) Role for CED-9 and Egl-1 as regulators of mitochondrial fission and fusion dynamics. Mol Cell 21:761–773.

[167] H. Li, Y. Chen, A. F. Jones, R. H. Sanger, L. P. Collis, R. Flannery, E. C. McNay, T. Yu, R. Schwarzenbacher, B. Bossy, E. Bossy-Wetzel, M. V. Bennett, M. Pypaert, J. A. Hickman, P. J. Smith, J. M. Hardwick and E. A. Jonas (2008) Bcl-xL induces Drp1-dependent synapse formation in cultured hippocampal neurons. Proceedings of the National Academy of Sciences of the United States of America 105:2169–2174.

[168] Y. B. Chen, M. A. Aon, Y. T. Hsu, L. Soane, X. Teng, J. M. McCaffery, W. C. Cheng, B. Qi, H. Li, K. N. Alavian, M. Dayhoff-Brannigan, S. Zou, F. J. Pineda, B. O'Rourke, Y. H. Ko, P. L. Pedersen, L. K. Kaczmarek, E. A. Jonas and J. M. Hardwick (2011) Bcl-xL regulates mitochondrial energetics by stabilizing the inner membrane potential. The Journal of cell biology 195:263–276.

[169] M. Veas-Perez de Tudela, M. Delgado-Esteban, C. Maestre, V. Bobo-Jimenez, D. Jimenez-Blasco, R. Vecino, J. P. Bolanos and A. Almeida (2015) Regulation of Bcl-xL-ATP Synthase Interaction by Mitochondrial Cyclin B1-Cyclin-Dependent Kinase-1 Determines Neuronal Survival. The Journal of neuroscience: the official journal of the Society for Neuroscience 35:9287–9301.

[170] A. Kretz, S. Kugler, C. Happold, M. Bahr and S. Isenmann (2004) Excess Bcl-XL increases the intrinsic growth potential of adult CNS neurons in vitro. Mol Cell Neurosci 26:63–74.

[171] H. Li, K. N. Alavian, E. Lazrove, N. Mehta, A. Jones, P. Zhang, P. Licznerski, M. Graham, T. Uo, J. Guo, C. Rahner, R. S. Duman, R. S. Morrison and E. A. Jonas (2013) A Bcl-xL-Drp1 complex regulates synaptic vesicle membrane dynamics during endocytosis. Nat Cell Biol 15:773–785.

[172] E. A. Jonas, J. A. Hickman, M. Chachar, B. M. Polster, T. A. Brandt, Y. Fannjiang, I. Ivanovska, G. Basanez, K. W. Kinnally, J. Zimmerberg, J. M. Hardwick and L. K. Kaczmarek (2004) Proapoptotic N-truncated BCL-xL protein activates endogenous mitochondrial channels in living synaptic terminals. Proceedings of the National Academy of Sciences of the United States of America 101:13590–13595.

[173] J. A. Hickman, J. M. Hardwick, L. K. Kaczmarek and E. A. Jonas (2008) Bcl-xL inhibitor ABT-737 reveals a dual role for Bcl-xL in synaptic transmission. J Neurophysiol 99:1515–1522.

[174] R. J. Clem, E. H. Cheng, C. L. Karp, D. G. Kirsch, K. Ueno, A. Takahashi, M. B. Kastan, D. E. Griffin, W. C. Earnshaw, M. A. Veliuona and J. M. Hardwick (1998) Modulation of cell death by Bcl-XL through caspase interaction. Proceedings of the National Academy of Sciences of the United States of America 95:554–559.

[175] N. S. Seng, J. Megyesi, A. Tarcsafalvi and P. M. Price (2016) Mimicking Cdk2 phosphorylation of Bcl-xL at Ser73 results in caspase activation and Bcl-xL cleavage. Cell Death Discov 2:1–6.

[176] N. Fujita, A. Nagahashi, K. Nagashima, S. Rokudai and T. Tsuruo (1998) Acceleration of apoptotic cell death after the cleavage of Bcl-XL protein by caspase-3-like proteases. Oncogene 17:1295–1304.

[177] R. Sugioka, S. Shimizu, T. Funatsu, H. Tamagawa, Y. Sawa, T. Kawakami and Y. Tsujimoto (2003) BH4-domain peptide from Bcl-xL exerts anti-apoptotic activity in vivo. Oncogene 22:8432–8440.

[178] M. Hirotani, Y. Zhang, N. Fujita, M. Naito and T. Tsuruo (1999) NH2-terminal BH4 domain of Bcl-2 is functional for heterodimerization with Bax and inhibition of apoptosis. The Journal of biological chemistry 274:20415–20420.

[179] G. Basanez, J. Zhang, B. N. Chau, G. I. Maksaev, V. A. Frolov, T. A. Brandt, J. Burch, J. M. Hardwick and J. Zimmerberg (2001) Pro-apoptotic cleavage products of Bcl-xL form cytochrome c-conducting pores in pure lipid membranes. The Journal of biological chemistry 276:31083–31091.

[180] B. Antonsson, F. Conti, A. Ciavatta, S. Montessuit, S. Lewis, I. Martinou, L. Bernasconi, A. Bernard, J. J. Mermod, G. Mazzei, K. Maundrell, F. Gambale, R. Sadoul and J. C. Martinou (1997) Inhibition of Bax channel-forming activity by Bcl-2. Science 277:370–372.

[181] M. Narita, S. Shimizu, T. Ito, T. Chittenden, R. J. Lutz, H. Matsuda and Y. Tsujimoto (1998) Bax interacts with the permeability transition pore to induce permeability transition and cytochrome c release in isolated mitochondria. Proceedings of the National Academy of Sciences of the United States of America 95:14681–14686.

[182] E. A. Jonas, J. M. Hardwick and L. K. Kaczmarek (2005) Actions of BAX on mitochondrial channel activity and on synaptic transmission. Antioxidants & redox signaling 7:1092–1100.

[183] S. Jiao and Z. Li (2011) Nonapoptotic function of BAD and BAX in long-term depression of synaptic transmission. Neuron 70:758–772.

[184] M. C. Wei, T. Lindsten, V. K. Mootha, S. Weiler, A. Gross, M. Ashiya, C. B. Thompson and S. J. Korsmeyer (2000) tBID, a membrane-targeted death ligand, oligomerizes BAK to release cytochrome c. Genes & development 14:2060–2071.

[185] L. Scorrano, M. Ashiya, K. Buttle, S. Weiler, S. A. Oakes, C. A. Mannella and S. J. Korsmeyer (2002) A distinct pathway remodels mitochondrial cristae and mobilizes cytochrome c during apoptosis. Dev Cell 2:55–67.

[186] N. Zamzami, C. El Hamel, C. Maisse, C. Brenner, C. Munoz-Pinedo, A. S. Belzacq, P. Costantini, H. Vieira, M. Loeffler, G. Molle and G. Kroemer (2000) Bid acts on the permeability transition pore complex to induce apoptosis. Oncogene 19:6342–6350.

[187] N. Plesnila, S. Zinkel, D. A. Le, S. Amin-Hanjani, Y. Wu, J. Qiu, A. Chiarugi, S. S. Thomas, D. S. Kohane, S. J. Korsmeyer and M. A. Moskowitz (2001) BID mediates neuronal cell death after oxygen/ glucose deprivation and focal cerebral ischemia. Proceedings of the National Academy of Sciences of the United States of America 98:15318–15323.

[188] X. M. Yin, Y. Luo, G. Cao, L. Bai, W. Pei, D. K. Kuharsky and J. Chen (2002) Bid-mediated mitochondrial pathway is critical to ischemic neuronal apoptosis and focal cerebral ischemia. The Journal of biological chemistry 277:42074–42081.

[189] G. L. Semenza (2011) Hypoxia-inducible factor 1: regulator of mitochondrial metabolism and mediator of ischemic preconditioning. Biochimica et biophysica acta 1813:1263–1268.

[190] M. C. Simon (2006) Mitochondrial reactive oxygen species are required for hypoxic HIF alpha stabilization. Adv Exp Med Biol 588:165–170.

[191] Y. Benita, H. Kikuchi, A. D. Smith, M. Q. Zhang, D. C. Chung and R. J. Xavier (2009) An integrative genomics approach identifies Hypoxia Inducible Factor-1 (HIF-1)-target genes that form the core response to hypoxia. Nucleic Acids Res 37:4587–4602.

[192] N. Chen, X. Chen, R. Huang, H. Zeng, J. Gong, W. Meng, Y. Lu, F. Zhao, L. Wang and Q. Zhou (2009) BCL-xL is a target gene regulated by hypoxia-inducible factor-1{alpha}. The Journal of biological chemistry 284:10004–10012.

[193] H. Zhang, M. Bosch-Marce, L. A. Shimoda, Y. S. Tan, J. H. Baek, J. B. Wesley, F. J. Gonzalez and G. L. Semenza (2008) Mitochondrial autophagy is an HIF-1-dependent adaptive metabolic response to hypoxia. The Journal of biological chemistry 283:10892–10903.

[194] G. Bellot, R. Garcia-Medina, P. Gounon, J. Chiche, D. Roux, J. Pouyssegur and N. M. Mazure (2009) Hypoxia-induced autophagy is mediated through hypoxia-inducible factor induction of BNIP3 and BNIP3L via their BH3 domains. Mol Cell Biol 29:2570–2581.

[195] K. Tracy, B. C. Dibling, B. T. Spike, J. R. Knabb, P. Schumacker and K. F. Macleod (2007) BNIP3 is an RB/E2F target gene required for hypoxia-induced autophagy. Mol Cell Biol 27:6229–6242.

[196] R. Fukuda, H. Zhang, J. W. Kim, L. Shimoda, C. V. Dang and G. L. Semenza (2007) HIF-1 regulates cytochrome oxidase subunits to optimize efficiency of respiration in hypoxic cells. Cell 129:111–122.

[197] T. Briston, J. Yang and M. Ashcroft (2011) HIF-1alpha localization with mitochondria: a new role for an old favorite? Cell Cycle 10:4170–4171.

[198] G. Hsiao, J. J. Lee, Y. C. Chen, J. H. Lin, M. Y. Shen, K. H. Lin, D. S. Chou and J. R. Sheu (2007) Neuroprotective effects of PMC, a potent alpha-tocopherol derivative, in brain ischemia-reperfusion: reduced neutrophil activation and anti-oxidant actions. Biochem Pharmacol 73:682–693.

[199] Y. Chang, C. Y. Hsieh, Z. A. Peng, T. L. Yen, G. Hsiao, D. S. Chou, C. M. Chen and J. R. Sheu (2009) Neuroprotective mechanisms of puerarin in middle cerebral artery occlusion-induced brain infarction in rats. J Biomed Sci 16:9.

[200] Y. Chang, G. Hsiao, S. H. Chen, Y. C. Chen, J. H. Lin, K. H. Lin, D. S. Chou and J. R. Sheu (2007) Tetramethylpyrazine suppresses HIF-1alpha, TNF-alpha, and activated caspase-3 expression in middle cerebral artery occlusion-induced brain ischemia in rats. Acta Pharmacol Sin 28:327–333.

[201] L. Chen, P. Feng, S. Li, D. Long, J. Cheng, Y. Lu and D. Zhou (2009) Effect of hypoxia-inducible factor-1alpha silencing on the sensitivity of human brain glioma cells to doxorubicin and etoposide. Neurochem Res 34:984–990.

[202] X. Zhang, K. Deguchi, T. Yamashita, Y. Ohta, J. Shang, F. Tian, N. Liu, V. L. Panin, Y. Ikeda, T. Matsuura and K. Abe (2010) Temporal and spatial differences of multiple protein expression in the ischemic penumbra after transient MCAO in rats. Brain Res 1343:143–152.

[203] T. Soucek, R. Cumming, R. Dargusch, P. Maher and D. Schubert (2003) The regulation of glucose metabolism by HIF-1 mediates a neuroprotective response to amyloid beta peptide. Neuron 39:43–56.

[204] M. A. Puchowicz, J. L. Zechel, J. Valerio, D. S. Emancipator, K. Xu, S. Pundik, J. C. LaManna and W. D. Lust (2008) Neuroprotection in diet-induced ketotic rat brain after focal ischemia. J Cereb Blood Flow Metab 28:1907–1916.

[205] O. Baranova, L. F. Miranda, P. Pichiule, I. Dragatsis, R. S. Johnson and J. C. Chavez (2007) Neuron-specific inactivation of the hypoxia inducible factor 1 alpha increases brain injury in a mouse model of transient focal cerebral ischemia. J Neurosci 27:6320–6332.

[206] J. Milosevic, M. Maisel, F. Wegner, J. Leuchtenberger, R. H. Wenger, M. Gerlach, A. Storch and J. Schwarz (2007) Lack of hypoxia-inducible factor-1 alpha impairs midbrain neural precursor cells involving vascular endothelial growth factor signaling. J Neurosci 27:412–421.

[207] S. Tomita, M. Ueno, M. Sakamoto, Y. Kitahama, M. Ueki, N. Maekawa, H. Sakamoto, M. Gassmann, R. Kageyama, N. Ueda, F. J. Gonzalez and Y. Takahama (2003) Defective brain development in mice lacking the Hif-1alpha gene in neural cells. Mol Cell Biol 23:6739–6749.

[208] S. N. Willis, L. Chen, G. Dewson, A. Wei, E. Naik, J. I. Fletcher, J. M. Adams and D. C. Huang (2005) Proapoptotic Bak is sequestered by Mcl-1 and Bcl-xL, but not Bcl-2, until displaced by BH3-only proteins. Genes & development 19:1294–1305.

[209] L. Ming, P. Wang, A. Bank, J. Yu and L. Zhang (2006) PUMA Dissociates Bax and Bcl-X(L) to induce apoptosis in colon cancer cells. The Journal of biological chemistry 281:16034–16042.

[210] J. Ding, B. H. Mooers, Z. Zhang, J. Kale, D. Falcone, J. McNichol, B. Huang, X. C. Zhang, C. Xing, D. W. Andrews and J. Lin (2014) After embedding in membranes antiapoptotic Bcl-XL protein binds both Bcl-2 homology region 3 and helix 1 of proapoptotic Bax protein to inhibit apoptotic mitochondrial permeabilization. The Journal of biological chemistry 289:11873–11896.

[211] S. Rajan, M. Choi, Q. T. Nguyen, H. Ye, W. Liu, H. T. Toh, C. Kang, N. Kamariah, C. Li, H. Huang, C. White, K. Baek, G. Gruber and H. S. Yoon (2015) Structural transition in Bcl-xL and its potential association with mitochondrial calcium ion transport. Sci Rep 5:10609.

[212] M. C. Maiuri, G. Le Toumelin, A. Criollo, J. C. Rain, F. Gautier, P. Juin, E. Tasdemir, G. Pierron, K. Troulinaki, N. Tavernarakis, J. A. Hickman, O. Geneste and G. Kroemer (2007) Functional and physical interaction between Bcl-X(L) and a BH3-like domain in Beclin-1. The EMBO journal 26:2527–2539.

[213] A. M. Petros, D. G. Nettesheim, Y. Wang, E. T. Olejniczak, R. P. Meadows, J. Mack, K. Swift, E. D. Matayoshi, H. Zhang, C. B. Thompson and S. W. Fesik (2000) Rationale for Bcl-xL/Bad peptide complex formation from structure, mutagenesis, and biophysical studies. Protein Sci 9:2528–2534.

[214] A. Chattopadhyay, C. W. Chiang and E. Yang (2001) BAD/BCL-[X(L)] heterodimerization leads to bypass of G0/G1 arrest. Oncogene 20:4507–4518.

[215] T. Moldoveanu, A. V. Follis, R. W. Kriwacki and D. R. Green (2014) Many players in BCL-2 family affairs. Trends Biochem Sci 39:101–111.

[216] X. Liu, S. Dai, Y. Zhu, P. Marrack and J. W. Kappler (2003) The structure of a Bcl-xL/Bim fragment complex: implications for Bim function. Immunity 19:341–352.

[217] S. Rajan, M. Choi, K. Baek and H. S. Yoon (2015) Bh3 induced conformational changes in Bcl-Xl revealed by crystal structure and comparative analysis. Proteins 83:1262–1272.

[218] A. V. Follis, J. E. Chipuk, J. C. Fisher, M. K. Yun, C. R. Grace, A. Nourse, K. Baran, L. Ou, L. Min, S. W. White, D. R. Green and R. W. Kriwacki (2013) PUMA binding induces partial unfolding within BCL-xL to disrupt p53 binding and promote apoptosis. Nat Chem Biol 9:163–168.

[219] Y. Hu, M. A. Benedict, D. Wu, N. Inohara and G. Nunez (1998) Bcl-XL interacts with Apaf-1 and inhibits Apaf-1-dependent caspase-9 activation. Proceedings of the National Academy of Sciences of the United States of America 95:4386–4391.

[220] G. Pan, K. O'Rourke and V. M. Dixit (1998) Caspase-9, Bcl-XL, and Apaf-1 form a ternary complex. The Journal of biological chemistry 273:5841–5845.

[221] L. Xue, F. Chu, Y. Cheng, X. Sun, A. Borthakur, M. Ramarao, P. Pandey, M. Wu, S. F. Schlossman and K. V. Prasad (2002) Siva-1 binds to and inhibits BCL-X(L)-mediated protection against UV radiation-induced apoptosis. Proceedings of the National Academy of Sciences of the United States of America 99:6925–6930.

[222] B. N. Chau, E. H. Cheng, D. A. Kerr and J. M. Hardwick (2000) Aven, a novel inhibitor of caspase activation, binds Bcl-xL and Apaf-1. Mol Cell 6:31–40.

[223] O. Kutuk, S. G. Temel, S. Tolunay and H. Basaga (2010) Aven blocks DNA damage-induced apoptosis by stabilising Bcl-xL. Eur J Cancer 46:2494–2505.

[224] G. Monaco, E. Decrock, H. Akl, R. Ponsaerts, T. Vervliet, T. Luyten, M. De Maeyer, L. Missiaen, C. W. Distelhorst, H. De Smedt, J. B. Parys, L. Leybaert and G. Bultynck (2012) Selective regulation of IP3-receptor-mediated Ca2+ signaling and apoptosis by the BH4 domain of Bcl-2 versus Bcl-Xl. Cell death and differentiation 19:295–309.

[225] G. Monaco, M. Beckers, H. Ivanova, L. Missiaen, J. B. Parys, H. De Smedt and G. Bultynck (2012) Profiling of the Bcl-2/Bcl-X(L)-binding sites on type 1 IP(3) receptor. Biochemical and biophysical research communications 428:31–35.

[226] S. C. Lo and M. Hannink (2006) PGAM5, a Bcl-XL-interacting protein, is a novel substrate for the redox-regulated Keap1-dependent ubiquitin ligase complex. The Journal of biological chemistry 281:37893–37903.

[227] S. K. Niture and A. K. Jaiswal (2011) Inhibitor of Nrf2 (INrf2 or Keap1) protein degrades Bcl-xL via phosphoglycerate mutase 5 and controls cellular apoptosis. The Journal of biological chemistry 286:44542–44556.

[228] G. Arena, V. Gelmetti, L. Torosantucci, D. Vignone, G. Lamorte, P. De Rosa, E. Cilia, E. A. Jonas and E. M. Valente (2013) PINK1 protects against cell death induced by mitochondrial depolarization, by phosphorylating Bcl-xL and impairing its pro-apoptotic cleavage. Cell death and differentiation 20:920–930.

[229] H. Huang, X. Hu, C. O. Eno, G. Zhao, C. Li and C. White (2013) An interaction between Bcl-xL and the voltage-dependent anion channel (VDAC) promotes mitochondrial Ca2+ uptake. The Journal of biological chemistry 288:19870–19881.

[230] M. G. Vander Heiden, X. X. Li, E. Gottleib, R. B. Hill, C. B. Thompson and M. Colombini (2001) Bcl-xL promotes the open configuration of the voltage-dependent anion channel and metabolite passage through the outer mitochondrial membrane. The Journal of biological chemistry 276:19414–19419.

[231] A. V. Follis, F. Llambi, L. Ou, K. Baran, D. R. Green and R. W. Kriwacki (2014) The DNA-binding domain mediates both nuclear and cytosolic functions of p53. Nat Struct Mol Biol 21:535–543.

[232] H. Endo, H. Kamada, C. Nito, T. Nishi and P. H. Chan (2006) Mitochondrial translocation of p53 mediates release of cytochrome c and hippocampal CA1 neuronal death after transient global cerebral ischemia in rats. The Journal of neuroscience: the official journal of the Society for Neuroscience 26:7974–7983.

11

Motor Cortex Hyperexcitability, Neuroplasticity, and Degeneration in Amyotrophic Lateral Sclerosis

Ilya S. Bakulin, Alexander V. Chervyakov,
Natalia A. Suponeva, Maria N. Zakharova and
Michael A. Piradov

Abstract

Neuronal hyperexcitability is a well-known phenomenon in amyotrophic lateral sclerosis and other neurodegenerative diseases. The use of transcranial magnetic stimulation in clinical and research practice has recently made it possible to detect motor cortex hyperexcitability under clinical conditions. Despite numerous studies, the mechanisms and sequelae of the development of hyperexcitability still have not been completely elucidated. In this chapter, we discuss the possibilities for detecting motor cortex hyperexcitability in patients with amyotrophic lateral sclerosis using transcranial magnetic stimulation. The potential relationship between hyperexcitability and neuronal degeneration or neuroplasticity processes is discussed using the data obtained by navigated transcranial magnetic stimulation and neuroimaging data, as well as the data of experimental studies.

Keywords: transcranial magnetic stimulation, amyotrophic lateral sclerosis, hyperexcitability, excitotoxicity, neuroplasticity

1. Introduction

Amyotrophic lateral sclerosis (ALS) is a fatal neurodegenerative disease affecting the upper and lower motor neurons. Despite the significant advance in molecular biology and genetics over the past years, many aspects of etiology and pathogenesis of ALS remain unstudied; neither biomarkers of the disease nor effective treatment methods have been designed [1].

A significant advance in understanding the pathophysiological mechanisms of the development of the neurodegenerative process of ALS has been made over the past years after novel neurophysiological and neuroimaging techniques were introduced into the research and clinical practice [2–4]. Transcranial magnetic stimulation (TMS) is a noninvasive brain stimulation method that is used to evaluate the functional status of the upper motor neuron in ALS patients. It has been shown in the recent studies that different TMS parameters are altered in ALS patients [4]. TMS is currently viewed as a valuable research and diagnostic tool in ALS.

Development of hyperexcitability of the primary motor cortex and the entire motor system is a well-studied phenomenon in ALS. Motor cortex hyperexcitability can be determined using TMS as reduced resting motor threshold and increased motor evoked potential (MEP) amplitude, decreased silent period, reduced effectiveness of short-interval intracortical inhibition (SICI), and increased intracortical facilitation (ICF) (see review [4]). Most authors attribute motor cortex hyperexcitability in ALS patients to enhanced glutamatergic neurotransmission in the neocortex and reduced gamma-aminobutyric acid (GABA)ergic inhibitory neurotransmission, thus suggesting that hyperexcitability provokes degeneration of motor neurons [5–7]. However, no direct evidence has been obtained yet that would unambiguously demonstrate the relationship between motor cortex hyperexcitability in ALS patients and its degeneration. There is an alternative opinion that hyperexcitability can potentially be related to neuroplasticity processes taking place in the motor cortex and compensation for the lost function.

We would like to discuss the potential relationship of motor cortex hyperexcitability with motor neuron degeneration and neuroplasticity in ALS patients, as well as the possible methods to solve this problem using modern neurophysiological and neuroimaging methods.

2. Motor cortex hyperexcitability in ALS

Although the term 'hyperexcitability' is widely used, it still does not have a commonly accepted definition. According to Bae et al. (2013), it 'means an increased or exaggerated response to a stimulus, which may usually have been expected to evoke a normal response' [7]. We deem that hyperexcitability is discussed in modern TMS studies more broadly: as the ability to respond to stimuli that normally do not evoke any response and, speaking more generally, as the predominance of excitation over inhibition.

Hyperexcitability in ALS patients can be determined using various methods at different levels of the motor system. It can be detected at the level of individual neurons and ion channels in cell cultures in transgenic animals, clinically (presenting as the well-known phenomena, such as fasciculation or cramps) or using the modern neurophysiological techniques such as electromyography (EMG) and TMS [7].

Motor cortex excitability is a complex integral parameter that depends on numerous factors. Hence, the hyperexcitability phenomenon is also a complex and multifactorial process that depends on glutamate synthesis and release, its reuptake and degradation, expression and functional status of several types of glutamate receptors, excitable properties of neuronal membranes, and the status of inhibitory GABAergic neurotransmission. A number of experimental studies demonstrated that all the aforementioned processes are disturbed in ALS [8, 9]. **Table 1** summarizes the results of some key studies.

Mechanism	Supporting facts
Decreased Glutamate reuptake	• A 70-80% decrease in expression of high-affinity astroglial glutamate transporter EAAT2 (excitatory amino acid transporter) in the motor cortex and spinal cord in ALS patients as a result of posttranslational modifications, oxidative stress, and other factors [10, 11] • Early reduction of glutamate transporter expression in mSOD1 transgenic animals [12] • Degeneration of motor neurons in the motor cortex and spinal cord as glutamate reuptake is inhibited *in vitro* in an organotypic cell culture [13] • The absence of compensatory increase in glutamate transporter expression by glial cells under excitotoxic conditions and oxidative stress [14]
Dysfunction of inhibitory GABAergic neurotransmission	• Degeneration of inhibitory interneurons in the motor cortex and spinal cord in ALS patients according to pathomorphological and animal model studies [15–17] • Decreased GABA level in the motor cortex according to the MR spectroscopy [18] and reduced ^{11}C-flumazenil binding according to the PET data [19] • Decreased level of mRNA of GABA(A) receptor subunits in a postmortem study [20]
Changes in excitability of motor neuron membranes	• Increased density and excitability of voltage-gated sodium channels in SOD1 transgenic animals [21, 22] • Decreased conductance of potassium channels Kv 1.2 • Hyperexcitability of individual motor neurons in a cell culture [23, 24]
Changes in expression and functions of glutamate receptors	• Decreased expression of the GluR2 subunit blocking calcium delivery to the cell in ALS patients with transgenic animals [25] • Disturbance of posttranslational modification of GluR2 subunit increasing permeability to calcium ions [25]

Table 1. Potential mechanisms of development of motor neuron hyperexcitability in ALS patients.

Today, TMS is the key and actually the only method for clinical investigation of motor cortex excitability. The use of the entire range of TMS parameters allows one to perform a relatively differentiated study of various factors contributing to motor cortex excitation [26]. TMS can be employed for assessing the functional status of the corticospinal tract due to the ability to excite motor cortex neurons by induced electrical current followed by propagation of excitation to alpha motor neurons of spinal cord. This causes contraction of muscle fibers within a certain motor unit, which can be recorded by cutaneous electrodes as a MEP [27]. TMS assesses the functional status of neuronal contours of the motor cortex [28].

Motor threshold is the key parameter used to assess motor cortex excitability. The motor threshold represents the density of corticospinal projections and can be regarded as a biomarker of neuronal membrane excitability [26]. Decreased motor threshold is considered to be one of the key signs of motor cortex hyperexcitability.

According to most studies, the motor threshold in ALS patients is increased, probably being indicative of degeneration of cortical motor neurons [29–35]. Meanwhile, a paradoxical decrease in the motor threshold when examining patients at the onset of the disease was shown in some studies [36–39]. The motor threshold is likely to decrease at the onset of ALS, probably until clinical signs appear, and subsequently increases as motor neurons die. A statistically significant direct correlation between the motor threshold and disease duration was demonstrated in some studies [29, 40].

Physiologically, the motor threshold is primarily determined by rapid AMPA receptor (AMPAR)-mediated glutamatergic neurotransmission in the neocortex and excitability of motor neuron membranes that depends on voltage-gated sodium channels [41]. In ALS, AMPA receptor-mediated glutamatergic neurotransmission increases and properties of sodium channels change (presenting as increased conductance) [23, 24, 42, 43]. Alteration in functional properties of potential-gated sodium channels has been revealed: more rapid recovery after inactivation, increased permeability to sodium, and increased density of ion channels [21]. Pieri et al. demonstrated a decrease in the action potential threshold, an increase in pulse frequency, and an increase in persistent sodium current in cortical motor neurons isolated in G93A mutant mice [22].

MEP amplitude is determined by the number of reduced motor units and the number of activated alpha motor neurons in the spinal cord. Increased stimulation intensity enhances MEP amplitude due to superimposition of late I-waves and I1-wave [28, 44]. Like the motor threshold, MEP amplitude is determined by the density of corticospinal projections. Meanwhile, MEP amplitude to a greater extent represents the function of neurons with lower excitability or those located farther from the stimulation site [4]. GABAergic drugs reduce MEP amplitude, which results from the scheme of generation of late I-waves modulated by inserted inhibitory GABAergic interneurons [41]. Noteworthy, the motor threshold and MEP amplitude are modulated by drugs belonging to different pharmacological classes, thus emphasizing the difference between the mechanisms of their formation.

Identically to the motor threshold, MEP amplitude in ALS patients changes in opposite directions depending on stage of the disease. MEP amplitude decreases in most cases, being accompanied by increased motor threshold and representing a decrease in motor neuron number and reduction of density of corticospinal projections [4]. On the contrary, some patients with the reduced motor threshold may have increased MEP amplitude and the ratio between MEP amplitude and M-response amplitude [45, 46]. The increased slope ratio of the amplitude vs intensity curve is additional evidence to motor cortex hyperexcitability in ALS patients as it demonstrates a more pronounced amplitude increment with increasing stimulation intensity compared to the norm. The increase in MEP amplitude and the slope ratio of the amplitude vs intensity curve in ALS patients is probably related to both enhanced glutamatergic and reduced inhibitory GABAergic neurotransmission in the neocortex [4].

The *cortical silent period* (cSP) represents inhibition of voluntary muscular activity during a certain period after a magnetic stimulus was applied [47]. It has been demonstrated that the first one-third of cSP is mostly controlled by inhibitory mechanisms at the spinal cord level, while the remaining two thirds are of cortical origin and are related to inhibitory neurotransmission through GABA(B) receptors [27].

It was demonstrated in most studies that patients with sporadic and familial ALS had either decreased cSP or no cSP at all, which is regarded as significant evidence attesting to intracortical inhibitory dysfunction in ALS patients [48–50].

Paired pulse stimulation is used to assess intracortical inhibition and excitation processes. The method involves sequential generation of two pulses: the conditioning (S1) and testing (S2) pulses. The physiological effects of paired pulse stimulation are determined by the intensity of S1 and the interval between S1 and S2 pulses. Application of the sub-threshold S1 pulse 1–6 ms before the supra-threshold S2 pulse reduces MEP amplitude compared to isolated application of a supra-threshold stimulus [51]. This phenomenon is known as SICI. Contrariwise, an increase of the interstimulus interval to 8–20 ms rises the amplitude of MEP to the testing pulse (ICF). Several protocols have been proposed where the conditioning pulse has the supra- and sub-threshold intensity. MEP amplitude increases at the long interstimulus interval (long-interval intracortical inhibition, LICI) and decreases at the short interval (short-interval intracortical facilitation, SICF) [27].

The neurophysiological mechanisms of formation of these phenomena remain insufficiently studied; however, it has been demonstrated rather convincingly that they have the predominantly intracortical origin. Thus, SICI and LICI protocols cause suppression of amplitude and the number of late descending waves [51, 52]. Intracortical inhibition processes are assumed to be caused by activation of neocortical inhibitory interneurons under the action of the conditioning pulse; SICI being mediated by inhibition through GABA(A) receptors and LICI, through GABA(B) receptors. The ICF phenomenon is presumably caused by activation of glutamatergic neurotransmission through NMDA glutamate receptors [26].

Disruption of intracortical inhibition and facilitation under paired-pulse stimulation is currently believed to be the most convincing evidence that motor cortex hyperexcitability develops in ALS patients and has been detected in numerous studies [6, 53, 54, 55]. It should be mentioned that a decrease in efficiency of SICI is revealed at the earliest stages of the disease, including asymptomatic SOD1 mutation carriers, and correlates with axonal degeneration of peripheral motor neurons [45]. Assessment of the disruptions of intracortical inhibition using the new threshold tracking technique is considered to be a potential diagnostic tool in ALS demonstrating high sensitivity and specificity [56, 57].

The role of inhibitory interneurons dysfunction in pathogenesis of ALS has been actively studied over the past years [58–60]. Degeneration of inhibitory interneurons both in the spinal cord and in the motor cortex was demonstrated in several pathomorphological studies carried out in the 1990s. Nihei et al. (1993) reported a reduced amount of parvalbumin-positive interneurons in the motor cortex in ALS patients [61]. In addition, Petri et al. (2003) demonstrated that the level of GABA(A) receptor alpha-1 subunit mRNA decreases in ALS patients

[20]. Dysfunction of inhibitory neurotransmission in the neocortex has also been confirmed in neuroimaging studies presenting as a decrease in GABA amount according to magnetic resonance spectroscopy [18] and decreased ^{11}C-flumazenil binding as shown by PET [19].

The TMS data additionally confirm that inhibitory neurotransmission in the neocortex is disrupted in ALS patients. It should be mentioned that TMS has been used to show the disturbance of inhibition in the motor cortex both mediated by GABA(A) (decreased SICI) and by GABA(B) receptors (decreased LICI and sCP), being indicative of degeneration of interneurons or GABA metabolism disruption rather than dysfunction of receptors of this mediator in the postsynaptic membrane.

Other factors that cause SICI disruption in ALS patients are being discussed. Thus, riluzole was reported to induce partial recovery of SICI in ALS patients, which gives grounds for suggesting that enhancement of glutamatergic neurotransmission plays a role in disturbance of intracortical inhibition in ALS patients. NMDA receptor antagonists, memantine and amantadine, were shown to increase SICI and decrease ICF in several pharmaco-TMS studies [41]. These data suggest that decreased intracortical inhibition in ALS patients can be related not only to reduction of inhibitory GABAergic neurotransmission but also to enhancement of glutamatergic neurotransmission through NMDAR.

Increased intracortical facilitation is another evidence for involvement of NMDAR in pathogenesis of ALS. This phenomenon is currently predominantly attributed to glutamatergic neurotransmission through NMDAR, which is confirmed, in particular, by its reduction due to antagonists of these receptors [41].

Hence, a large body of data attesting to the development of motor cortex hyperexcitability in ALS patients can currently be obtained by TMS. Signs attesting to degeneration of the upper motor neuron are detected simultaneously (**Table 2**). Importantly, some TMS parameters (MEP threshold and amplitude) can change in opposite directions and attest to motor cortex hyperexcitability at onset of the disease and degeneration as the disease progresses. Meanwhile, such signs of hyperexcitability as decreased cSP and efficiency of SICI are detected even in patients with pronounced degeneration of motor neurons. This phenomenon in ALS patients was referred to as 'dying but overactive' [7]; it can cause difficulties for interpretation of TMS results in a specific patient.

Hyperexcitability	Degeneration
• Resting motor threshold decreased	• Resting motor threshold increased
• MEP amplitude increased	• CMCT increased
• SICI reduced and ICF increased	• MEP amplitude decreased
• SP decreased	• Central conduction failure (triple stimulation technique)

Table 2. Motor cortex hyperexcitability and degeneration in ALS: TMS findings.

Table 3 summarizes the TMS data on the potential mechanisms responsible for the signs of motor cortex hyperexcitability in ALS patients. It should be mentioned that the variety of TMS procedures makes it possible not only to reveal the dysfunction of individual mediator systems but also to perform differentiated evaluation of neurotransmission through different types of glutamate and GABA receptors in ALS patients.

Sign	Mechanism
Decreased motor threshold	• Increased glutamatergic neurotransmission through AMPAR • Increased sodium current due to an increase in density and/or alteration in functional properties of sodium channels
Increased MER amplitude	• Increased glutamatergic neurotransmission through AMPAR • Decreased inhibitory GABAergic neurotransmission
Decreased silent period	• Decreased inhibitory GABAergic neurotransmission through GABA(B) receptors
Decreased SICI	• Decreased inhibitory GABAergic neurotransmission through GABA(A) receptors • Increased glutamatergic neurotransmission through NMDAR
Increased ICF	• Increased glutamatergic neurotransmission through NMDAR

Table 3. Potential mechanisms of formation of TMS signs of motor cortex hyperexcitability in ALS.

Based on TMS findings, it is rather promising and reasonable to suggest that motor cortex hyperexcitability and the underlying molecular events (e.g., excitotoxicity) cause degeneration of motor neurons in ALS patients. We attempt to discuss the specific potential mechanisms underlying motor cortex hyperexcitability in ALS and present the evidence for its pathogenetic relationship with degeneration of motor neuron.

3. What does motor cortex hyperexcitability mean?

3.1. Is hyperexcitability bad?

The evidence that motor cortex hyperexcitability plays a role in pathogenesis of ALS is still rather sparse [62]. Hyperexcitability is registered at different stages of the disease, including the pre-symptomatic ones [23, 45]. However, this fact tells nothing about its role in pathogenesis of the disease. It is still unclear when true onset of neurodegeneration occurs; however, the results of studies using transgenic animals demonstrate that the pathological process in ALS may start at the earliest stages of embryogenesis (e.g., at the stage when neural networks are formed) [63]. In this situation, all the objectively detectable alterations may be either primary or secondary (i.e., emerge as one of nonspecific stages of neurodegeneration or via the compensatory mechanism).

The enhancement of excitatory glutamatergic neurotransmission and reduction of inhibitory GABAergic neurotransmission in the neocortex, which underlie hyperexcitability in ALS patients, are believed to damage motor neurons via the excitotoxicity mechanism [4, 7]. The role of excitotoxicity as one of the universal mechanisms causing neuronal death in various nervous system diseases has currently been demonstrated [8, 9, 64]. High sensitivity of motor neurons to excitotoxicity can be related to high expression of glutamate receptors and low expression of calcium-binding proteins [9].

An important argument in favor of the role of hyperexcitability and the underlying molecular processes in ALS pathogenesis is that this phenomenon can be early detected using TMS in asymptomatic SOD1 mutation carriers. Vucic et al. (2008) demonstrated a decrease in SICI in three SOD1 mutation carriers who were asymptomatic at the time the study was performed but developed clinical signs of the disease during a prospective study within 3 years. It is interesting that no neurophysiological signs of motor cortex excitability were revealed in 14 other asymptomatic carriers and they did not present with any clinical manifestations of the disease within the entire study period [45]. Early development of signs of hyperexcitability of neurons of the motor cortex, spinal cord, and even the extramotor areas such as hippocampus (e.g., see [23]) were demonstrated in a large series of experimental studies using a culture of neurons isolated from transgenic animals. Additional evidence is that signs of motor cortex hyperexcitability in ALS patients can be detected before the pyramidal pathways are affected and EMG signs of degeneration of the lower motor neuron emerge. A recent study carried out by Menon et al. (2015) showed that 24 patients with ALS had a statistically significant decrease in motor threshold, duration of cSP and intracortical inhibition, while simultaneously having an increased MER amplitude and intracortical facilitation at onset of the disease [5]. No signs of alterations in central motor conduction time (CMCT) were detected in these patients, thus attesting to the fact that the conduction function of the pyramidal pathway was retained and there were signs of denervation and reinnervation process according to the EMG data. The results of this study demonstrated that motor cortex hyperexcitability precedes degeneration of both the upper and the lower motor neurons and is the earliest neurophysiological signs of neurodegeneration. This supports the hypothesis proposed by Charkot back in 1869 that the upper motor neuron is the first one to be affected in ALS patients ('dying-forward') [65].

The certain effectiveness of riluzole in treating ALS also indirectly confirms the pathogenetic role of hyperexcitability and excitotoxicity. Despite the diversity of its mechanisms of action, riluzole is primarily considered to be a medication reducing excitotoxicity [66]. It has been demonstrated that riluzole can partially normalize SICI and reduce excitability of peripheral nerve axons in ALS patients [67].

The indirect evidence to the pathogenetic role of excitotoxicity was also obtained in studies on using therapeutic repetitive magnetic stimulation in ALS. High-frequency repetitive TMS increases neuronal excitability in the stimulated area (see reviews [68] and [69]). It has been demonstrated in a small study conducted by Di Lazzaro et al. (2004) that high-frequency stimulation may accelerate onset of the disease, while low-frequency stimulation may inhibit it [70]. Hence, high-frequency stimulation may increase excitotoxic degeneration of motor neurons and motor cortex excitability, having an unfavorable effect on the course of the disease.

3.2. Is hyperexcitability good?

Excitotoxicity and hyperexcitability have been for a long time regarded only as damaging phenomena facilitating neuronal death. However, findings obtained in a number of studies suggest that hyperexcitability can also have a compensatory effect, at least at early stages. Furthermore, molecular alterations that accompany excitotoxicity are similar to the processes taking place when neuroplasticity is ensured. We present the results of some studies confirming the validity of this alternative view of the hyperexcitability problem in patients with ALS and other neurodegenerative diseases.

3.2.1. Motor cortex excitability and neuroplasticity

The term 'neuroplasticity' means brain's ability to alter structurally and functionally in response to internal and external factors. This ability is currently attributed both to strengthening or weakening of the existing neural connections and to the formation of new connections or destruction of the old ones [71]. Starting with the first description of cellular mechanisms of neuroplasticity, this universal property of neural tissue is inseparably associated with alteration in neuronal excitability. Long-term potentiation was shown to be predominantly of postsynaptic origin and is mostly connected to the glutamatergic system [72–74].

A series of studies have shown the alteration in motor cortex excitability and reorganization of the cortical representation of muscles after motor learning and acquisition of new skills [75, 76]. The TMS data confirmed that there is a relationship between neuroplastic alterations and an increase in motor cortex excitability [77–79]. Thus, Tyč and Boyadjian (2011) performed TMS mapping of cortical representation of the deltoid and brachioradialis muscles in healthy volunteers before and after a 6-week training (playing darts three to four times a week). The boundaries of cortical representation of the muscles under study were expanded after training, which was accompanied by an increase in the slope ratio of the amplitude-intensity curve, being indicative of the increase in motor cortex excitability [80]. According to Perez et al. (2004), a 32-minute training causes statistically significant increase in the slope ratio of the amplitude-intensity curve and a decrease in intracortical inhibition [81]. Increased motor cortex excitability presenting as increased MER amplitude and reduced motor threshold is observed in healthy volunteers not only after actual training but also after they had imagined the movements [82]. Professional sportsmen and musicians were found to have increased motor cortex excitability and increased ability of the motor cortex to undergo plastic alterations [83, 84].

To sum up, the aforementioned facts indicate that motor cortex excitability and glutamatergic neurotransmission increase during neuroplastic alterations.

3.2.2. *Hyperexcitability and neuroplasticity in pathology*

The most forcible evidence for the possible relationship between hyperexcitability and neuroplasticity was observed in patients with Alzheimer's disease (AD). Neurodegeneration in this disease is not limited to the structures involved in the cognitive function and affects other brain regions as well, including the primary motor cortex. At the late stages of the disease, AD patients often have motor disorders, including spasticity and pathologic plantar responses, attesting to involvement of the upper motor neuron [85]. Furthermore, lesions of the motor cortex, predominantly giant pyramidal cells of Betz, were detected in AD patients in pathomorphological studies [86]. In this connection, investigation of the structural and functional status of the motor cortex in AD patients is of interest as a model of clinically asymptomatic neurodegeneration of the motor cortex.

In AD patients, identically to those with ALS, motor cortex hyperexcitability can be recorded using TMS. It has been demonstrated in many studies that the motor threshold decreases in AD patients. Decreased intracortical inhibition and short cSP duration were also detected in some studies (although not all of them) (see reviews [87, 88]). There is controversy in data on disrupted inhibitory neurotransmission in AD patients; however, decreased SICI in AD is most probably not associated with dysfunction of the GABAergic system [89]. The enhanced glutamatergic neurotransmission is currently the predominant conception of the development of motor cortex hyperexcitability in AD patients.

It is interesting to mention that motor cortex hyperexcitability in AD patients is predominantly attributed to neuroplasticity processes. Hyperexcitability is believed to develop via the compensatory mechanism as a response to disruption of associative connections [90].

Motor cortex hyperexcitability in AD patients is accompanied by reorganization of the cortical representation of muscles according to TMS mapping presenting as displacement of the center of gravity of the cortical representation in the frontomedial direction with respect to localization of hot spots in patients without motor disorders [90]. Ferreri et al. (2011) believe that this may attest to plastic brain alterations aimed at maintaining normal motor activity as the neuron number decreases progressively [91]. fMRI studies in patients at early stages of AD, identically to those with ALS, showed areas with increased activation, which is also regarded as a result of compensatory changes [92]. In their recent study, Guerra et al. (2015) demonstrated the relationship between motor cortex hyperexcitability and neuroplasticity. Examination of seven patients with vascular dementia and nine AD patients showed a statistically significant decrease in motor threshold compared to healthy volunteers of comparable age. Parameters related to motor cortex excitability (the area of cortical representation of muscles and the area of active cortical points) showed a statistically significant correlation with neuroplastic reorganization of the motor cortex assessed based on the distance between the center of gravity of the maps and hot spot localization. The authors drew a conclusion that motor cortex hyperexcitability may promote neuroplasticity [93].

As opposed of the cortical motor zones, most AD patients at the dementia stage have decreased connectivity and activation of the hippocampus, medial temporal, and prefronal cortex when performing cognitive tasks involving short-term memory [94]. Meanwhile, activity of these areas is increased in AD patients at the moderate cognitive impairment stage and in asymptomatic carriers of mutations in the presenilin-1 gene [95–97]. This is believed to result from turning on of the compensatory mechanisms. It should be mentioned that transgenic animals at the presymptomatic stage and stage of initial manifestations (which approximately corresponds to the moderate cognitive impairment stage in humans) showed an increased expression of a number of genes promoting synaptic plasticity [98]. In particular, transgenic mice showed enhanced expression of the AMPAR subunit genes at the early stages of the pathological process [99]. Furthermore, experimental studies revealed an increase in synaptic plasticity and hyperexcitability in hippocampal neurons, which preceded β-amyloid deposition [100, 101]. Schneider et al. (2001) reported that hippocampal neurons in transgenic mice with presenilin mutation are characterized not only by hyperexcitability and reduced threshold to excitotoxic damage but also by facilitation of long-term synaptic potentiation [102]. In their pathomorphological study, Bell et al. (2007) showed that patients with moderate cognitive impairments had increased density of presynaptic boutons in glutamatergic synapses, while the density of presynaptic boutons in AD patients was reduced [103]. On the contrary, expression of the genes involved in synaptic plasticity and energy exchange was shown to decrease at the late stages of the disease [98, 104]. These data give grounds for assuming that the increase in neuronal excitability in AD patients at early stages of the disease may occur via the compensatory mechanism.

3.2.3. Compensatory hyperexcitability in ALS: evidence from fundamental research

Several recently published studies using transgenic animals expressing mSOD1 have compromised the conception of the pathological role of excitability of motor neurons in ALS. Saxena et al. (2013) demonstrated that hyperexcitability can be a defense mechanism preventing degeneration of motor neurons. Thus, reduced excitability of motor neurons decreased accumulation of mutant SOD1, whereas increased excitability was accompanied by the greater number of intracellular aggregates and quicker death of motor neurons. It was also demonstrated that mutant protein accumulation increases after AMPAR blockade and decreases when AMPA is introduced. Stronger excitatory stimulation may contribute to the decrease in severity of endoplasmic stress and accumulation of abnormal proteins, thus exhibiting protective properties. Interestingly, mutant SOD1 accumulation was first detected in the least excitable fast fatiguing (FF) motor neurons of the spinal cord [105]. Leroy et al. (2014) studied the excitability of various populations of spinal cord motor neurons isolated from G93A mutant mice [106]. In this study, the electrophysiological signs of hyperexcitability were revealed only in degeneration-resistant motor neurons. The authors believe that their findings indicate that hyperexcitability does not cause degeneration; instead, it can be a defense mechanism [106].

3.2.4. Neuroplasticity in ALS: evidence from fMRI studies

Nowadays, fMRI is the key method for studying neuroplasticity in ALS patients. Numerous studies have revealed the changes in activation patterns of various brain regions in ALS both in rest and using various paradigms [2]. In this publication, the changes in activation patterns in ALS patients performing motor tasks are of special interest.

In the study performed by Konrad et al. (2002), ALS patients and healthy volunteers underwent fMRI as they performed a motor paradigm (bending fingers) [107]. Significant changes in the patterns of cortex activation were observed: a forward displacement of the activation cluster, into the supplementary motor area, and an increase in its volume. Activation volume in the inferior frontal gyrus (Brodmann area 6) in the contralateral hemisphere and parietal lobes increased bilaterally. The authors have put forward a hypothesis that these changes represent the structural and functional rearrangement of the motor system induced by degeneration of the upper and lower motor neuron [107]. Lule et al. (2007) reported that an increase in activation of the primary motor and premotor cortex in ALS patients is revealed not only when performing the movement but also when imaging it [108]. Stanton et al. (2007) detected that activation in the sensorimotor cortex (Brodmann areas 1, 2, and 4), the inferior parietal lobule, and the superior temporal gyrus increased when the ALS patients performed a motor task, while activation in the dorsolateral prefrontal cortex decreased [109]. It is noteworthy that these changes were observed when comparing ALS patients not only to healthy volunteers but also to patients with peripheral nerve disorders [109]. This confirms that involvement of the upper motor neuron plays a crucial role in development of these changes and does not give grounds for considering them as just a response to the development of muscle fatigue.

Thus, an analysis of the results of fMRI with the motor paradigm in ALS patients demonstrates that the activation areas expand when a motor task is being performed. Interestingly, the changes in activation during fMRI can have a prognostic value. Poujois et al. (2013) reported that activation in the somatosensory and parietal cortex increases in ALS patients performing a simple motor task compared to the control group. The dynamic follow-up for 1 year has shown that activity of the contralateral parietal lobe has a statistically significant negative correlation with the rate of disease progression ($p = 0.001$) [110].

These findings give grounds for suggesting that expansion of activation areas as an ALS patient performs a motor task has the compensatory mechanism and is probably aimed at maintaining the motor function in response to progressive degeneration of cortical motor neurons. Meanwhile, certain researchers believe that the activation areas can increase due to degeneration of inhibitory interneurons [2]. The relationship between alterations in activation patterns in ALS patients according to fMRI data and changes in motor cortex excitability according to TMS data has not been studied yet. It should be mentioned that the positive prognostic significance of neuroplastic alterations demonstrated by Poujois et al. (2013) is in contrast with the views about the negative role of hyperexcitability in this disease.

4. Navigated TMS mapping in ALS

Navigated TMS (nTMS) is today considered to be the most promising method to answer the question about the relationship between hyperexcitability and neuroplastic alterations in the motor cortex under kinetic conditions. On the one hand, nTMS is a neuroimaging technique and allows visualization of the location of cortical representation of certain muscles on individual MR images and provides an opportunity to assess the changes in their size and displacement with respect to anatomical landmarks. On the other hand, nTMS is a neurophysiological method that allows one to assess various parameters showing the excitability and degeneration of the motor cortex. The nTMS method uses the brain of a person being examined as a landmark when applying stimuli for an individual MR model; the stimuli can be accurately applied to a certain area with allowance for the area of interest, the individual anatomy, and topography of the gyri [111].

In our recent study, we mapped the cortical representation of m. abductor pollicis brevis (APB) in 30 ALS patients and 24 healthy volunteers [29]. It was demonstrated that ALS patients exhibit a statistically significant increase in the resting motor threshold and a decrease in the MEPs amplitude, as well as a statistically significant reduction of the volume of cortical representation of APB ($p < 0.001$). The latter observation agrees with the results of the findings of Carvalho et al. (1999) who demonstrated a progressive decrease in size of the cortical representation in ALS patients [112]. This phenomenon is probably based on the neurodegenerative process that reduces motor cortex excitability and decreases the number of cortical motor neurons. According to our data, the volume of cortical representation statistically significantly correlates with disease duration and negatively correlates with strength of the corresponding muscle and disease severity according to ALS Functional Rating Scale Revised (ALS FRS-R). These data give grounds for hypothesizing that the size of cortical representation can be regarded as a neurophysiological marker of disease severity, which opens new avenues for using it both in fundamental research and in clinical trials of new therapy methods. Further studies are needed to determine the sensitivity and specificity of this marker compared to other neurophysiological parameters and to determine its diagnostic significance.

The capabilities of navigated TMS made it possible not only to determine the size of cortical representation but also to accurately localize the maps within the anatomic landmarks. In most ALS patients, the maps were localized within the precentral gyrus (Brodmann area 4); some active sites, similar to those in healthy volunteers, were detected within the postcentral gyrus (Brodmann area 1) and the premotor cortex.

Meanwhile, we detected expanded boundaries of individual maps of the APB in some ALS patients, usually presenting as a displacement of the greatest portion of the map toward the postcentral gyrus. It was found by analyzing these cases that the aforementioned reorganization is mostly typical of patients at onset of the disease or when the disease course is relatively benign (**Figures 1** and **2**). It is important to mention that the motor threshold in these cases remained within the normal values or was decreased.

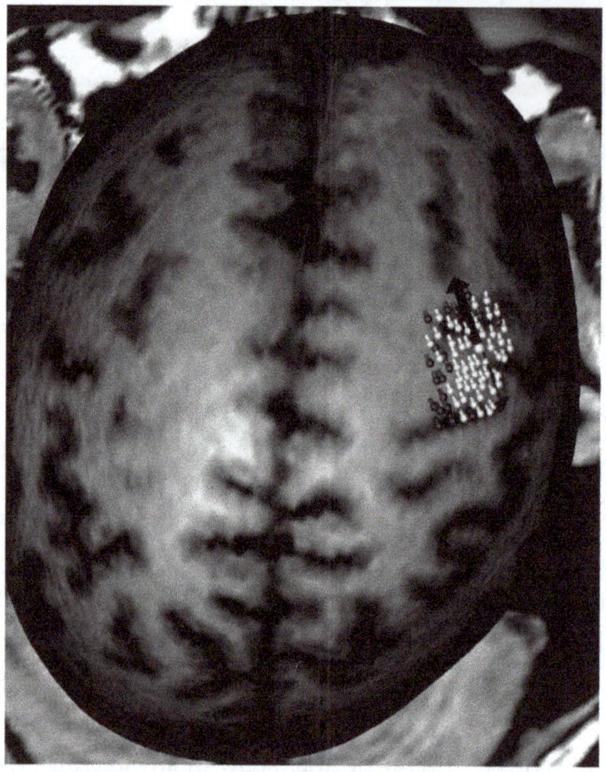

Figure 1. Map of cortical representation of the APB in a healthy volunteer (28 years old, motor threshold—43%). Here and in other figures, the points whose stimulation provides MEPs with amplitude over 50 μV from the contralateral APB are shown in white.

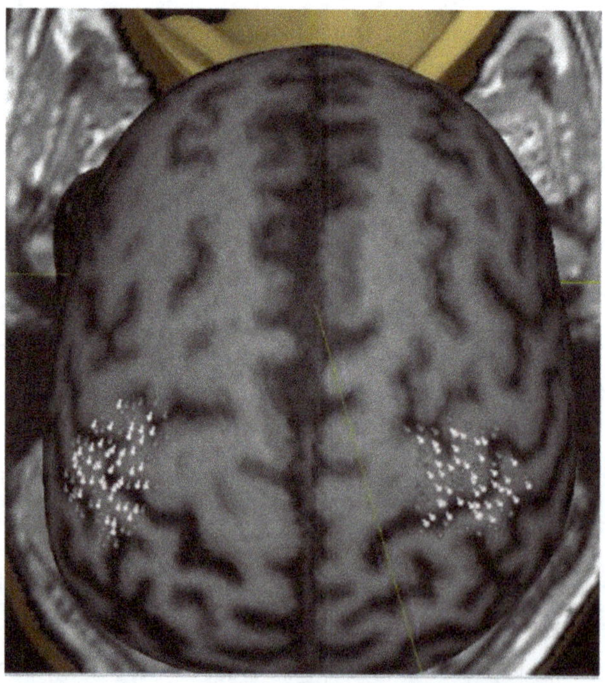

Figure 2. Maps of cortical representation of the APB in ALS patient with the relatively benign course of the disease (54 years old, right-side motor threshold—31%, left-side motor threshold—35%, duration of the disease—25 months, APB strength is bilaterally reduced to MRC score 4).

Although we have not performed mathematical analysis of the relationship between motor cortex excitability and reorganization of cortical representation, we suppose that hyperexcitability can be one of the mechanisms of the aforementioned neuroplastic alterations. Thus, a statistically significant relationship between the passive threshold as an excitability marker and the volume of cortical representation has been revealed. So the largest cortical representation was revealed in patients with lower thresholds. This made it possible to rule out the possible role of higher-intensity stimuli in expansion of the map boundaries in ALS patients compared to the control group. Indeed, the motor threshold in some patients was 100% and we used this intensity in mapping. However, only single MEPs were detected in the aforementioned cases and the size of cortical representation was very small (**Figure 3**).

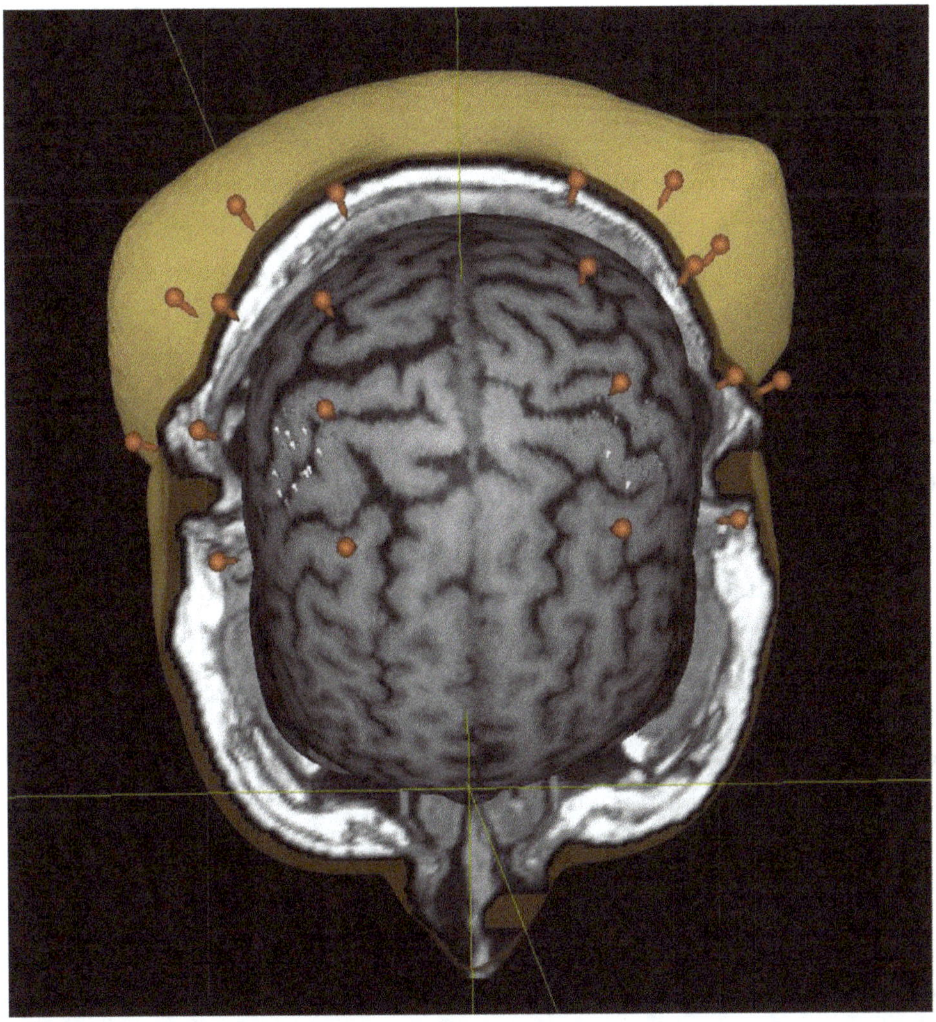

Figure 3. Maps of cortical representation of the APB in a 62-year-old female patient with ALS. Upper-limb form of the disease; disease duration—8 months. ALS-FRS-R—38. APB strength is bilaterally reduced to MRC score 2. Motor threshold on the right and left sides—100%. The volume of cortical representation is significantly decreased.

Our findings agree with the fMRI data described above that attest to expansion of the activation areas in ALS patients performing a motor task. Like fMRI, visual assessment of nTMS mapping data allows one to detect displacement of cortical representation. Our preliminary data demonstrate that displacement of the boundaries of cortical representation as a result of neuroplastic alterations can be caused by decreased motor cortex excitability. Hence, the phenomenon of motor cortex hyperexcitability can have the compensatory function in ALS patients.

5. Conclusions and future perspectives

Motor cortex hyperexcitability in ALS patients is a well-studied phenomenon that can be of significant interest as a biomarker of neurodegeneration. However, despite the large number of studies, the reasons and sequelae currently remain poorly studied. Since motor cortex hyperexcitability in ALS patients was first described, this phenomenon has been attributed to the development of excitotoxicity and weakening of inhibitory neurotransmission in the neocortex, thus ensuring its pathogenetic role in the development of neurodegeneration. However, no direct evidence to the fact that motor cortex hyperexcitability in ALS patients attests to development of excitotoxicity and precedes its degeneration has been obtained yet. Meanwhile, hyperexcitability can be one of the mechanisms of neuroplastic alterations, thus having the compensatory (sanogenetic) rather than pathogenetic value. This theory has been supported by the data on interaction between decreased motor cortex excitability and neuroplasticity in the norm and in some pathologic conditions such as Alzheimer's disease and vascular dementia. Furthermore, expansion of the cortical representation of certain muscles was demonstrated for ALS patients in fMRI and nTMS studies, which can be a manifestation of neuroplasticity and related to increased motor cortex excitability.

It should be mentioned that hyperexcitability is not a specific sign of ALS and is also revealed in other neurodegenerative diseases. More and more data supporting the similarity between pathophysiology of neurodegeneration in various diseases and its relationship with intracellular accumulation of abnormal proteins have been obtained. This may result in dysfunction of synaptic connections and a compensatory increase in expression of the genes ensuring increased excitability and synaptic plasticity.

A hypothesis can be put forward based on these data that hyperexcitability plays different roles at different stages of the disease (**Figure 4**). At onset of the disease, this phenomenon can develop via the compensatory mechanism in response to reduced number of functioning motor neurons and disruption of synaptic connections. Hence, increased hyperexcitability can be regarded as a method for maintaining functioning of the system as the number of its components decreases. In addition, hyperexcitability can have a protective effect at the cellular level as it prevents accumulation of pathologically altered proteins. As the disease progresses, hyperexcitability may start to have a pathological effect and induce excitotoxicity. Does this mean that our effect on motor cortex excitability in ALS patients needs to be differentiated depending on disease stage? Further research involving various methods and focusing on patients at different stages of the disease needs to be carried out to answer this question.

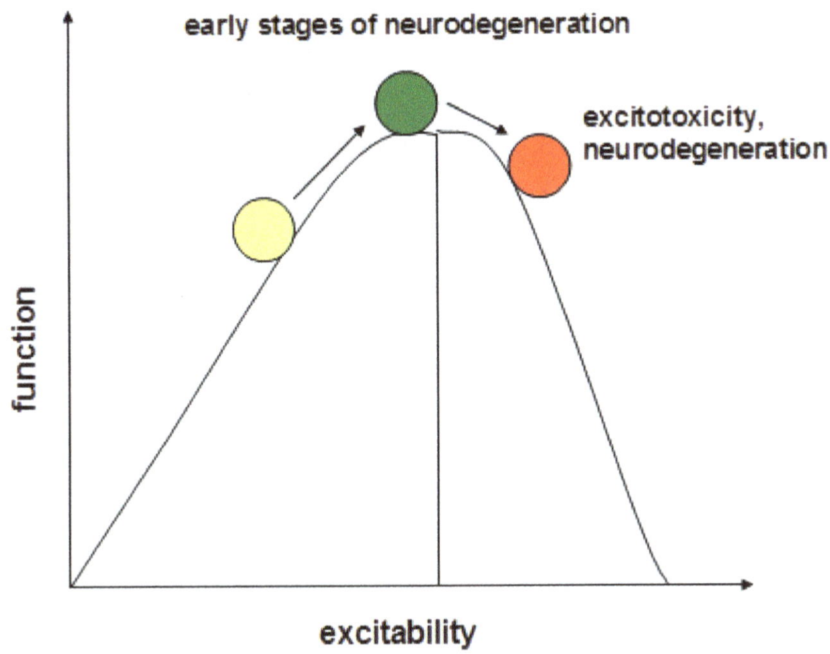

Figure 4. A link between excitability and function.

Author details

Ilya S. Bakulin, Alexander V. Chervyakov*, Natalia A. Suponeva, Maria N. Zakharova and Michael A. Piradov

*Address all correspondence to: tchervyakovav@gmail.com

Research Center of Neurology, Moscow, Russia

References

[1] Turner MR, Bowser R, Bruijn L, Dupuis L, Ludolph A, McGrath M. Mechanisms, models and biomarkers in amyotrophic lateral sclerosis. Amyotroph Lateral Scler Frontotemporal Degener. 2013;14(1):19–32. DOI: 10.3109/21678421.2013.778554.

[2] Chiò A, Pagani M, Agosta F, Calvo A, Cistaro A, Filippi M. Neuroimaging in amyotrophic lateral sclerosis: insights into structural and functional changes. Lancet Neurol. 2014;13(12):1228–40. DOI: 10.1016/S1474-4422(14)70167-X.

[3] Bede P, Hardiman O. Lessons of ALS imaging: Pitfalls and future directions - A critical review. Neuroimage Clin. 2014; 27(4):436–43. DOI: 10.1016/j.nicl.2014.02.011.

[4] Vucic S, Ziemann U, Eisen A, Hallett M, Kiernan MC. Transcranial magnetic stimulation and amyotrophic lateral sclerosis: pathophysiological insights. J Neurol Neurosurg Psychiatry. 2013;84(10):1161–70. DOI: 10.1136/jnnp-2012-304019.

[5] Menon P, Kiernan MC, Vucic S. Cortical hyperexcitability precedes lower motor neuron dysfunction in ALS. Clin Neurophysiol. 2015;126(4):803–9. DOI: 10.1016/j.clinph.2014.04.023.

[6] Zanette G, Tamburin S, Manganotti P, Refatti N, Forgione A, Rizzuto N. Different mechanisms contribute to motor cortex hyperexcitability in amyotrophic lateral sclerosis. Clin Neurophysiol. 2002;113(11):1688–97.

[7] Bae JS, Simon NG, Menon P, Vucic S, Kiernan MC. The puzzling case of hyperexcitability in amyotrophic lateral sclerosis. J Clin Neurol. 2013;9(2):65–74. DOI: 10.3988/jcn.2013.9.2.65.

[8] King AE, Woodhouse A, Kirkcaldie MT, Vickers JC. Excitotoxicity in ALS: Overstimulation, or overreaction? Exp Neurol. 2016;275(1):162–71. DOI: 10.1016/j.expneurol.2015.09.019.

[9] Blasco H, Mavel S, Corcia P, Gordon PH. The glutamate hypothesis in ALS: pathophysiology and drug development. Curr Med Chem. 2014;21(31):3551–75.

[10] Fray AE, Ince, PG, Banner SJ, Milton ID, Usher PA, Cookson MR, Shaw PJ. The expression of the glial glutamate transporter protein EAAT2 in motor neuron disease: an immunohistochemical study. Eur. J. Neurosci. 1998;10(8):2481–2489.

[11] Sasaki S, Komori T, Iwata M. Excitatory amino acid transporter 1 and 2 immunoreactivity in the spinal cord in amyotrophic lateral sclerosis. Acta Neuropathol. 2000;100(2):138–44.

[12] Howland DS, Liu J, She Y, Goad B, Maragakis NJ, Kim B, Erickson J, Kulik J, DeVito L, Psaltis G, DeGennaro LJ, Cleveland DW, Rothstein JD. Focal loss of the glutamate transporter EAAT2 in a transgenic rat model of SOD1 mutant-mediated amyotrophic lateral sclerosis (ALS). Proc. Natl. Acad. Sci. U. S. A. 2002;99(3):1604–1609.

[13] Velasco I, Tapia R, Massieu L. Inhibition of glutamate uptake induces progressive accumulation of extracellular glutamate and neuronal damage in rat cortical cultures. J. Neurosci. Res. 1996;44(6):551–561.

[14] Benkler C, Ben-Zur T, Barhum Y, Offen D. Altered astrocytic response to activation in SOD1(G93A) mice and its implications on amyotrophic lateral sclerosis pathogenesis. Glia. 2013;61(3):312–326. DOI: 10.1002/glia.22428.

[15] Ince P, Stout N, Shaw P, Slade J, Hunziker W, Heizmann CW, Baimbridge KG. Parvalbumin and calbindin D-28k in the human motor system and in motor neuron disease. Neuropathol. Appl. Neurobiol. 1993;19(4):291–299.

[16] Stephens B, Guiloff RJ, Navarrete R, Newman P, Nikhar N, Lewis P. Widespread loss of neuronal populations in the spinal ventral horn in sporadic motor neuron disease. A morphometric study. J. Neurol. Sci. 2006;244(1-2):41–58.

[17] McGown A, McDearmid JR, Panagiotaki N, Tong H, Al Mashhadi S, Redhead N, Lyon AN, Beattie CE, Shaw PJ, Ramesh TM. Early interneuron dysfunction in ALS: insights from a mutant sod1 zebrafish model. Ann. Neurol. 2013;73(2):246–258. DOI: 10.1002/ana.23780.

[18] Foerster BR, Callaghan BC, Petrou M, Edden RA, Chenevert TL, Feldman EL. Decreased motor cortex γ-aminobutyric acid in amyotrophic lateral sclerosis. Neurology. 2012;78(20):1596–600. DOI: 10.1212/WNL.0b013e3182563b57.

[19] Turner MR, Hammers A, Al-Chalabi A, Shaw CE, Andersen PM, Brooks DJ, Leigh PN. Distinct cerebral lesions in sporadic and 'D90A' SOD1 ALS: studies with [11C]flumazenil PET. Brain. 2005;128(Pt 6):1323–9.

[20] Petri S, Krampfl K, Hashemi F, Grothe C, Hori A, Dengler R, Bufler J. Distribution of GABAA receptor mRNA in the motor cortex of ALS patients. J Neuropathol Exp Neurol. 2003;62(10):1041–51.

[21] Kuo JJ, Siddique T, Fu R, Heckman CJ. Increased persistent Na(+) current and its effect on excitability in motoneurones cultured from mutant SOD1 mice. J Physiol. 2005; 563(3):843–854.

[22] Pieri M, Carunchio I, Curcio L, Mercuri NB, Zona C. Increased persistent sodium current determines cortical hyperexcitability in a genetic model of familial amyotrophic lateral sclerosis. Exp Neurol. 2009;215(2):368–379. DOI: 10.1016/j.expneurol.2008.11.002.

[23] van Zundert B, Peuscher MH, Hynynen M, Chen A, Neve RL, Brown RH, Jr, Constantine-Paton M, Bellingham MC. Neonatal neuronal circuitry shows hyperexcitable disturbance in a mouse model of the adult-onset neurodegenerative disease amyotrophic lateral sclerosis. J Neurosci. 2008;28(43):10864–10874. DOI: 10.1523/JNEUROSCI.1340-08.2008.

[24] Pambo-Pambo A, Durand J, Gueritaud J-P. Early excitability changes in lumbar motoneurons of transgenic $SOD1^{G85R}$ and $S0D1^{G93A\text{-}Low}$ mice. J Neurophysiol. 2009;102(6):3627–3642. DOI:10.1152/jn.00482.2009.

[25] Kawahara Y, Ito K, Sun H, Aizawa H, Kanazawa I, Kwak S. Glutamate receptors: RNA editing and death of motor neurons. Nature. 2004;427(6977):801.

[26] Di Lazzaro V, Ziemann U. The contribution of transcranial magnetic stimulation in the functional evaluation of microcircuits in human motor cortex. Front Neural Circuits. 2013;13(7):18. DOI: 10.3389/fncir.2013.00018.

[27] Rossini PM, Burke D, Chen R, Cohen LG, Daskalakis Z, Di Iorio R et al. Non-invasive electrical and magnetic stimulation of the brain, spinal cord, roots and peripheral

nerves: basic principles and procedures for routine clinical and research application. An updated report from an I.F.C.N. Committee. Clin Neurophysiol. 2015;126(6):1071–107. DOI: 10.1016/j.clinph.2015.02.001.

[28] Di Lazzaro V. Biological effects of non-invasive brain stimulation. Handb Clin Neurol. 2013;2013(116):367-74. DOI: 10.1016/B978-0-444-53497-2.00030-9.

[29] Chervyakov AV, Bakulin IS, Savitskaya NG, Arkhipov IV, Gavrilov AV, Zakharova MN, Piradov MA. Navigated transcranial magnetic stimulation in amyotrophic lateral sclerosis. Muscle Nerve. 2015;51(1):125–31. DOI: 10.1002/mus.24345.

[30] de Carvalho M, Turkman A, Swash M. Motor responses evoked by transcranial magnetic stimulation and peripheral nerve stimulation in the ulnar innervation in amyotrophic lateral sclerosis: the effect of upper and lower motor neuron lesion. J Neurol Sci. 2003;210(1–2):83–90.

[31] Miscio G, Pisano F, Mora G, Mazzini L. Motor neuron disease: usefulness of transcranial magnetic stimulation in improving the diagnosis. Clin Neurophysiol. 1999;110(5):975–81.

[32] Eisen A, Shytbel W, Murphy K, Hoirch M. Cortical magnetic stimulation in amyotrophic lateral sclerosis. Muscle Nerve. 1990;13(2):146–51.

[33] Mills KR. The natural history of central motor abnormalities in amyotrophic lateral sclerosis. Brain. 2003;126(Pt 11):2558–66.

[34] Triggs WJ, Menkes D, Onorato J, Yan RS, Young MS, Newell K et al. Transcranial magnetic stimulation identifies upper motor neuron involvement in motor neuron disease. Neurology. 1999;53(3):605–11.

[35] Urban PP, Wicht S, Hopf HC. Sensitivity of transcranial magnetic stimulation of cortico-bulbar vs. cortico-spinal tract involvement in Amyotrophic Lateral Sclerosis (ALS). J Neurol. 2001;248(10):850–5.

[36] Vucic S, Cheah BC, Kiernan MC. Defining the mechanisms that underlie cortical hyperexcitability in amyotrophic lateral sclerosis. Exp Neurol. 2009;220(1):177–82. DOI: 10.1016/j.expneurol.2009.08.017.

[37] Caramia MD, Cicinelli P, Paradiso C, Mariorenzi R, Zarola F, Bernardi G, Rossini PM. Excitability changes of muscular responses to magnetic brain stimulation in patients with central motor disorders. Electroencephalogr Clin Neurophysiol. 1991;81(4):243–50.

[38] Vucic S, Kiernan MC. Novel threshold tracking techniques suggest that cortical hyperexcitability is an early feature of motor neuron disease. Brain. 2006;129(Pt 9):2436–46.

[39] Mills KR, Nithi KA. Corticomotor threshold is reduced in early sporadic amyotrophic lateral sclerosis. Muscle Nerve. 1997;20(9):1137–41.

[40] Khedr EM, Ahmed MA, Hamdy A, Shawky OA. Cortical excitability of amyotrophic lateral sclerosis: transcranial magnetic stimulation study. Neurophysiol Clin. 2011;41(2):73–9. DOI: 10.1016/j.neucli.2011.03.001.

[41] Ziemann U, Reis J, Schwenkreis P, Rosanova M, Strafella A, Badawy R, Müller-Dahlhaus F. TMS and drugs revisited 2014. Clin Neurophysiol. 2015;126(10):1847–68. DOI: 10.1016/j.clinph.2014.08.028.

[42] Carriedo SG, Sensi SL, Yin HZ, Weiss JH. AMPA exposures induce mitochondrial Ca(2+) overload and ROS generation in spinal motor neurons in vitro. J Neurosci. 2000;20(1):240–50.

[43] Saba L, Viscomi MT, Caioli S, Pignataro A, Bisicchia E, Pieri M, Molinari M, Ammassari-Teule M, Zona C. Altered Functionality, Morphology, and Vesicular Glutamate Transporter Expression of Cortical Motor Neurons from a Presymptomatic Mouse Model of Amyotrophic Lateral Sclerosis. Cereb Cortex. 2016;26(4):1512-28. pii: bhu317.

[44] Paulus W, Classen J, Cohen LG, Large CH, Di Lazzaro V, Nitsche M, Pascual-Leone A, Rosenow F, Rothwell JC, Ziemann U. State of the art: pharmacologic effects on cortical excitability measures tested by transcranial magnetic stimulation. Brain Stimul. 2008;1(3):151–63. DOI: 10.1016/j.brs.2008.06.002.

[45] Vucic S, Nicholson GA, Kiernan MC. Cortical hyperexcitability may precede the onset of familial amyotrophic lateral sclerosis. Brain. 2008;131(6):1540-50. DOI: 10.1093/brain/awn071.

[46] Vucic S, Kiernan MC. Cortical excitability testing distinguishes Kennedy's disease from amyotrophic lateral sclerosis. Clin Neurophysiol. 2008;119(5):1088–96. DOI: 10.1016/j.clinph.2008.01.011.

[47] Wilson SA, Lockwood RJ, Thickbroom GW, Mastaglia FL. The muscle silent period following transcranial magnetic cortical stimulation. J Neurol Sci. 1993;114(2):216–22.

[48] Zanette G, Tamburin S, Manganotti P, Refatti N, Forgione A, Rizzuto N. Changes in motor cortex inhibition over time in patients with amyotrophic lateral sclerosis. J Neurol. 2002;249(12):1723–8.

[49] Siciliano G, Manca ML, Sagliocco L, Pastorini E, Pellegrinetti A, Sartucci F et al. Cortical silent period in patients with amyotrophic lateral sclerosis. J Neurol Sci. 1999;169(1–2): 93–7.

[50] Prout AJ, Eisen AA. The cortical silent period and amyotrophic lateral sclerosis. Muscle Nerve. 1994;17(2):217–23.

[51] Kujirai T, Caramia MD, Rothwell JC, Day BL, Thompson PD, Ferbert A et al. Corticocortical inhibition in human motor cortex. J Physiol. 1993;471(1):501-19.

[52] Nakamura H, Kitagawa H, Kawaguchi Y, Tsuji H. Intracortical facilitation and inhibition after transcranial magnetic stimulation in conscious humans. J Physiol. 1997;498 (Pt 3):817–23.

[53] Vucic S, Cheah BC, Yiannikas C, Kiernan MC. Cortical excitability distinguishes ALS from mimic disorders. Clin Neurophysiol. 2011;122(9):1860–6. DOI: 10.1016/j.clinph.2010.12.062.

[54] Ziemann U, Winter M, Reimers CD, Reimers K, Tergau F, Paulus W. Impaired motor cortex inhibition in patients with amyotrophic lateral sclerosis. Evidence from paired transcranial magnetic stimulation. Neurology. 1997;49(5):1292–8.

[55] Yokota T, Yoshino A, Inaba A, Saito Y. Double cortical stimulation in amyotrophic lateral sclerosis. J Neurol Neurosurg Psychiatry. 1996;61(6):596–600.

[56] Menon P, Geevasinga N, Yiannikas C, Howells J, Kiernan MC, Vucic S. Sensitivity and specificity of threshold tracking transcranial magnetic stimulation for diagnosis of amyotrophic lateral sclerosis: a prospective study. Lancet Neurol. 2015;14(5):478–84. DOI: 10.1016/S1474-4422(15)00014-9.

[57] Geevasinga N, Menon P, Yiannikas C, Kiernan MC, Vucic S. Diagnostic utility of cortical excitability studies in amyotrophic lateral sclerosis. Eur J Neurol. 2014;21(12): 1451–7. DOI: 10.1111/ene.12422.

[58] Clark R, Blizzard C, Dickson T. Inhibitory dysfunction in amyotrophic lateral sclerosis: future therapeutic opportunities. Neurodegener Dis Manag. 2015;5(6):511–25. DOI: 10.2217/nmt.15.49.

[59] Martin LJ, Chang Q. Inhibitory synaptic regulation of motoneurons: a new target of disease mechanisms in amyotrophic lateral sclerosis. Mol Neurobiol. 2012;45(1):30–42. DOI: 10.1007/s12035-011-8217-x.

[60] Turner MR, Kiernan MC. Does interneuronal dysfunction contribute to neurodegeneration in amyotrophic lateral sclerosis? Amyotroph Lateral Scler 2012;13(3):245–50. DOI: 10.3109/17482968.2011.636050.

[61] Nihei K, McKee AC, Kowall NW. Patterns of neuronal degeneration in the motor cortex of amyotrophic lateral sclerosis patients. Acta Neuropathol. (Berl.) 1993;86(1):55–64.

[62] Leroy F, Zytnicki D. Is hyperexcitability really guilty in amyotrophic lateral sclerosis? Neural Regen Res. 2015;10(9):1413–5. DOI: 10.4103/1673-5374.165308.

[63] van Zundert B, Izaurieta P, Fritz E, Alvarez FJ. Early pathogenesis in the adult-onset neurodegenerative disease amyotrophic lateral sclerosis. J Cell Biochem. 2012;113(11): 3301–12. DOI: 10.1002/jcb.24234.

[64] Jia M, Njapo SA, Rastogi V, Hedna VS. Taming glutamate excitotoxicity: strategic pathway modulation for neuroprotection CNS Drugs. 2015;29(2):153–62. DOI: 10.1007/s40263-015-0225-3.

[65] Bromberg MB. The cart or the horse first? Did Charcot have it right? Clin Neurophysiol. 2015;126(4):647–8. DOI: 10.1016/j.clinph.2014.07.019.

[66] Bellingham MC. A review of the neural mechanisms of action and clinical efficiency of riluzole in treating amyotrophic lateral sclerosis: what have we learned in the last decade? CNS Neurosci Ther. 2011;17(1):4–31. DOI: 10.1111/j.1755-5949.2009.00116.x.

[67] Vucic S, Lin CS, Cheah BC, Murray J, Menon P, Krishnan AV, Kiernan MC. Riluzole exerts central and peripheral modulating effects in amyotrophic lateral sclerosis. Brain. 2013;136(Pt 5):1361–70. DOI: 10.1093/brain/awt085.

[68] Chervyakov AV, Chernyavsky AY, Sinitsyn DO, Piradov MA. Possible mechanisms underlying the therapeutic effects of transcranial magnetic stimulation. Front Hum Neurosci. 2015;9:303. DOI: 10.3389/fnhum.2015.00303.

[69] Tang A, Thickbroom G, Rodger J. Repetitive Transcranial Magnetic Stimulation of the Brain: Mechanisms from Animal and Experimental Models. Neuroscientist. [Epub ahead of print]. pii: 1073858415618897.

[70] Di Lazzaro V, Oliviero A, Saturno E, Pilato F, Dileone M, Sabatelli M, Tonali PA. Motor cortex stimulation for amyotrophic lateral sclerosis. Time for a therapeutic trial? Clin Neurophysiol. 2004;115(6):1479–85.

[71] Nitsche MA, Müller-Dahlhaus F, Paulus W, Ziemann U. The pharmacology of neuroplasticity induced by non-invasive brain stimulation: building models for the clinical use of CNS active drugs. J Physiol. 2012;590(Pt 19):4641–62. DOI: 10.1113/jphysiol.2012.232975.

[72] Malenka RC, Kauer JA, Zucker RS, Nicoll RA. Postsynaptic calcium is sufficient for potentiation of hippocampal synaptic transmission. Science. 1988;242(4875):81–84.

[73] Malinow R, Malenka RC. AMPA receptor trafficking and synaptic plasticity. Annu Rev Neurosci. 2002;25(1):103–126.

[74] Liao D, Hessler NA, Malinow R. Activation of postsynaptically silent synapses during pairing-induced LTP in CA1 region of hippocampal slice. Nature. 1995;375(6530):400–404.

[75] Chernikova LA, Kremneva EI, Cherviakov AV, Saenko IV, Konovalov RN, Piramidov MA, Kozlovskaia IB. New approaches in the study of neuroplasticity process in patients with central nervous system lesion Fiziol Cheloveka. 2013;39(3):54–60. Russian.

[76] Bezzola L., Merillat S., Jäncke L. Motor training-induced neuroplasticity. The Journal of Gerontopsychology and Geriatric Psychiatry. 2012;25(4):189–197.

[77] Koeneke S, Lutz K, Herwig U, Ziemann U, Jäncke L. Extensive training of elementary finger tapping movements changes the pattern of motor cortex excitability. Exp Brain Res. 2006;174(2):199–209.

[78] Svensson P, Romaniello A, Wang K, Arendt-Nielsen L, Sessle BJ. One hour of tongue-task training is associated with plasticity in corticomotor control of the human tongue musculature. Exp Brain Res. 2006;173(1):165–73.

[79] Classen J, Liepert J, Hallett M, Cohen L. Plasticity of movement representation in the human motor cortex. Electroencephalogr Clin Neurophysiol Suppl. 1999;51(1):162–73.

[80] Tyč F, Boyadjian A. Plasticity of motor cortex induced by coordination and training. Clin Neurophysiol. 2011;122(1):153–62. DOI: 10.1016/j.clinph.2010.05.022.

[81] Perez MA, Lungholt BK, Nyborg K, Nielsen JB. Motor skill training induces changes in the excitability of the leg cortical area in healthy humans. Exp Brain Res. 2004;159(2): 197–205.

[82] Mokienko OA, Chervyakov AV, Kulikova SN, Bobrov PD, Chernikova LA, Frolov AA, Piradov MA. Increased motor cortex excitability during motor imagery in brain-computer interface trained subjects. Front Comput Neurosci. 2013;7:168. DOI: 10.3389/fncom.2013.00168.

[83] Rosenkranz K, Williamon A, Rothwell JC. Motorcortical excitability and synaptic plasticity is enhanced in professional musicians. J Neurosci. 2007;27(19):5200–6.

[84] Pearce AJ, Thickbroom GW, Byrnes ML, Mastaglia FL. Functional reorganisation of the corticomotor projection to the hand in skilled racquet players. Exp Brain Res. 2000;130(2):238–43.

[85] Funkenstein HH, Albert MS, Cook NR, West CG, Scherr PA, Chown MJ, Pilgrim D, Evans DA. Extrapyramidal signs and other neurological findings in clinically diagnosed Alzheimer's disease. Arch Neurol. 1993;50(1):51–6.

[86] Rogers J, Morrison JH. Quantitative morphology and regional and laminar distribution of senile plaques in Alzheimer's disease. J Neurosci. 1985;5(10):2801–8.

[87] Pennisi G, Ferri R, Lanza G, Cantone M, Pennisi M, Puglisi V, Malaguarnera G, Bella R. Transcranial magnetic stimulation in Alzheimer's disease: a neurophysiological marker of cortical hyperexcitability. J Neural Transm (Vienna). 2011;118(4):587–98. DOI: 10.1007/s00702-010-0554-9.

[88] Guerra A, Assenza F, Bressi F, Scrascia F, Del Duca M, Ursini F, Vollaro S, Trotta L, Tombini M, Chisari C, Ferreri F. Transcranial magnetic stimulation studies in Alzheimer's disease. Int J Alzheimers Dis. 2011; 2011:263817. DOI: 10.4061/2011/263817.

[89] Di Lazzaro V, Oliviero A, Pilato F, Saturno E, Dileone M, Marra C, Daniele A, Ghirlanda S, Gainotti G, Tonali PA. Motor cortex hyperexcitability to transcranial magnetic stimulation in Alzheimer's disease. J Neurol Neurosurg Psychiatry. 2004; 75(4):555–9.

[90] Ferreri F, Pauri F, Pasqualetti P, Fini R, Dal Forno G, Rossini PM. Motor cortex excitability in Alzheimer's disease: a transcranial magnetic stimulation study. Ann Neurol. 2003;53(1):102–8.

[91] Ferreri F, Pasqualetti P, Määttä S, Ponzo D, Guerra A, Bressi F, Chiovenda P, Del Duca M, Giambattistelli F, Ursini F, Tombini M, Vernieri F, Rossini PM. Motor cortex excitability in Alzheimer's disease: a transcranial magnetic stimulation follow-up study. Neurosci Lett. 2011;492(2):94–8. DOI: 10.1016/j.neulet.2011.01.064.

[92] Vidoni ED, Thomas GP, Honea RA, Loskutova N, Burns JM. Evidence of altered corticomotor system connectivity in early-stage Alzheimer's disease. J Neurol Phys Ther. 2012;36(1):8–16. DOI: 10.1097/NPT.0b013e3182462ea6.

[93] Guerra A, Petrichella S, Vollero L, Ponzo D, Pasqualetti P, Määttä S et al. Neurophysiological features of motor cortex excitability and plasticity in Subcortical Ischemic Vascular Dementia: a TMS mapping study. Clin Neurophysiol. 2015; 126(5):906–13. DOI: 10.1016/j.clinph.2014.07.036.

[94] Dickerson BC, Sperling RA. Large-scale functional brain network abnormalities in Alzheimer's disease: insights from functional neuroimaging. Behav. Neurol. 2009;21(1): 63–75. DOI: 10.3233/BEN-2009-0227.

[95] Dickerson BC, Salat DH, Greve DN, Chua EF, Rand-Giovannetti E, Rentz DM, Bertram L, Mullin K, Tanzi RE, Blacker D, Albert MS, Sperling RA. Increased hippocampal activation in mild cognitive impairment compared to normal aging and AD. Neurology. 2005;65(3):404–411.

[96] Hamalainen A, Pihlajamaki M, Tanila H, Hanninen T, Niskanen E, Tervo S, Karjalainen PA, Vanninen RL, Soininen H. Increased fMRI responses during encoding in mild cognitive impairment. Neurobiol Aging. 2007;28(12):1889–1903.

[97] Kircher TT, Weis S, Freymann K, Erb M, Jessen F, Grodd W, Heun R, Leube DT. Hippocampal activation in patients with mild cognitive impairment is necessary for successful memory encoding. J. Neurol. Neurosurg. Psychiatry 2007;78(8):812–818.

[98] Saura CA, Parra-Damas A, Enriquez-Barreto L. Gene expression parallels synaptic excitability and plasticity changes in Alzheimer's disease. Front Cell Neurosci. 2015;9:318. DOI: 10.3389/fncel.2015.00318.

[99] Palop JJ, Chin J, Roberson ED, Wang J, Thwin MT, Bien-Ly N, Yoo J, Ho KO, Yu GQ, Kreitzer A, Finkbeiner S, Noebels JL, Mucke L. Aberrant excitatory neuronal activity and compensatory remodeling of inhibitory hippocampal circuits in mouse models of Alzheimer's disease. Neuron. 2007;55(5):697–711.

[100] Busche MA, Eichhoff G, Adelsberger H, Abramowski D, Wiederhold KH, Haass C, Staufenbiel M, Konnerth A, Garaschuk O. Clusters of hyperactive neurons near amyloid plaques in a mouse model of Alzheimer's disease. Science. 2008;321(5896): 1686–1689. DOI: 10.1126/science.1162844.

[101] Jolas T, Zhang XS, Zhang Q, Wong G, Del Vecchio R, Gold L, Priestley T. Long-term potentiation is increased in the CA1 area of the hippocampus of APP (swe/ind) CRND8 mice. Neurobiol. Dis. 2002;11(3):394–409.

[102] Schneider I, Reverse D, Dewachter I, Ris L, Caluwaerts N, Kuiperi C, Gilis M, Geerts H, Kretzschmar H, Godaux E, Moechars D, Van Leuven F, Herms J. Mutant presenilins disturb neuronal calcium homeostasis in the brain of transgenic mice, decreasing the threshold for excitotoxicity and facilitating long-term potentiation. J Biol Chem. 2001;276(15):11539–44.

[103] Bell KF, Bennett DA, Cuello AC. Paradoxical upregulation of glutamatergic presynaptic boutons during mild cognitive impairment. J Neurosci. 2007;27(40):10810–7.

[104] Cantanelli P, Sperduti S, Ciavardelli D, Stuppia L, Gatta V, Sensi SL. Age-dependent modifications of AMPA receptor subunit expression levels and related cognitive effects in 3xTg-AD mice. Front Aging Neurosci. 2014;6:200. DOI: 10.3389/fnagi.2014.00200.

[105] Saxena S, Roselli F, Singh K, Leptien K, Julien JP, Gros-Louis F, Caroni P. Neuroprotection through excitability and mTOR required in ALS motoneurons to delay disease and extend survival. Neuron. 2013;80(1):80–96. DOI: 10.1016/j.neuron.2013.07.027.

[106] Leroy F, Lamotte d'Incamps B, Imhoff-Manuel RD, Zytnicki D. Early intrinsic hyperexcitability does not contribute to motoneuron degeneration in amyotrophic lateral sclerosis. Elife. 2014;3: e04046. doi: 10.7554/eLife.04046.

[107] Konrad C, Henningsen H, Bremer J, Mock B, Deppe M, Buchinger C et al. Pattern of cortical reorganization in amyotrophic lateral sclerosis: a functional magnetic resonance imaging study. Exp Brain Res. 2002;143(1):51–6.

[108] Lulé D, Diekmann V, Kassubek J, Kurt A, Birbaumer N, Ludolph AC, Kraft E. Cortical plasticity in amyotrophic lateral sclerosis: motor imagery and function. Neurorehabil Neural Repair. 2007;21(6):518–26.

[109] Stanton BR, Williams VC, Leigh PN, Williams SC, Blain CR, Jarosz JM, Simmons A. Altered cortical activation during a motor task in ALS. Evidence for involvement of central pathways. J Neurol. 2007;254(9):1260–7.

[110] Poujois A, Schneider FC, Faillenot I, Camdessanché JP, Vandenberghe N, Thomas-Antérion C, Antoine JC. Brain plasticity in the motor network is correlated with disease progression in amyotrophic lateral sclerosis. Hum Brain Mapp. 2013; 34(10):2391–401. DOI: 10.1002/hbm.22070.

[111] Ruohonen J, Karhu J. Navigated transcranial magnetic stimulation. Neurophysiol Clin. 2010;40(1):7–17. DOI: 10.1016/j.neucli.2010.01.006.

[112] de Carvalho M, Miranda PC, Luís ML, Ducla-Soares E. Cortical muscle representation in amyotrophic lateral sclerosis patients: changes with disease evolution. Muscle Nerve. 1999;22(12):1684–92.

Permissions

All chapters in this book were first published in SP, by InTech Open; hereby published with permission under the Creative Commons Attribution License or equivalent. Every chapter published in this book has been scrutinized by our experts. Their significance has been extensively debated. The topics covered herein carry significant findings which will fuel the growth of the discipline. They may even be implemented as practical applications or may be referred to as a beginning point for another development.

The contributors of this book come from diverse backgrounds, making this book a truly international effort. This book will bring forth new frontiers with its revolutionizing research information and detailed analysis of the nascent developments around the world.

We would like to thank all the contributing authors for lending their expertise to make the book truly unique. They have played a crucial role in the development of this book. Without their invaluable contributions this book wouldn't have been possible. They have made vital efforts to compile up to date information on the varied aspects of this subject to make this book a valuable addition to the collection of many professionals and students.

This book was conceptualized with the vision of imparting up-to-date information and advanced data in this field. To ensure the same, a matchless editorial board was set up. Every individual on the board went through rigorous rounds of assessment to prove their worth. After which they invested a large part of their time researching and compiling the most relevant data for our readers.

The editorial board has been involved in producing this book since its inception. They have spent rigorous hours researching and exploring the diverse topics which have resulted in the successful publishing of this book. They have passed on their knowledge of decades through this book. To expedite this challenging task, the publisher supported the team at every step. A small team of assistant editors was also appointed to further simplify the editing procedure and attain best results for the readers.

Apart from the editorial board, the designing team has also invested a significant amount of their time in understanding the subject and creating the most relevant covers. They scrutinized every image to scout for the most suitable representation of the subject and create an appropriate cover for the book.

The publishing team has been an ardent support to the editorial, designing and production team. Their endless efforts to recruit the best for this project, has resulted in the accomplishment of this book. They are a veteran in the field of academics and their pool of knowledge is as vast as their experience in printing. Their expertise and guidance has proved useful at every step. Their uncompromising quality standards have made this book an exceptional effort. Their encouragement from time to time has been an inspiration for everyone.

The publisher and the editorial board hope that this book will prove to be a valuable piece of knowledge for researchers, students, practitioners and scholars across the globe.

List of Contributors

Stefan Golaszewski
Department of Neurology and Neuroscience Institute, Paracelsus Medical University, Salzburg, Austria

Meghan A. Van Zandt and Janice R. Naegele
Wesleyan University, Middletown, CT, USA

Robert J Oliver and Nora I Perrone-Bizzozero
Department of Neurosciences, University of New Mexico School of Medicine, Albuquerque, NM, USA

Dylan Kiltschewskij
School of Biomedical Sciences and Pharmacy, Faculty of Health, The University of Newcastle, Callaghan, Australia
Priority Research Centre for Brain and Mental Health Research, Hunter Medical Research Institute, New Lambton, Australia

Murray J. Cairns
School of Biomedical Sciences and Pharmacy, Faculty of Health, The University of Newcastle, Callaghan, Australia
Priority Research Centre for Brain and Mental Health Research, Hunter Medical Research Institute, New Lambton, Australia
Schizophrenia Research Institute, Sydney, Australia

Marlos Vasconcelos Rocha
Department of Cognitive Neurology, University Hospital Professor Edgard Santos, Salvador, Bahia, Brazil
Program of Mood and Anxiety Disorders (CETHA), Federal University of Bahia, Bahia, Brazil
Fabiana Nery, Amanda Galvão-de-Almeida, Lucas de Castro Quarantini and Ângela Miranda-Scippa
Program of Mood and Anxiety Disorders (CETHA), Federal University of Bahia, Bahia, Brazil
Department of Neuroscience and Mental Health, Federal University of Bahia, Salvador, Bahia, Brazil

Ignacio González-Burgos Nallely Vázquez-Hernández and Néstor I. Martínez-Torre
Laboratorio de Psicobiología, División de Neurociencias, Centro de Investigación Biomédic de Occidente, Instituto Mexicano del Seguro Social, Jalisco, México

Masako Isokawa
Department of Health and Biomedical Sciences, The University of Texas Rio Grande Valley, One West University Boulevard, Brownsville, TX, USA

Dulce A. Velázquez-Zamora and David González-Tapia
Laboratorio de Psicobiología, División de Neurociencias, Centro de Investigación Biomédic de Occidente, Instituto Mexicano del Seguro Social, Jalisco, México
Universidad Politécnica de la Zona Metropolitana de Guadalajara, Tlajomulco de Zúñiga, Jalisco, México

Ping Hu
State Key Laboratory of Optoelectronic Materials and Technologies, School of Materials Science and Engineering, Sun Yat-Sen University, Guangzhou, People's Republic of China
School of Mathematics and Physics, University of South China, Hengyang, People's Republic of China

Shuxiang Wu and Shuwei Li
State Key Laboratory of Optoelectronic Materials and Technologies, School of Materials Science and Engineering, Sun Yat-Sen University, Guangzhou, People's Republic of China

Karolina A Bearss
Department of Psychology, Centre for Vision Research, York University, Toronto, ON, Canada

Joseph FX DeSouza
Department of Psychology, Centre for Vision Research, York University, Toronto, ON, Canada
Biology and Interdisciplinary Studies, York University, Toronto, ON, Canada

Han-A Park and Elizabeth A. Jonas
Department of Internal Medicine, Section of Endocrinology, Yale University, New Haven, CT, USA

Ilya S. Bakulin, Alexander V. Chervyakov, Natalia A. Suponeva, Maria N. Zakharova and Michael A. Piradov
Research Center of Neurology, Moscow, Russia

Index